HIMSS Dictionary of Healthcare Information Technology Terms, Acronyms and Organizations

Second Edition

- Authoritative, Timely Definitions
- Comprehensive Acronym Listings
- Organizations and Associations Linked to Healthcare IT
- Healthcare Credentials

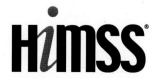

HIMSS Mission

To lead healthcare transformation through the effective use of health information technology.

Printed in the U.S.A. 5 4 3 2 1

Requests for permission to reproduce any part of this work should be sent to:

Permissions Editor
HIMSS
230 E. Ohio St., Suite 500
Chicago, IL 60611-3270
cmclean@himss.org

ISBN: 978-0-9800697-5-4

For more information about HIMSS, please visit www.himss.org.

Contents

Foreword to the Second Edition

*By Raymond D. Aller, MD, FHIMSS**

My colleagues tell me that one of the most daunting aspects of dealing with health information technology and informatics is the bewildering array of terminology used to describe and characterize this field of endeavor. In some respects, this represents a microcosm of the English language. English is unique among modern languages in the sheer number of entities it contains—some estimates place the number of words in English at well over a million. This is more than five times the number of words in any other language. A century ago, the language of diplomacy was French, the language of medicine was Latin, the language of chemistry and engineering was German. Today, English has become dominant in all these fields. I've recently been reading texts that present the same information in two languages, in adjacent columns. I'm struck that the English version is notably shorter than the foreign language text. English has such a large number of unique words that gradations of meaning can be conveyed with a single word—while (say) the speaker of French must use two to three words to say the same thing.

When I began medical school, we were advised (correctly) that the first two years would be largely an intense vocabulary lesson. I still learn new words every day—and, where I need a word to describe a concept, I sometimes invent one. But the worlds of both information technology and medicine outdo me.

Words permit us to precisely characterize a concept and communicate with others in a field of endeavor without resorting to multisyllabic circumlocutions. Information technology in general has created a vast number of new concepts, and clinical information technology and clinical informatics have been particularly prolific. Not surprisingly, the nexus of medicine (with a huge vocabulary) and information systems (with a rapidly growing and volatile terminology) makes for an explosion of expressions.

Given this plethora of words and terms, how does the ordinary health professional have any hope of coping? We believe that the compendium you now hold in your hands can be of assistance. This book focuses on terms emerging from the nexus of information technology and healthcare. For general information technology terms, we refer you to other sources, such as *Newton's Telecom Dictionary* (print only); *Online Dictionary for Library and Information Science* (print and online); and *Jones Media and Information Technology Encyclopedia* (online only). Given a concept that you want to express in a word, we refer you to the various online reverse-dictionaries, including www.onelook.com/reverse-dictionary.shtml or www.wordtree.com.

---

* Dr. Aller practices clinical informatics, laboratory medicine and public health in Southern California and in Haiti. He can be reached at raller@usc.edu.

A particularly common source of obscure and unclear terms are the acronyms so prolific in the language of both medicine and information technology. The same acronym may refer to several different concepts. These have become so problematic in hospital charts that hospitals now publish lists of "approved" abbreviations. In one hospital, we saw an apparent outbreak of Crimean hemorrhagic fever; upon investigation, these indeed were patients with "CHF," but congestive heart failure was the intended meaning.

When we operate at the intersection of two complex disciplines, the numbers of acronyms proliferate. For example, one's professional affiliations (organizational memberships, etc.) are often indicated by a string of acronyms following the name. In the first edition of this book, a daunting string followed my name: MD, FHIMSS, FACMI, HFAPI, FCAP. In a mere 32 characters, I provided (to the cognoscenti) knowledge of my professional degree, medical specialty, and distinctive recognition within three professional societies of clinical informatics. However, to the less initiated, I obfuscated my message in a meaningless alphabet soup. We must always be vigilant to use acronyms selectively, and only where absolutely necessary. For this reason, we have included a new term in this edition: "TLAlgia." This term is composed of "TLA" (meaning "three-letter acronym") and "-algia" (meaning "pain")—thus, "pain induced by excessive use of three-letter acronyms." Beware!

In this second edition, we provide 575 new entries, for a total of 2,700 words, acronyms and terms. Also, there are two new appendices: a list of healthcare credentials and their acronyms, and NAHIT's Key Health Information Technology Terms.

One of the troublesome aspects of this endeavor—and of any complex domain where "newbie" practitioners attempt to use a complex lexicography to describe an even more complex realm—is that words are misused, or come through usage to assume two or three mutually exclusive meanings. In some cases, we have listed multiple meanings of a term; be aware that when you use that term, the listener may be thinking of a different definition than you are.

With all of these caveats in mind, dive in, speak and write this new language we have invented at the intersection of medicine and information technology.

Introduction

HIMSS Dictionary of Healthcare Information Technology Terms, Acronyms and Organizations, Second Edition, is a collaborative project led by HIMSS Standards Task Force in response to a need to define terms and acronyms used in the Healthcare Information Technology (HIT) Community. This extensive resource includes terms and acronyms used in the industry, as well as in legislation, white papers, presentations, reports, directories, committee work and HIT standards. Because of the growth of the HIT industry, this second edition contains a 27 percent increase in terms and acronyms from the first edition.

This dictionary is a compilation of well used terms from multiple sources consisting of healthcare informatics,* information technology, providers, payers and HIT standards work. The editing was carefully done to avoid listing clinical-only acronyms and terms, such as chest x-ray (CXR), as excellent dictionaries for these terms already exist.

Rather than applying strict dictionary definitions, the dictionary is a reference tool for the use of HIT terms. The terms are cross-referenced by acronym in an A-to-Z format. Most terms have one definition; for those terms with two definitions, the first definition is the preferred. All terms have a source, located in the References section of this dictionary.

This expanded edition includes four appendices. Because the terms 'Electronic Health Record' and 'Interoperability' have multiple definitions, each has an appendix including those definitions. 'Healthcare Credentials' lists most of the academic and certification credentials used in healthcare today. And the fourth appendix has the terms from the National Alliance for Health Information Technology Report, which defined key HIT terms using a consensus-based process.

We would appreciate your feedback on this dictionary, especially on the terms and acronyms, so that we can improve future editions. Please send your comments to us at dictionary@himss.org.

**HIMSS Standards Task Force and
the Dictionary Editing Work Group**

---

* Includes clinical, medical and nursing informatics

Acknowledgments

HIMSS sincerely thanks many people who, during the months in which this dictionary was developed, provided us with useful and helpful assistance. Without their expertise and consideration, this dictionary would likely not have become a reality.

Raymond D. Aller, MD, FHIMSS,
  FACMI, HFAPI, FCAP
Director
Automated Disease Surveillance
  Section, LA County

Michael W. Davis
Executive Vice President
HIMSS Analytics

J. Michael Fitzmaurice, PhD, FACMI
Senior Science Advisor for
  Information Technology
Office of the Director
Agency for Healthcare Research
  and Quality

David E. Garets, FHIMSS
President/CEO
HIMSS Analytics

Erik Pupo
Health Interoperability Architect
Vangent Inc.

Anthony Stever
Consultant
AWS Consulting

Asif Syed, MD
Senior Clinical Terminology Consultant
Clinical Informatics Department
American Medical Association

LuAnn Whittenburg, RN, MSN,
  APRN, BC
ISO/TC 215 Health Informatics,
  US Expert
Technical Advisory Group Health
  Informatics Member
Virginia Medical Reserve Corps

Terms and Acronyms

A

AA Attribute authority. Authority which assigns privileges by issuing attribute certificates.[121]

Abbreviated term Term resulting from the omission of any part of a term while designating the same concept.[3]

ABC Activity based costing. An accounting technique that allows an organization to determine the actual cost associated with each product and service produced by the organization, without regard to the organizational structure.[1]

ABC codes Terminology to describe alternative medicine, nursing, and other integrative healthcare interventions that include relative value units and legal scope of practice information.[52]

Abend Abnormal end to a program.[7]

Abort 1. Terminate. 2. In data transmission, an abort is a function invoked by a sending station to cause the recipient to discard or ignore all bit sequences transmitted by the sender since the preceding flag sequence.[7]

Abstract class Virtual common parent to two or more classes which cannot itself be instantiated.[116]

Abstract message Includes the data fields that will be sent within a message, the valid response messages, and the treatment of application level errors.[16]

Abstract syntax A formal description method that allows data types relevant to an application to be specified in terms of other data types, including basic data types, such as integer and octet string.[3]

Abstract syntax notation *See* **ASN.**

Acceptable risk The level of risk management finds acceptable to a particular information asset. Acceptable risk is based on empirical data and supportive technical opinion that the overall risk is understood, and that the controls placed on the asset, or environment, will lower the potential for its loss. Any remaining risk is recognized and accepted as an accountability issue.[118]

Acceptable use policy *See* **AUP.**

Acceptance testing A user-run testing event that demonstrates the application's ability to meet the business objectives and system requirements.[6]

Access Providing a person the opportunity to approach, inspect, review, or make use of data, information, or an information system.[1]

Access control 1. A security policy to authenticate who can have access to what data or information, or policies and procedures preventing access by those who are not authorized to have it; a process that determines which data elements can be read, written, or erased by certain users of a system. 2. The prevention of use of a resource by unauthorized entities.[1]

Access control decision function *See* **ACDF.**

Access control enforcement function *See* **AEF.**

Access control information *See* **ACI.**

Access control lists *See* **ACL.**

Access control policy A set of rules, part of a security policy, by which human customers or representatives are authenticated, and by which access by the customers to applications and other services and security objects is granted or denied.[4]

Access control service *See* **ACS.**

Access decision function The combining of security functions with decision algorithms creating an access control matrix.[1]

Access level A level associated with an individual who may be accessing information, or with the information that may be accessed (e.g., a classification level).[1]

Access mode   A distinct operation recognized by protection mechanisms as a possible operation on data or information. 'Read' and 'write' are possible modes of access to a computer file; 'execute' is an additional mode of access to a program; and 'create' and 'delete' are access modes for directory objects.[1]

Access point   A wireless networking radio transceiver that allows an appropriately equipped computer or other device to connect to a data network.[1]

Access provider   *See* **ISP**.

Access to radiology information   *See* **ARI**.

Accessibility   Ability of a patient or population to utilize needed healthcare services unrestricted by geographic, economic, social, cultural, organizational, or linguistic barriers.[123]

Accountability 1.   Property that allows auditing of IT system activities to be traced to persons or processes that may then be held responsible for their actions. Accountability includes authenticity and nonrepudiation. **2.** The relationship between two parties that provides authorization for an action to be carried out.[97,4]

Accounting of disclosures   Refers to the right of individuals, with limitations, to a listing of the uses and disclosures of their identifiable health information for a period of time not to exceed six years prior to the date of the request.[48]

Accreditation   Formal declaration by a designated approving authority that an information system approved to operate in a particular security mode using a prescribed set of safeguards at an acceptable level of risk.[97]

ACDF   Access control decision function. Specialized function that makes access control decisions by applying access control policy rules to an access request, access control decision information (of initiators, targets, access requests, or that retained from prior decisions), and the context in which the access request is made.[125]

ACG   Ambulatory care group. Preventative, diagnostic, therapeutic, surgical, and/or reha-

bilitative outpatient care, where the duration of treatment is less than 24 hours.[2] Note: Sometimes called *adjusted clinical groups*.

ACI   Access control information. Information used for access control purposes, including contextual information.[125]

ACID   The basic properties of a database transaction: atomicity, consistency, isolation, and durability. Either all steps in a transaction succeed, or the entire transaction is rolled back; partial completion should never be observed.[7]

ACK   General acknowledgment message.[16]

ACL   Access control lists. An ordered list of rules that control file permissions.[42]

ACS   Access control service. Includes embedded security management capabilities (provided as precursor information to this construct), and all other user-side access control and decision making capabilities (policy enforcement point, policy decision point, PIP, PAP, obligation service, etc.), needed to enforce use-side system-object security and privacy policy. The ACS is responsible for creating trustworthy credentials forwarded in cross-domain assertions regarding security information and attributes. Access control services may be hierarchical and nested, distributed or local.[48]

Active server pages   *See* **ASP**.

Activities of daily living   *See* **ADLs**.

Activity   An action for the creation, the acquisition, or the furnishing of a 'product' (e.g., register a patient).[4]

Activity based costing   *See* **ABC**.

Actor   A system or application responsible for certain information or tasks (e.g., the order placer actor). Each actor supports a specific set of Integrating the Healthcare Enterprise (IHE) transactions to communicate with other actors. A vendor product may include one or more actors.[56]

Acute care   An abrupt onset of disease lasting for a short period of time; some authorities say three months or shorter duration.[32]

Acute Physiologic and Chronic Health Evaluation   *See* **APACHE**.

AD Addendum. A portion added on to a document.[32]

Addendum *See* **AD**.

Address The unique location of: **1.** an Internet server; **2.** a specific file (e.g., a Web page); or **3.** an e-mail user.[32]

Address class One of four TCP/IP network types: Class A, B, C, or D. Only A, B, and C are used in association with IP addressing. Class A: 1-126; Class B: 128-191; Class C: 192-223.[1]

Address resolution Conversion of an IP address to the corresponding low-level physical address.[1]

Address resolution protocol *See* **ARP**.

ADE Adverse drug event. An injury resulting from the use of a drug. Under this definition, the term ADE includes harm caused by the drug (adverse drug reactions and overdose) and harm from the use of the drug (including dose reductions and discontinuations of drug therapy). Adverse drug events may result from medication errors, but most do not.[96]

Ad-hoc query A query that is not determined prior to the moment it is run against a data source.[1]

ADLs Activities of daily living. Activities that are considered a normal part of everyday life. Some of these are bathing, dressing, eating, toileting, and transferring (e.g., moving from and into a chair). These activities are used to measure the degree of impairment, and can effect the eligibility for certain types for insurance benefits.[102]

Administrative code sets Code sets that characterize a general business situation, rather than a medical condition or service. Under HIPAA, these are sometimes referred to as non-clinical, or non-medical, code sets. Compare to code sets and medical code sets.[10]

Administrative record A record concerned with administrative matters, such as length of stay, details of accommodation, and billing.[4]

Administrative safeguards Administrative actions and policies and procedures to manage the selection, development, implementation, and maintenance of security measures to protect electronic protected health information; and to manage the conduct of the covered entity's workforce in relation to the protection of that information.[118]

Administrative services only *See* **ASO**.

Administrative simplification Title II, Subtitle F, of HIPAA, which authorizes the U.S. Department of Health and Human Services (HHS) to: (1) adopt standards for transactions and code sets that are used to exchange health data; (2) adopt standard identifiers for health plans, healthcare providers, employers, and individuals for use on standard transactions; and (3) adopt standards to protect the security and privacy of personally identifiable health information.[102]

Administrative users access level The special rights given to the team of users who maintain and support a network.[1]

Admission date The date the patient was admitted for inpatient care, outpatient service, or start of care.[102]

Admitted term Term accepted as a synonym for a preferred term by an authoritative body.[3]

ADPAC Automated data processing application coordinator. The person assigned by a service to coordinate computer activities for that service.

ADR Adverse drug reaction. 1. Response to a drug which is noxious and unintended, and which occurs at doses normally used in humans for prophylaxis, diagnosis, or therapy of disease; or for the modification of physiological function. Note that there is a causal link between a drug and an adverse drug reaction. In summary, an adverse drug reaction is harm directly caused by the drug at normal doses, during normal use.[96] **2.** A complication caused by use of a drug in the usual (i.e., correct) manner and dosage.[18]

ADR ADT response message. Admission, discharge, and transfer response message.[16]

ADSL Asymmetric digital subscriber line. A high-speed line that allows voice and data to travel concurrently over a local copper loop (or pair), with speeds ranging from 2–8 Mbps downstream, and 640–960 kpbs upstream.[1]

ADT Admission, discharge, and transfer message for patients in a healthcare facility.[102]

ADT response message   *See* **ADR**.

Adult learning theory   Based on the premise that in order for adults to learn, there must be a perceived need, practical application, and relevance to their situation.[6]

Advance directives   Documentation allowing a person to give directions regarding his or her own healthcare in the event that person loses decision-making capacity. It may include a Living Will and a Durable Power of Attorney for healthcare.[102]

Adverse drug event   *See* **ADE**.

Adverse drug reaction   *See* **ADR**.

Adverse event   *See* **AE**.

AE   **Adverse event. 1.** Untoward incidents, therapeutic misadventures, iatrogenic injuries, or other adverse occurrences, directly associated with care or services provided within the jurisdiction of a medical center, outpatient clinic, or other medical facility. **2.** An injury caused by medical management, rather than by the underlying condition of the patient.[97]

AEF   **Access control enforcement function.** Specialized function that is part of the access path between an initiator and a target on each access control request; enforces the decision made by the access control decision function.[125]

Affinity domain policy   Clearly defines the appropriate uses of the XDS affinity domain. Within this policy is a defined set of acceptable use privacy consent policies that are published and understood.[56]

Agency specific data   All data pertinent to the agency where care is provided, and which are used for patient care, such as procedures, hours of operations, visiting hours, standards of care, pharmacy formulary, etc.[6]

Aggregate   The collection or gathering of elements into a mass or whole.[6]

Aggregate data   Data that are the result of applying a process to summarize atomic data elements. *See also* **Atomic data**.[1]

Aggregation logics   Logic for aggregating detailed data into categories.[28]

AHT   **Average handling time.** The average duration of a call handled by a customer service associate.[15]

AIS privileges   **Automated information system** permissions to perform specified functions within a computer system.[1]

Alert   Written or acoustic signals to announce the arrival of messages and results, and to avoid possible undesirable situations, such as contradictions, conflicts, erroneous entry, tasks that are not performed in time or an exceptional result. A passive alert will appear on the screen in the form of a message. An active alert calls for immediate attention, and the appropriate person is immediately notified (e.g., by electronic pager). *See also* **Decision support**.[4]

Alerting system   Computer-based   system that automatically generates alerts and advice as a consequence of monitoring, or other information processing activities.[4]

Algorithm   **1.** A precise statement of a method of calculation. Sometimes expressed in programming language. **2.** A predetermined set of instructions for solving a problem in a finite number of steps.[4,6]

Alias   **1.** A link to another file in a file system. **2.** An indirect, usually unexpected effect on other data, when a variable or reference is changed.[7]

Alias domain name   The practice of establishing an e-mail protocol within another e-mail protocol, to allow for the local identification of users within a larger enterprise.[1]

ALOS   **Average length of stay.** The American Hospital Association computes the average length of hospital stay by dividing the number of inpatient days by the number of admissions.

Alpha/beta testing   A pre-production development stage comprised of an initial trial (alpha test) by a select set of users. This initial test is to ensure that the system is stable enough for a rigorous trial (beta test) by additional users, or in a variety of settings. *See also* **Beta testing**.[6]

Alphanumeric   Describes use of numbers, the letters of the alphabet, and punctuation markers. Normally used to describe the typewriter-style keyboard used by computers.[4]

ALU **Arithmetic logic unit.** Portion of the CPU that performs the following arithmetic operations: add, subtract, multiply, divide, and negate.[1]

Ambulatory care Medical care, including diagnosis, observation, treatment, and rehabilitation that is provided on an outpatient basis. Ambulatory care is given to persons who are able to ambulate or walk about.[102]

Ambulatory care group *See* **ACG.**

Ambulatory care information system Information system to deal with the care of outpatients.[4]

Ambulatory EHR The EMR that supports the ambulatory/clinic/physician office environments. Provides all of the functions of an EMR; clinical documentation, order entry, clinical data repository, practitioner order entry, physician clinical documentation, etc.[2]

Ambulatory medical record *See* **AMR.**

Amendments and corrections In the final Privacy Rule, an amendment to a record would indicate that the data is in dispute while retaining the original information, while a correction to a record would alter or replace the original record.[10]

American Standard Code for Information Interchange *See* **ASCII.**

Amplifier A device used to increase the strength of broadband signals to travel further distances.[1]

AMR **Ambulatory medical record.** An electronic medical record used in the outpatient or ambulatory care setting.[45]

Analog Representing data by measurement of a continuous physical variable, as voltage or pressure, as opposed to 'digital,' which represents data as discrete units.[7]

Analog signal A continuous transmission signal that carries information in the form of varying waveforms/frequencies. *See also* **Digital signal.**[1]

Analog-to-digital conversion Analog-to-digital conversion is an electronic process in which a continuous variable analog is changed, without altering its essential content, into a multi-level digital signal.[1]

Ancillary service Service in a hospital or healthcare facility which is not part of the healthcare domain (e.g., laundry, transportation, cleaning, materials).[4]

Ancillary service information system Information system designed to provide support for the management, monitoring, planning, scheduling, and request processing of ancillary service functions.[4]

Anonymized data Originally identifiable data which have been permanently stripped of identifiers.[8]

Anonymous file transfer protocol *See* **Anonymous FTP.**

Anonymous FTP **Anonymous file transfer protocol.** An FTP session that allows users to access designated public system resources or files.[1]

Anti-tearing The process or processes that prevent data loss when a smart card is withdrawn from the contacts during a data operation.[1]

Anti-virus software *See* **Virus scanner.**

APACHE The Acute Physiologic and Chronic Health Evaluation (APACHE) scoring system has been widely used in the United States. APACHE II is the most widely studied version of this instrument (a more recent version, APACHE III, is proprietary, whereas APACHE II is publicly available); it derives a severity score from such factors as underlying disease and chronic health status. Other points are added for 12 physiologic variables (e.g., hematocrit, creatinine, Glasgow Coma Score, mean arterial pressure) measured within 24 hours of admission to the ICU. The APACHE II score has been validated in several studies involving tens of thousands of ICU patients.[14]

APC **Ambulatory payment class.** A payment type for outpatient PPS claims.[5]

API **Application program interface. 1.** A set of standard software that interrupts calls, functions, and data formats that can be used by an application program to access network services, devices, applications, or operating systems. **2.** A set of pre-made functions used to build programs. APIs ask the operating system or another application to perform specific tasks. There is an API for almost everything, including messaging APIs for e-mail, telephony APIs for calling systems, Java APIs, and graphics APIs, such as DirectX.[12] *See also* **Socket, SSL**.[1]

APN Appendix.[32]

Application A program or set of programs that perform a task. The use of information resources (information and information technology) to satisfy a specific set of user requirements.[1]

Application architecture Defines how applications are designed and how they cooperate; promotes common presentation standards to facilitate rapid training and implementation of new applications and functions. Good application architecture enables a high level of system integration, reuse of components, and rapid deployment of applications in response to changing business requirements.[8]

Application integrator Software that is used between different managed care applications to provide data conversion and transmission, without the need for special programming to interface two or more applications, thereby reducing the cost of systems interface.[1]

Application layer The seventh and highest layer of the OSI model. Provides resources for the interaction that takes place between a user and application. *See also* **OSI**.[1]

Application metadata Data about a data dictionary concerning the structure and contents of application menus, forms, and reports.[1]

Application program interface *See* **API**.

Application protocol services These are services supporting application level protocols. Simple object access protocol (SOAP) will be supported. Other remoting protocols, such as remote method invocation, DICOM, etc., can be plugged into the application protocol service.[8]

Application role A characteristic of an application that defines a portion of its interfaces. It is defined in terms of the interactions (messages) that the role sends or receives in response to trigger events. Thus, it is a role played by a healthcare information system component when sending or receiving health information technology messages; a set of responsibilities with respect to an interaction.[8]

Application server **1.** Program on a distributed network that provides business logic and server side execution environment for application programs. **2.** A computer that handles all operations between a company's back-end applications or databases, and the users' computers' Web browsers. **3.** The device that connects end users to software applications and databases that are managed by the server.[8,2]

Application service provider *See* **ASP**.

Appointment system System for the planning of appointments between resources, such as clinicians, facilities, and patients. Note: Used in order to minimize waiting time, prioritize appointments, and optimize the utilization of resources.[4]

Archetype A named content type specification with attribute declarations.[33]

Archetype instance Metadata class instance of an archetype model, specifying the clinical concept and the value constraints that apply to one class of record component instances in an electronic health record extract.[116]

Archetype model Information model of the metadata to represent the domain-specific characteristics of electronic health record entries, by specifying values or value constraints for classes and attributes in the electronic health record reference model.[116]

Archetype repository Persistent repository of archetype definitions accessed by a client authoring tool, or by a run-time component within an electronic health record service.[116]

Architecture **1.** Architecture is a term applied to both the process and the outcome of specifying the overall structure, logical components, and the logical interrelationships of a computer, its operating system, a network, or other conception. **2.** A framework from which applications, databases, and workstations can be developed in a coherent manner, and in which every part fits together without containing a mass of design details. Normally used to describe how a piece of hardware or software is constructed and which protocols and interfaces are required for communications. Network architecture specifies the function and data transmission needed to convey information across a network.[8,4]

Archive Long-term, physically separate storage.[114]

Archiving Moving rarely or never accessed computer files to an off-line storage device, such as magnetic tape or optical disk system. Archiving is a good practice to provide backup of important files, as well as to save critical space on the system hard disk.[1]

Arden syntax A language created to encode actions within a clinical protocol into a set of situation-action rules for computer interpretation, and to facilitate exchange between different institutions.[13]

Argument 1. The values that a formula uses; they may be entered by the user, or be functions provided by the software. 2. The part of a command that specifies what the command is to do.[11,4]

ARI Access to radiology information. Specifies a number of query transactions providing access to radiology information, including images and related reports, in a DICOM format, as they were acquired or created. Such access is useful, both to the radiology department and to other departments, such as pathology, surgery, and oncology. See also **Profile**.[56]

Arithmetic logic unit See **ALU**.

ARP Address resolution protocol. Used in TCP/IP networks to provide the physical address (MAC address) or a device from the assigned Internet provider (IP) address.[1]

ARPANET Developed by the (Defense) Advanced Research Projects Agency (DARPA), this distributed network grew into the Internet.[18]

Array A set of sequentially indexed elements having the same intrinsic data type. Each element of an array has a unique identifying index number.[12]

Artificial intelligence A computer application that has been designed to mimic the actions of an intelligent human in a given situation, and to be capable of substituting for a human.[11]

ASA Average speed to answer. The average amount of time (measured in seconds) from when a caller calls customer service, to when he or she begins speaking to a customer service associate.[140]

ASCII American Standard Code for Information Interchange. Extensively used bit standard information processing code that represents 128 possible standard characters used by PCs. In an ASCII file, each alphabetic, numeric, or special character is represented with a 7-bit number (a string of seven 0s or 1s), which yields the 128 possible characters.[1]

ASMOP A simple matter of programming. An expression used to convey the sense 'yes, it's possible, but it would require an unknown, but most likely large, expenditure of resources.'[7]

ASN Abstract syntax notation. A metadata standard to define standards, mainly used in the area of telecommunications.[119]

ASO Administrative services only. An arrangement whereby a self-insured entity contracts with a third party administrator (TPA) to administer a health plan.[10]

ASP Active server pages. A protocol for creating and displaying Web pages.[99]

ASP Application service provider. A company that provides some type of specialty automation service or access, under a service agreement for a customer, with the business model of being able to provide expertise and reliability at a desired lower cost than the customer could provide for itself within a local data center.[1]

Assembler A tool that reads source code written in assembly language and produces executable machine code; possibly together with information needed by linkers, debuggers, and other tools. See also Compiler.[7]

Assembly services A business request may include calls to various components providing multiple result sets. These result sets will be assembled together in the appropriate output format by the assembly service. This service will use assembly templates to carry out its function.[8]

Association Linking a document with the program that created it so that both can be opened with a single command (e.g., double-clicking a 'doc' file opens Word for Windows and loads the selected document).[105]

Assurance Measure of confidence that the security features, practices, procedures, and architecture of an IT system accurately mediate and enforce the security policy.[97]

Asymmetric cryptographic algorithm   Algorithm for performing encipherment or the corresponding decipherment, in which the keys used for encipherment and decipherment differ.[121]

Asymmetric digital subscriber line   *See* **ADSL.**

Asymmetric keys   Independent review and examination of records and activities to assess the adequacy of system controls; to ensure compliance with established policies and operational procedures; and to recommend necessary changes in controls, policies, or procedures.[114]

Asymmetric multiprocessing   Multiprocessing technique in which certain tasks are dedicated to specific processors. One processor executes the operating system, while another processor handles applications.[1]

Asynchronous communication   Communication in which the reply is not made immediately after the message is sent, but when the recipient is available. E-mail is an example of asynchronous communication.[11]

Asynchronous transfer mode   *See* **ATM.**

ATM   Asynchronous transfer mode. Asynchronous transfer mode is a high-performance, cell-oriented, switching and multiplexing technology that utilizes fixed-length packets to carry different types of traffic. *See also* **Frame relay, SONET**.[34]

ATNA   Audit trail and node authentication. Establishes the characteristics of a Basic Secure Node: **1.** It describes the security environment (user identification, authentication, authorization, access control, etc.). **2.** It defines basic security requirements for the communications of the node. **3.** It defines basic auditing requirements for the node. The profile also establishes the characteristics of the communication of audit messages between the Basic Secure Nodes and Audit Repository Nodes that collect audit information. *See also* **Profile**.[56]

Atomic concept   **1.**   Primitive   concept. **2.** Concept in a formal system whose definition is not a compositional definition.[98,126]

Atomic data   Data elements that represent the lowest level of possible detail in a data warehouse.[1]

Atomic level data   The elemental, precise data captured at the source in the course of clinical care, which can be manipulated in a variety of ways. These data are collected once, but used many times.[6]

Atomicity   The entire sequence of actions must be either completed or aborted. The transaction cannot be partially successful.[7]

Attachment unit interface   *See* **AUI**.

Attack   The act of aggressively trying to bypass security controls in a computer system.[1]

Attempted security violation   An unsuccessful action to gain unauthorized access to computer resources.[1]

Attenuation   The measurement of how much a signal weakens over distance on a transmission medium. The longer the medium, the more attenuation becomes a problem without the regeneration of the signal. Signal regeneration is usually accomplished through the use of hubs (baseband) and amplifiers (broadband).[1]

Attester   Party (person) who certifies and records legal responsibility for a particular unit of information.[116]

Attribute   **1.** An attribute expresses characteristics of a basic elemental concept. Attributes are also known as roles or relationship types. Semantic concepts form relationships to each other through attributes. **2.** Abstractions of the data captured about classes. Attributes capture separate aspects of the class and take their values independent of one another. **3.** Piece of information describing a particular entity.[16,19]

Attribute authority   *See* **AA**.

Attribute certificate   Data structure, digitally signed by an attribute authority, that binds some attribute values with identification about its holder.[121]

Attribute relationship   An attribute relationship consists of two semantic concepts related to each other through an attribute. When an attribute-value pair has been assigned to a concept, that relationship becomes part of the concept's logical definition. For this reason, attribute relationships are called 'defining characteristics' of semantic concepts.[19]

Attribute type The last part of an attribute name (suffix). Attribute type suffixes are rough classifiers for the meaning of the attribute. *See* **Data type** for contrast in definition.[16]

Attribute-value pair The combination of an attribute with a value that is appropriate for that attribute. Assigning attribute-value pairs to semantic concepts is known as 'authoring' or 'modeling,' and is part of the process of semantic content development. Attributes and values are always used together as attribute-value pairs. Sometimes the entire relationship is referred to as an object-attribute-value triple, or 'OAV' triple.[19]

Audit Independent review and examination of records and activities to assess the adequacy of system controls; to ensure compliance with established policies and operational procedures; and to recommend necessary changes in controls, policies, or procedures.[114]

Audit data Chronological record of system activities to enable the reconstruction and examination of the sequence of events and changes in an event.[114]

Audit trail **1.** Chronological record of system activity which enables the reconstruction of information regarding the creation, distribution, modification, and deletion of data. **2.** Documentary evidence of monitoring each operation of individuals on health information. May be comprehensive or specific to the individual and information. Audit trails are commonly used to search for unauthorized access by authorized users.[8,1]

Audit trail and node authentication *See* **ATNA**.

Auditing Specific activities that make up an audit (*see* **Audit**). This can be manual, automated, or a combination.[48]

AUI **Attachment unit interface.** Connector port on network devices.[1]

AUP **Acceptable use policy.** Set of rules and guidelines that specify, in more or less detail, the expectations in regard to appropriate use of systems or networks.[48]

Authenticate To verify the identity of a user, user device, other entity, or the integrity of data stored, transmitted, or exposed to unauthorized modification in an information system.[1]

Authentication Security measure, such as the use of digital signatures, to establish the validity of a transmission, message, or originator, or a means of verifying an individual's authorization to receive specific categories of information. The process of proving that a user or system is really who or what it claims to be. It protects against the fraudulent use of a system, or the fraudulent transmission of information.[1]

Authenticity Ability to verify; confidence in the validity of a transmission, a message, or message originator.[48]

Authority certificate Certificate issued to a certification authority or to an attribute authority.[121]

Authorization **1.** Process of determining what activities are permitted, usually in the context of authentication. **2.** The permission to perform certain operations, or use certain methods or services.[8]

Authorization decision Evaluating applicable policy, returned by the PDP to the PEP. A function that evaluates to 'Permit,' 'Deny,' 'Indeterminate,' or 'Not Applicable,' and (optionally) a set of obligations (OASIS XACML).[48]

Authorized access Mechanisms by which access to data is granted by challenges to the requesting entity, to assure proper authority based on the identity of the individual, level of access to the data, and rights to manipulation of that data.[48]

Automated data processing application coordinator *See* **ADPAC**.

Availability Assurance that the systems responsible for delivering, storing, and processing information are accessible when needed, by those who need them, and that the information it provides will be of acceptable integrity.[118]

Average handling time *See* **AHT**.

Average length of stay *See* **ALOS**.

Average speed to answer *See* **ASA**.

AVR **Analysis visualization reporting.** To analyze, display, report, and map accumulated data, and share data and technologies for analysis and visualization with other public health partners.[46]

B

b/w Between.[32]

B/W Black and white. Indicates a print image is being formulated to be readable in pure black and white, without the use of color (and perhaps without the use of grayscale).

B2B Business-to-business. Healthcare eCommerce applications that support online business enhancements to standardize previous processes that involved paper, fragmented interfaces, or delay. The electronic commerce is conducted between the business of the hospital (or other healthcare entity) and the business of the supplier.[1]

B2C Business-to-consumer. 1. The electronic commerce that is conducted between the business of the hospital (or other healthcare entity) and the consumer or patient. **2.** eCommerce transactions conducted over the Internet. **3.** Healthcare eCommerce applications that support online business enhancements to standardize previous processes that involved paper, fragmented interfaces, or delay.[1]

Back door Unauthorized, undocumented code in a program that gives special privileges. *See also* **Trap doors**.[1]

Backbone The high-speed, high-performance main transmission path in a network; a set of paths that local or regional networks connect to as a node for interconnection.[1]

Background Application that is executing without user input on a multi-tasking machine.[1]

Background process A secondary process which runs concurrently behind the active process appearing on the computer terminal.[4]

Backup Creation or duplication of files from a hard disk drive to a tape medium for storage, security, or safekeeping.[1]

Backup domain controller *See* **BDC**.

Bandwidth The total range of frequency capacity that can pass over a network. The capacity of a channel to carry information as measured by the difference between the highest and lowest frequencies that can be transmitted by that channel.[1]

Banyan VINES A networking operating system that allows users of PC desktop operating systems, such as OS/2, Windows, DOS, and Macintosh, to share information and resources with each other and with host computing systems.[1]

Bar chart A graphic display of data in the form of a bar showing the number of units (e.g., frequency) in each category.[123]

Bar code One-dimensional pattern of thick and thin parallel lines printed on objects and containing coded information, which can be read by a light pen or similar device and translated into an electronic form.[4]

Bar code Two-dimensional: Array of coded bars and/or dots in a two-dimensional array, read by a laser, camera, or other imaging device, and translated into electronic form. There are several commonly used symbologies. Not only do these permit the storage and scanning of far more information than a one-dimensional bar code, but also typically include error checking and redundancy. Depending on the symbology, a small 2-D bar code can store 200+ characters of information, and still be ready, even if 30% or more of the bar code is smudged or missing.[99]

Bar coding A code consisting of a group of printed and variously patterned bars and spaces, and sometimes numerals, that are designed to be scanned and read into computer memory as identification for the object it labels. Bar coding is used by materials management, nursing, and pharmacy, in inpatient and outpatient settings.[2]

Baseband The use of an entire bandwidth for digital bi-directional data transmission. Only one transmission at a time is possible in baseband networks. An Ethernet network is a baseband network.[1]

Baseline Compiled performance statistics for use in the planning and analysis of systems and networks.[1]

BASIC Beginner's All-purpose Symbolic Instruction Code. A family of high-level programming languages. Originally devised as an easy-to-use programming language, it became widespread on home microcomputers in the 1980s, and remains popular to this day in a handful of heavily evolved dialects.[33]

Basic input output system *See* **BIOS**.

BAT Filename extension for a batch file.[1]

Batch Amount of material which is uniform in character and quantity, as shown by compliance with production and quality assurance test requirements, and produced during a defined validated process of manufacture.[117]

Batch mode A non-interactive mode of using a computer in which customers submit jobs for processing and receive results on completion.[4]

Batch processing Batch processing is the sequential execution of a series of programs ('jobs') on a computer. In many companies, the batch jobs are scheduled on a timetable (e.g., 'end of day' and 'end of quarter') and can be initiated automatically by, for example, the IBM mainframe Job Control Language, or manually by an operator.[7]

Baud A measure of signal changes per second in a modem or other communications device.[1]

BBS **Bulletin board service.** A noncommercial dial-up service usually run by a user group or software company. One can exchange messages with other users, and upload or download software.[1]

BDC **Backup domain controller.** Secondary Windows NT server that contains a copy of the security database. Authenticates users of the PDC (primary domain controller) are unavailable.[1]

Beaconing Token-ring network signaling process that informs computers on the network that a serious error has occurred. A problem area ablation process.[1]

Beaming Transfer of data or software programs between devices, such as personal digital assistants (PDAs), personal computers, and printers using either infrared or radio-wave transmission.[107]

Bedside workstation Workstation in a patient room or examining room.[4]

Beginner's All-purpose Symbolic Instruction Code *See* **BASIC**.[1]

Benchmarking A process of searching out and studying the best practices that produce superior performance. Benchmarks may be established within the same organization (internal benchmarking), outside of the organization, with another organization that produces the same service or product (external benchmarking), or with reference to a similar function or process in another industry (functional benchmarking).[123]

Best of breed Information technology strategy approach throughout the organization that can be defined as a system that is using vendors who concentrate on category/niche (business office, financial, medical records) or application-specific software; as opposed to vendors who supply hospital information systems that support a broad range of applications across many business categories.[2]

Best practice A way or method of accomplishing a business function, or process, that is considered to be superior to all other known methods.[123]

Best practices Best practices are the most up-to-date patient care interventions, which result in the best patient outcomes and minimize patient risk of death or complications.[138]

Beta testing The final stage in the testing of new software before its commercial release, conducted by testers other than its developers.[35]

BGI **Binary gateway interface.** Provides a method of running a program from a Web server. Uses a binary Dynamic Link Library (DLL), which is loaded into memory when the server starts.[1]

BGP **Border gateway protocol.** Used to advertise the networks that can be reached within an autonomous system. Newer than the EGP (exterior gateway protocol).[1]

Binary A base two numbering system consisting of two numbers (0 and 1), called bits.[1]

Binary gateway interface *See* **BGI**.

Binding 1. The linking of a protocol driver to a network adapter. 2. An affirmation by a certificate authority/attribute authority (or its acting registration authority) of the relationship between a named identity and its public key or biometric template.[1,114]

BinHex A file conversion format that converts binary files to ASCII test files.[1]

Bioinformatics An academic field involving the application of informatics to the biological sciences.[58]

Biomedical informatics An academic field involving the application of informatics in medicine.

Biometric Pertaining to the use of specific attributes that reflect unique personal characteristics, such as a fingerprint, an eye blood-vessel print, or a voice print, to validate the identity of a person.[3]

Biometric authentication Use of technology to identify a person through recognition of specific or unique physical characteristics, such as retina, fingerprints, or voice patterns.[114]

Biometric identification Use of physiological characteristics, such as fingerprints or voiceprint, for identification.[11]

Biometric identifier An identifier based on some physical characteristic, such as a fingerprint.[5]

Biometric information The stored electronic information pertaining to a biometric. This information can be in terms of raw or compressed pixels, or in terms of some characteristic.[114]

Biometric system An automated system capable of the following: capturing a biometric sample from the end user, extracting biometric data from that sample, comparing the extracted biometric data with data contained in one or more references, deciding how well the samples match, indicating whether or not an identification or verification of identity has been achieved.[114]

BIOS **Basic input output system.** The first operating system code that executes open computer boot-up. It is contained in flash memory or ROM firmware on the motherboard.[1]

Biosense A syndromic surveillance and situational awareness program being developed by the Centers for Disease Control and Prevention (CDC). Focuses on collecting data from many hospitals in the community, as well as other data sources, to develop an understanding of the current state of community health.[99]

Biosurveillance Surveillance programs in areas such as human health, hospital preparedness, state and local preparedness, vaccine research and procurement, animal health, food and agriculture safety, and environmental monitoring that integrate those efforts into one comprehensive system. *See also* **Surveillance**.[48]

Biosurveillance Use Case This HITSP Interoperability Specification (IS02) is designed to meet the specific requirements of the Biosurveillance Use Case, defined as implementation of near real-time, nationwide public health event monitoring to support early detection, situational awareness, and rapid response management across care delivery, public health, and other authorized government agencies.

Bioterrorism Terrorism using germ warfare; an intentional human release of a naturally-occurring, or human-modified, toxin or biological agent.[7]

Bit **Binary digit.** First termed by John Tukey in 1949. Smallest unit of information associated with computers and information processing.[1]

Bit depth The number of bits used to represent each pixel in an image, determining its color or tonal range.[1]

Bitmap An image stored as a pattern of pixels corresponding bit-by-bit with the associated image. Used by computers because of its simplicity.[1] Also called *bit-mapped data.*

Bitpipe Online resource for technical white papers, product literature, Web casts, and case studies.[36]

Bits per second *See* **BPS**.

Block algorithms Formulas that encrypt data one block at a time.[1]

Blog A Web site, usually maintained by an individual with regular entries of commentary, descriptions of events, or other material such as graphics or video.

Bluetooth A protocol designed for short-range wireless communication, or networking, among a variety of devices.[107]

Boolean logic Form of logic seen in computer applications in which all values are expressed either as true or false. Symbols used to designate this are often called Boolean operators. They consist of equal to (=), more than (>), less than (<), and any combination of these, plus the use of 'AND,' 'OR,' and 'NOT.'[11]

Boot partition Partition that contains the operating system files.[1]

Border gateway protocol *See* **BGP.**

Bounce Act of gracefully shutting down a system and subsequent restarting or rebooting. Ensures system changes are active and program areas are cleared due to the reboot process.[1]

Bound applications Programs compiled to run under DOS or OS/2.[1]

Bourne shell Original and most widely used interactive command interpreter and programming language. UNIX shell.[1]

BPS **Bits per second.** The basic unit of speed associated with data transmission.[1]

Breach of security Any action by an authorized or unauthorized user that violates access rules and regulations, and results in a negative impact upon the data in the system or the system itself; or that causes data or services within a system to suffer unauthorized disclosure, modification, destruction, or denial of service.[1]

Breakthrough use case A use case selected for implementation which crosses boundaries and levels, intended to stimulate investment and deliver both immediate and long-term benefits.[48]

Bridge Computer or device that connects or relates two or more similar networks or local area networks (LAN) that use the same protocols.[1]

Bridging router *See* **Brouter.**

Broadband The use of all bands of overall bandwidth for unidirectional data transmission. Multiple transmissions can occur at the same time in broadband networks.[1]

Broadcast A packet delivery technique that sends and delivers a single message for all nodes on a network.[1]

Broadcast storm Result of the number of broadcast messages on the network, reaching or surpassing the bandwidth capability of the network.[1]

Broker Application system that acts as a intermediary between two collaborating systems or services.[8]

Brouter **Bridging router.** A device that provides both bridging and routing functions. Acts as a bridge for some protocols, and a router for the rest.[1]

Browser A program that enables users to access information on the Internet through the World Wide Web. A software tool that supports graphics and hyperlinks, and is needed to navigate the Web.[1]

Buffer Temporary storage holding areas for input or output data, mainly used to compensate for differences in data flows.[1]

Bug Unwanted or unintended programming mistake or hardware error condition that causes system failure, error, malfunction, or unpredictable system actions.[1]

Bulletin board service *See* **BBS.**

Bus **1.** A structure that is used for connecting processors and peripherals, either within a system or in a local area network (LAN). **2.** The internal wiring between and within the CPU and other motherboard subsystems.[4,1]

Business associate An individual or corporate 'person' who performs on behalf of the department any function or activity involving the use or disclosure of protected health information (PHI), and who is not a member of the department's workforce. The definition of 'function or activity' includes: claims processing or administration, data analysis, utilization review, quality assurance, billing, legal, actuarial, accounting, consulting, data processing, management, administrative, accreditation, financial services, and similar services for which the department might contract are included, if access to PHI is involved. Business associates do not include licensees or providers, unless the licensee or provider also performs some 'function or activity' on behalf of the Department of Homeland Security.[118]

Business associate agreement Agreement between a covered entity and its business associate, in which the business associate agrees to restrict its use and disclosure of the covered entities' protected health information.[48]

Business intelligence system Business intelligence (BI) is a broad category of business processes, application software, and other technologies for gathering, storing, analyzing, and providing access to data to help users make better business decisions. It can be described as the process of enhancing data into information, and then into knowledge. Business intelligence is carried out to gain sustainable competitive advantage, and is a valuable core competence in some instances. *See also* **Decision support system**.[7]

Business-to-business *See* **B2B**.

Business-to-consumer *See* **B2C**.

Byte Series of either 0 or 1 bits used to represent a character and recognized by the computer as a single entity.[1]

C

C, programming language A standardized imperative computer programming language, developed in the early 1970s by Dennis Ritchie, for use on the UNIX operating system. It has since spread to many other operating systems, and is one of the most widely used programming languages. C is prized for its efficiency, and is the most popular programming language for writing system software, though it is also used for writing applications. It is also commonly used in computer science education, despite not being designed for novices.[7]

C+/C++ An established programming language found in many operating systems, including UNIX. C++ is a daughter program based on objects, and is quickly becoming a favored programming language as object-oriented technology gains popularity.[107] *See also* **Java**.

CA Certification authority. The official responsible for performing the comprehensive evaluation of the technical and nontechnical security features of an IT system and other safeguards, made in support of the accreditation process, to establish the extent that a particular design and implementation meet a set of specified security requirements.[97]

caBIG™ The Cancer Biomedical Informatics Grid.[37]

Cache 1. An area of temporary computer memory storage space that is reserved for data recently read from disk, which allows the processor to quickly retrieve it, if it is needed again. A part of random access memory (RAM). **2.** A small, fast memory holding recently-accessed data, designed to speed up further access.[1,8]

Caching services This service is used to manage the cache, and will provide functions related to cache responses based on configured settings. These settings may include time to live, persistence, cache cycling, parameter/role/facility based caching, etc.[8]

CAD Computer aided design. The use of a wide range of computer-based tools that assist engineers and architects in their design activities. It involves both software and special-purpose hardware.[7]

CAL Computer assisted learning. Refers to a system of educational instruction, performed almost entirely by computer. Such systems typically incorporate functions, such as assessing student capabilities with a pre-test; presenting educational materials in a navigable form; providing repetitive drills to improve the student's command of knowledge; possibly, providing game-based drills to increase learning enjoyment; assessing student progress with a post-test; routing students through a series of courseware instructional programs; and recording student scores and progress for later inspection by a courseware instructor. *See also* **CBL**.[7]

Call back A procedure in which a data processing system identifies a calling terminal, disconnects the call, and dials the calling terminal to authenticate the calling terminal.[3]

Canon Group (The) A group of leading health informaticists who convened in the early 1990s and defined the need for a concept-oriented (ontologically based) medical terminology.[38]

Canonical Of, or relating to, a set of core, standard, irreducible, or foundational concepts, works, or documents.[38]

CAP Capitation. Pre-established payment of a set dollar amount to a provider on a per member basis, for certain contracted services, for a given period of time. Amount of money paid to provider depends on number of individuals registered to his/her patient list, not on volume or type of service provided.[15]

Capability Nonfunctional, observable system qualities that do not represent specific functions and cannot be satisfied by any one component. These are emerging properties that are observed in a collection of components working together.[8]

Capacity The ability to run a number of jobs per unit of time.[8]

Capture The method of taking a biometric sample from an end user.[114]

Card reader Equipment capable of reading the information on a smart card, such as that in the magnetic stripe or chip.[1]

Care 1. Suffering of mind: grief. 2. (a) A disquieted state of mixed uncertainty, apprehension, and responsibility; (b) a cause for such anxiety. 3. (a) painstaking or watchful attention; (b) maintenance. 4. Regard coming from desire or esteem. 5. Charge, supervision (under a doctor's care). 6. A person or thing that is an object of attention, anxiety, or solicitude.[32]

Care coordination A central, ongoing component of an effective system of care for children and youth with special healthcare needs and their families. Care coordination engages families in development of a care plan and links them to health and other services that address the full range of their needs and concerns. Principles of care coordination reflect the central role of families and the prioritization of child and family concerns, strengths and needs in effective care of children with special healthcare needs. Activities of care coordination may vary from family to family, but start with identification of individual child and family needs, strengths and concerns, and aim simultaneously at meeting family needs, building family capacity and improving systems of care.[132]

Care management A set of activities which assures that every person served by the treatment system has a single approved care (service) plan that is coordinated, not duplicative, and designed to assure cost effective and good outcomes. Care managers will oversee a patient's journey through treatment.[133]

Care plan. *See* Patient plan of care.

Care transitions Movement of patients between different formal or informal healthcare providers over the course of an illness, encompassing the set of actions or processes designed to ensure the patient has continuity of care. Every change from provider or setting is another care transition.[128]

Cardiac catheterization workflow *See* **CATH**.

Cardinality 1. The number of rows in a table, or the number of indexed entries in a defined index. 2. The number of elements in a set. *See also* **Multiplicity**.[16]

Carrier sense multiple access with collision detection *See* **CSMA/CD**.

CAS **Computer-assisted surgery.**

Case management A collaborative process involving the patient/member and his or her family, the healthcare provider, and the health plan's case management nurse.[15]

Casemix 1. The 'mix' of cases treated by a provider, based on the average 'weight' (based on a relative scale) of case types treated. Originally used with DRGs, with weights calculated by the Centers for Medicare & Medicaid Services based on historical cost data, casemix was a rough measure of the complexity and severity of the cohort of patients treated by a particular provider. 2. Grouping of patients according to disease or procedure categories with homogeneous cost, following a scoring system using mean values by hospital, in relation with the means obtained from national statistics.[4]

Casemix index A composite 'score' derived from the average 'weight' assigned by Medicare to individual DRGs. Initially based on costs by case type, the casemix index was used to establish base rates for payment that were then adjusted as the index changed for a given provider.[1]

Casemix systems An early form of analytic decision support system, which, for the first time, combined clinical and financial data for analysis. Sparked by the introduction of prospective payment (DRGs), the first system was developed at Rush-Presbyterian-St. Luke's and was popularized by a system developed by New England Medical Center.[1]

Case-sensitive Programming languages that distinguish between uppercase and lowercase letters.[1]

CAT-1-5 Categories 1-5. Categories of unshielded twisted pair cable (UTP). Allows voice grade only transmission rates below 100 Mbps up to 100 meters, or 328 feet in length per segment.[1]

Categories 1-5 *See* **CAT-1-5.**

Categorization Process by which individual information products can be associated with other products, using vocabularies designed to help citizens locate and access information. There can be multiple attributes assigned to a product (e.g., multiple categorizations). Categorization is used to provide context to a specific product, and to define relationships across a group of information products.[17]

CATH Cardiac catheterization workflow. Establishes the continuity and integrity of basic patient data in the context of the cardiac catheterization procedure. This profile deals specifically with consistent handling of patient identifiers and demographic data, including that of emergency patient presentation where the actual patient identity may not be established until after the beginning of the procedure, or even a significant time after the completion of the procedure. It also specifies the scheduling and coordination of procedure data across a variety of imaging, measurement, and analysis systems, and its reliable storage in an archive form where it is available to support subsequent workflow steps, such as reporting. It also provides central coordination of the completion status of steps of a potentially multi-phase (diagnostic and interventional) procedure. *See also* **Profile.**[56]

Cause-and-effect diagram A display of the factors that are thought to affect a particular problem or system outcome. The tool is often used in a quality improvement program to group people's ideas about the causes of a particular problem in an orderly way. (Also known as the fishbone diagram because of the shape that it takes when illustrating the primary and secondary causes.)[123]

CBL Computer-based learning. Refers to the use of computers as a key component of the educational environment. While this can refer to the use of computers in a classroom, the term more broadly refers to a structured environment, in which computers are used for teaching purposes. The concept is generally seen as being distinct from the use of computers in ways where learning is at least a peripheral element of the experience (e.g., computer games and Web browsing).[7]

CBSA Core-based statistical area. Defined by the Census Bureau as a geographic area with an urbanized population of at least 50,000, or an urban cluster with a population of at least 10,000, plus the adjacent counties that have a high degree of social and economic integration with the core as measured through commuting ties.[2]

CCC Clinical Care Classification (CCC) System is a concept-oriented nursing terminology framework and coding structure for the electronic documentation and classification of the nursing process. The nomenclature is discrete atomic level data elements about the nursing process, encompassing nursing assessment, diagnosis, intervention, actions, and actual and expected outcomes to measure patient outcomes over time, across population groups and geographic locations. Recognized by the American Nurses Association. (Formerly Home Health Care Classification - HHCC.)[27]

CCD Continuity of care document. A specification is an XML-based markup standard (developed between HL7 and ASTM) intended to specify the encoding, structure and semantics of a patient summary clinical document for message exchange.[16]

CCoM Clinical context management. Coordinates different healthcare applications on a desktop, creating a user-driven, patient-centered information workspace.[7]

CCOW Clinical context object workgroup. Using a technique called 'context management,' CCOW provides the clinician with a unified view on the information held in separate and disparate healthcare applications referring to the same patient, encounter, or user. This means that when a clinician signs onto one application within the group of disparate applications tied together by the CCOW environment, that same sign-on is simultaneously executed on all other applications within the group. Similarly, when the clinician selects a patient, the same patient is selected in all the applications. CCOW then builds a combined view of the patient on one screen. CCOW works for both client-server and Web-based applications. The acronym CCOW is a reference to the standards committee within the HL7 group that developed the standard.[16]

CCR   Continuity of care record. 1. A standard specification developed jointly by ASTM International, the Massachusetts Medical Society (MMS), the Healthcare Information and Management Systems Society (HIMSS), the American Academy of Family Physicians (AAFP), and the American Academy of Pediatrics (AAP). It is intended to foster and improve continuity of patient care, reduce medical errors, and assure at least a minimum standard of health information transportability when a patient is referred or transferred to, or is otherwise seen by another provider. **2.** A new XML document standard for a summary of personal health information that clinicians can send when a patient is referred, and that patients can carry with them to promote continuity, quality, and safety of care.[39]

CD   Committee draft. The second internal technical committee balloting stage for international standards from ISO.[3]

CD   Compact disc. Optical disc used to store digital data, originally developed for storing digital audio files.[7]

CDA   Clinical document architecture. An XML-based document markup standard that specifies the structure and semantics of clinical documents for the purpose of exchange. Known earlier as the patient record architecture, CDA provides an exchange model for clinical documents, such as discharge summaries and progress notes, and brings the healthcare industry closer to the realization of an electronic medical record. By leveraging the use of XML, the HL7 Reference Information Model (RIM), and coded vocabularies, the CDA makes documents both machine-readable (so they are easily parsed and processed electronically) and human-readable so they can be easily retrieved and used by the people who need them.[16]

CDFS   CD-ROM file system. 32-bit file system used in conjunction with CD-ROMs on Windows 95 and Windows NT machines.[1]

CDMA   Code division multiple access. A wireless technology that includes digital voice service with 9.6 Kpbs to 14.4 Kpbs data services, and includes enhanced calling features, such as caller ID, but lacks an 'always-on' data connection feature.[1]

CDPD   Cellular digital packet data. A TCP/IP-based industry standard for data, which is compatible with nearly all TCP/IP applications. Data packets can follow the user from cell to cell of calling regions, keeping an 'always-on' data connection alive while the user is in motion.[1]

CDR   Clinical data repository. 1. A structured, systematically collected storehouse of patient-specific clinical data. **2.** A centralized database that allows organizations to collect, store, access, and report on clinical, administrative, and financial information collected from various applications within or across the healthcare organization that provides health organizations an open environment for accessing/viewing, managing, and reporting enterprise information.[12]

CD-ROM   Compact disk read-only memory. Read-only optical disk storage used for imaging, reference, and database application with massive amounts of data and for multi-media.[1]

CD-ROM file system   *See* **CDFS**.

CDT-2   Current Dental Terminology. Official coding system for dentists.[40]

CDW   Clinical data warehouse. Grouping of data accessible by a single data management system, possibly of diverse sources, pertaining to a health system or subsystem, enabling secondary data analysis for questions relevant to understanding the functioning of that health system and, hence, can support proper maintenance and improvement of that health system.[94]

CE   Coded element. A data type that transmits codes and the text associated with the code.[16]

Cellular digital packet data   *See* **CDPD**.

Central processing unit   *See* **CPU**.

Central processing unit   *See* **Microprocessor**.

CERT   Computer emergency response team. A team of system specialists and other professionals, such as lawyers, who investigate computer break-ins and attacks.[1]

Certificate   Public key certificate.[121]

Certificate authority An independent licensing agency that vouches for a patient/person's identity in encrypted electronic communication. Acting as a type of electronic notary public, a certified authority verifies and stores a sender's public and private encryption keys and issues a digital certificate, or 'seal of authenticity,' to the recipient.[8]

Certificate distribution Act of publishing certificates and transferring certificates to security subjects.[121]

Certificate extension Extension fields (known as extensions) in X.509 certificates that provide methods for associating additional attributes with users or public keys, and for managing the certification hierarchy. Note: Certificate extensions may be either critical (i.e., a certificate-using system has to reject the certificate if it encounters a critical extension it does not recognize) or noncritical (i.e., it may be ignored if the extension is not recognized).[121]

Certificate generation Act of creating certificates.[121]

Certificate issuer Authority trusted by one or more relying parties to create and assign certificates and which may, optionally, create the relying parties' keys.[121] Note 1: Adapted from ISO 9594-8:2001. Note 2: Authority in the CA term does not imply any government authorization, but only denotes that it is trusted. Note 3: Certificate issuer may be a better term, but CA is very widely used.

Certificate management Procedures relating to certificates (i.e., certificate generation, certificate distribution, certificate archiving, and revocation).[121]

Certificate policy *See* **CP**.

Certification 1. Comprehensive evaluation of the technical and nontechnical security features of an IT system and other safeguards, made in support of the accreditation process, to establish the extent that a particular design and implementation meets a set of specified security requirements. **2.** Procedure by which a third party gives assurance that all, or part of, a data processing system conforms to security requirements.[97,121]

Certification authority *See* **CA**.

Certification practices statement *See* **CPS**.

Certification profile Specification of the structure and permissible content of a certificate type.[121]

Certification revocation Act of removing any reliable link between a certificate and its related owner (or security subject owner) because the certificate is not trusted any more, even though it is unexpired.[121]

CF Conditional formatting/coded formatted element. 1. A tool that allows a user to apply formats to a cell or range of cells, and have that formatting change, depending on the value of the cell or the value of a formula. **2.** Coded element with formatted values data type. This data type transmits codes and the formatted text associated with the code.[41,16]

CGI Common gateway interface. A standard or protocol for external gateway programs to interface with information servers, such as HTTP servers. Part of the overall HTTP protocol.[1]

Challenge handshake authentication protocol *See* **CHAP**.

Changing or moving Presenting new directions and developing new behaviors and attitudes based on new information. A learning process and social support is critical to this phase.[6]

Channel A path for the transmission of signals between a transmitting and receiving device.[1]

Channel sharing unit/data service unit *See* **CSU/DSU**.

CHAP Challenge handshake authentication protocol. An authentication protocol used to logon a user to an Internet access provider.[1]

Character A member of a set of elements that is used for representation. Organization or control of data.[3]

Character-based terminal A type of computer terminal and system that supports only alphabetical or numeric characters, with the visual displays and 'mouse'-driven, bit-map software that most systems now utilize; the opposite of graphical user interface (GUI).[1]

Characteristic Abstraction of a property of an object or of a set of objects.[98]

Charge posting *See* **CHG**.

Check digit The resultant representation of a checksum operation.[1]

CHG Charge posting. Specifies the exchange of information from the department system scheduler/order filler actor to the charge processor actor regarding charges associated with particular procedures, as well as communication between the ADT/patient registration and charge processor actors about patient demographics, accounts, insurance, and guarantors. The charge posted transaction contains all of the required procedure data to generate a claim. Currently, these interfaces contain fixed field formatted or HL7-style data. The goal of including this transaction in the IHE Technical Framework is to standardize the charge posted transaction to a charge processor, thus reducing system interface installation time between clinical systems and charge processors. Additionally, the charge posted transaction reduces the need of the billing system to have knowledge of the radiology internals. The result is that the charge processor will receive more complete, timely, and accurate data. *See also* **Profile**.[56]

Chief information officer *See* **CIO**.

Chief medical information officer *See* **CMIO**.

Chief nursing information officer *See* **CNIO**.

Chief security officer *See* **CSO**.

Chief technology officer *See* **CTO**.

Child Document subordinate to another, such as a parent document.[16]

CHIN Community health information network. The service model for delivery of medical information across a local community, shared between providers, that was promulgated in the early 1990s. The movement failed to take hold due to concerns about aligning costs with benefits, with confidentiality of patient and propriety information, and for other factors.[99] *See* **RHIO**.[1]

Chip A small piece of thin semiconductor material, such as silicon, that has been chemically processed to have a specific set of electrical characteristics, such as circuits, storage, and/or logic elements.[1]

Chronic care model Model developed by Edward Wagner and colleagues that provides a solid foundation from which healthcare teams can operate. The model has six dimensions: community resources and policies; health system organization of healthcare; patient self-management supports; delivery system redesign; decision support; and clinical information system. The ultimate goal is to have activated patients interact in a productive way with well-prepared healthcare teams. Three components that are particularly critical to this goal are adequate decision support, which includes systems that encourage providers to use evidence-based protocols; delivery system redesign, such as using group visits and same-day appointments; and use of clinical information systems, such as disease registries, which allow providers to exchange information and follow patients over time.[138]

Chronic disease A sickness that is long-lasting or recurrent. Examples include diabetes, asthma, heart disease, kidney disease and chronic lung disease.[138]

Chronic disease management *See* **disease management**.

CIO Chief information officer. The senior officer responsible for information systems within an organization.[1]

Cipher text Data produced through the use of encipherment, the semantic content of which is not available.[121]

Circuit switched A type of network connection that establishes a continuous electrical connection between calling and called users for their exclusive use until the connection is released (e.g., telephone system); ideal for communications that require data to be transmitted in real time. *See also* **Packet switching**.[1]

CIS Clinical information system. A system dedicated to collecting, storing, manipulating, and making available clinical information important to the delivery of healthcare. Clinical information systems may be limited in scope to a single area (e.g., lab system, ECG management system) or they may be comprehensive and cover virtually all facets of clinical information (e.g., electronic patient; the original discharge summary residing in the chart, with a copy of the report sent to the admitting physician, another copy existing on the transcriptionist's machine).[8]

CISC Complex instruction set computer processor. CISC computers use microprocessors with a large number of execution steps and many clock cycles to operate. Intel computers are CISC computers.[1]

Claim attachment Any variety of hardcopy forms or electronic records needed to process a claim, in addition to the claim itself.[10]

Claim status category codes A national administrative code set that indicates the general category of the status of healthcare claims. This code set is used in the X12 248 claim status notification transaction, and is maintained by the healthcare code maintenance committee.[10]

Claim status codes A national administrative code set that identifies the status of healthcare claims. This code set is used in the X12 277 claim status notification transaction, and is maintained by the healthcare code maintenance committee.[10]

Class A term used in programs written in the object-oriented paradigm. A class description will contain the code which describes the features (i.e., the data [properties] and behaviors [methods] of an object).[4]

Classification The systematic placement of things or concepts into categories which share some common attribute, quality, or property. A classification structure is a listing of terms that depicts hierarchical structures.[4]

Clear text Unencoded text that can easily be read. *See also* **Plain text**.[1]

Clearance level The security level of an individual who may access information.[1]

Clickable image Any image that has instructions embedded on it so that clicking on it initiates some kind of action or result. On a Web page, a clickable image is any image that has a URL embedded in it.[1]

Client An individual who requests or receives services in healthcare. May be used in place of the word 'patient.'[118]

Client A single term used interchangeably to refer to the user, the workstations, and the portion of the program that runs on the workstation. If the client is on a local area network (LAN), it can share resources with another computer (server).[8]

Client application A system entity, usually a computer process acting on behalf of a human user, that makes use of a service provided by a server.[114]

Client information Personal information relating to healthcare.[118]

Client records All personal information that has been collected, compiled, or created about clients which may be maintained in one or more locations and in various forms, reports, or documents, including information that is stored or transmitted by electronic media.[118]

Client registry A client registry is the area where a patient/person's information (i.e., name, date of birth, Social Security number, health access number) is securely stored and maintained.[8]

Client/server model 1. A client application is one that resides on a user's computer, but sends requests to a remote system to execute a designated procedure using arguments supplied by the user. The computer that initiates the request is the client, and the computer responding to the request is the server. **2.** A model for computing that splits the processing between clients and servers on a network, assigning functions to the machine most able to perform the function.[1]

Clinical algorithm Flow charts to which a diagnostician or therapist can refer a decision on how to manage a patient with a specific clinical program.[14]

Clinical Care Classification System CCC. Two interrelated taxonomies of nursing diagnoses and outcomes, and of nursing interventions and actions.[52]

Clinical context management *See* **CCoM**.

Clinical context object workgroup *See* **CCOW**.

Clinical data All relevant clinical and socioeconomic data disclosed by the patient and others, as well as observations, findings, therapeutic interventions, and prognostic statements, generated by the members of the healthcare team.[1]

Clinical data information systems Automated systems that serve as a tool to inform clinicians about tests, procedures, and treatment in an effort to improve quality of care through real-time assistance in decision making, and to increase efficiency and decrease unnecessary utilization.[1]

Clinical data repository See **CDR**.

Clinical data warehouse See **CDW**.

Clinical decision support system **1.** An application that uses pre-established rules and guidelines that can be created and edited by the healthcare organization, and integrates clinical data from several sources to generate alerts and treatment suggestions. For example, all patients who have a potassium below 2.5% should not have a cardiac glycoside. The physician would enter into the system the prescription for a cardiac glycoside, and the system would pop up an alert to the fact that the patient should not be given this medication due to the low level of potassium in his or her blood. **2.** Computer system designed to help health professionals make clinical decisions.[2,4]

Clinical document architecture See **CDA**.

Clinical documentation system An application that allows clinicians to chart treatment/therapy/health assessment results for a patient. This application provides the flow sheets and care plan documentation for a patient's course of therapy.[2]

Clinical informatics Broadly defined as the use of computers and information technology in the provision of patient care.

Clinical information or data Information/data related to the health and healthcare of an individual, collected from or about an individual receiving healthcare services.[1]

Clinical laboratory information system Information system that manages clinical laboratory data to support laboratory management, laboratory data collection and processing, patient care, and medical decision making. Note: May be part of a hospital information system, or may be independent.[4]

Clinical observation Clinical information, excluding information about treatment and intervention. Note: Clinical information that does not record an intervention is, by nature, a clinical observation.[4]

Clinical observation access service See **COAS**.

Clinical pathway A patient care management tool that organizes, sequences, and times the major interventions of nursing staff, physicians, and other departments for a particular case type, subset, or condition.[123]

Clinical performance measure This is a method or instrument to estimate or monitor the extent to which the actions of a healthcare practitioner or provider conform to practice guidelines, medical review criteria, or standards of quality.[102]

Clinical practice guidelines A set of systematically developed statements, usually based on scientific evidence, to assist practitioners and patient decision making about appropriate healthcare for specific clinical circumstances.[123]

Clinical protocol A set of rules defining a standardized treatment program or behavior in certain circumstances.[4]

Clinical record See **EHR**.[4]

Clinical status Description of the individual by means of results for a specified set of measurable quantities.[4]

Clinical terminology Terminology required directly or indirectly to describe health conditions and healthcare activities.[59]

Clinical terminology system A collection of words or phrases organized together to represent the entities and relationships that characterize the knowledge within a given biomedical domain.[108]

Clinical trials Research studies that involve patients. Biotechnology companies typically use clinical trials to assess the efficacy and safety of new therapies and to answer scientific questions. Typically, there are three phases during a clinical trial. Phase I is designed to evaluate the safety of the product in humans; phase II analyzes the effects of dose escalation, and phase III definitively evaluates the clinical efficacy of the product.[104]

Clinical/medical code sets   Identify medical conditions and the procedures, services, equipment, and supplies used to deal with them. Nonclinical or nonmedical or administrative code sets identify, or characterize, entities and events in a manner that facilitates an administrative process.[10]

Clipboard   An area used to temporarily store cut or copied information; can store text, graphics, objects, and other data. Clipboard contents are erased when new information is placed on the clipboard or when the computer is shut down.[1]

Clipper chip   A data encryption chip used by the federal government in data communications equipment, such as computers, modems, fax machines, and phones for protection from hackers, intruders, and criminals.[1]

Clock speed   Measure, referred to in MHz (mega-Hertz), is an indicator of the speed of computer operations.[4]

Clone   A computer, software product, or device, that works the same as another, better-known product.[2]

Closed card system   A smart card system in which the cards can only be used in a specified environment, such as a college campus.[1]

Closed loop medication administration The process for administering medication to patients in a hospital where the medication order is created by the physician, validated and dispensed by the pharmacist, and administered by the nurse to the patient at point of care, where the clinical decision support system monitors the process for the five rights of administration—right patient, right time, right drug, right dose, and right route. The identification of the nurse, patient, and medication is facilitated by either bar codes or radio frequency identification (RFID) tags that are scanned during the administration process. If the medication passes the five rights check, it is administered to the patient and recorded on the electronic medication administration record for the patient. Overriden (given in spite of alerts) or failed medication administration processes are logged to audit functions for evaluation by clinicians to

manage and monitor this process for continuing improvement.[2]

Cluster   Disk storage unit of 1,024 bytes.[1]

CM   Composite message/composite data type. A field that is a combination of other meaningful data fields. Each portion is called a component.[16]

CMD   Cmd. Similar to a .bat (batch file) or an .exe. A way of giving command line (like DOS) prompts to the computer (e.g., to map the drive).[7]

CMET   Common message element type. Reusable data types which can be included in any number of messages without repeating the common internal structure.[16]

CMIO   Chief medical information officer. Responsible for the development of clinical information systems that assist clinicians in the delivery of patient care, promoting quality care, positive outcomes, and efficient use of clinical human resources.[32]

CMYK   Printing processes, such as offset lithography, use CMYK (cyan, magenta, yellow, black) inks; digital art must be converted to CMYK color for print.[57]

CNCL   Cancelled.

CNIO   Chief nursing information officer. Responsible for ensuring appropriate selection, implementation, and use of clinical IT throughout nursing areas. The scope of the position encompasses all aspects of clinical coordination and oversight for the integration of technology with nursing practice.[32]

COA   Compliance oriented architecture. The virtues of service-oriented architectures (SOAs) applied to the specific business challenge of compliance; the result is a flexible architecture that can meet compliance challenges now and in the future. Compliance requirements can be expressed as a set of core services.

COAS   Clinical observation access service. Standardizes access to clinical observations in multiple formats, including numerical data stored by instruments or entered from observations.

Coaxial cable   Network/communications cable medium, consisting of an inner conductor encased in a clear/white insulation and a braided outer conductor, surrounded by black PVC insulation.[1]

COB Close of business.[99]

COB Coordination of benefits. The process by which a payer handles claims that may involve other insurance companies (i.e., situations where an insured individual is covered by more than one insurance plan).

Code Concept identifier that is unique within a coding system.[126]

Code 128 A one-dimensional bar code symbology, using four different bar widths, used in Blood Banking and other health and non-healthcare applications.[99]

Code division multiple access *See* **CDMA**.

Code meaning Element within a coded set.[117]

Code set 1. A set of elements which is mapped on to another set according to a coding scheme. **2.** Clinical or medical code sets identify medical conditions, and the procedures, services, equipment, and supplies used to deal with them. Nonclinical or nonmedical or administrative code sets identify, or characterize, entities and events in a manner that facilitates an administrative process.[3,9]

Code set maintaining organization Under the Health Insurance Portability and Accountability Act (HIPAA), this is an organization that creates and maintains the code sets adopted by the Secretary for use in the transactions for which standards are adopted.[10]

Code value Result of applying a coding scheme to a code meaning.[117]

Codec Compression/decompression. An algorithm or specialized computer program that reduces the number of bytes consumed by large files and programs.[57]

Coded element *See* **CE**.

Coded formatted elements *See* **CF**.

Coded with exceptions *See* **CWE**.

Coding The activity of using a coding scheme to map from one set of elements to another set of elements. The products of classification and

coding are often used for similar purposes and sometimes considered as the same; however, coding and classification are distinct concepts.[4]

Coding scheme The collection of rules that maps the elements of one set onto the elements of a second set.[3]

Coding system Combination of a set of concepts (coded concepts), a set of code values, and at least one coding scheme mapping code values to coded concepts.[126]

Collect and communicate audit trails Define and identify security-relevant events and the data to be collected and communicated, as determined by policy, regulation, or risk analysis.[48]

Collect/collection The assembling of personal information through interviews, forms, reports, or other information sources.[48]

Collision detection The ability of a transmitting node to detect traffic on an Ethernet (baseband) shared network. If a transmitting station detects silence, it will transmit data. If a collision takes place, the transmitting station will wait a random amount of time before attempting to re-transmit the entire message. *See also* **CSMA/CD**.[1]

Comm closet Room or location where network electronic equipment resides and where drops terminate. Also known as a *wiring closet*.[1]

Command A sequence of words and/or symbols that instructs the computer to perform a specific task.[4]

Command interpreter Program that accesses and executes user input.[1]

Commission on Systemic Interoperability The Commission on Systemic Interoperability was authorized by the Medicare Modernization Act, and held its first meeting on January 10, 2005. The Commission is developing a strategy to make healthcare information instantly accessible at all times by consumers and their healthcare providers. It released its report and disbanded in October 2005.

Committee draft *See* **CD**.

Common gateway interface *See* **CGI**.

Common message element type *See* **CMET**.

Common object request broker architecture *See* **CORBA**.

Common services A type of software service that can be shared across multiple applications. These include services such as messaging, security, logging, auditing, mapping, etc. Common services are part of the Health Information Access Layer.[8]

Common vulnerabilities and exposures *See* **CVE**.

Common weakness enumeration *See* **CWE**.

Communication bus Part of the Health Information Access Layer (HIAL) that allows applications to communicate according to standard messages and protocols.[8]

Communication network Configuration of hardware, software, and transmission facilities for transmission and routing of data carrying signals between electronic devices.[4]

Communications security *See* **COMSEC**.

Communities of interest Inclusive term to describe collaborative groups of users who must exchange information in pursuit of shared goals, interests, missions, or business process and must have a shared vocabulary for the information exchanged. Communities provide an organization and maintenance construct for data.[18]

Community health information network *See* **CHIN**.

Compact disc *See* **CD**.

Compact disk read-only memory *See* **CD-ROM**.

Comparability The ability of different parties to share precisely the same meaning for data.[45]

Comparison The process of comparing a biometric with a previously stored reference.[114]

Compatibility Suitability of products, processes, or services for use together under specific conditions to fulfill relevant requirements without causing unacceptable interactions.[4]

Competence Demonstrated performance and application of knowledge to perform a required skill or activity to a specific, predetermined standard.[123]

Compiler 1. Programs written in high-level languages are translated into assembly language or machine language by a compiler. Assembly language programs are translated into machine language by a program called an assembler. Every CPU has its own unique machine language. Programs must be rewritten or recompiled, therefore, to run on different types of computers. 2. A program that translates a program written in a high-level programming language to a machine-language program which can then be executed. *See also* **Assembler**.[7,4]

Complex instruction set computer processor *See* **CISC**.

Compliance Adherence to those policies, procedures, guidelines, laws, regulations, and contractual arrangements to which the business process is subject.[118]

Compliance date Under the Health Insurance Portability and Accountability Act (HIPAA), this is the date by which a covered entity must comply with a standard, an implementation specification, or a modification. This is usually 24 months after the effective date of the associated final rule for most entities; by 36 months after the effective date for small health plans. For future changes in the standards, the compliance date would be at least 180 days after the effective date, but can be longer for small health plans and for complex changes.[10]

Component An object-oriented term used to describe the building block of GUI applications. A software object that contains data and code. A component may or may not be visible.[4]

Component object model Used by developers to create reusable software components, link components together to build applications, and take advantage of Windows services.[12]

Composite message *See* **CM**.

Compression/decompression *See* **Codec**.

Compromise Disclosure of information to unauthorized persons, or a violation of the security policy of a system in which unauthorized intentional or unintentional disclosure, modification, destruction, or loss of an object may have occurred.[114]

Computed tomography *See* **CT**.

Computer emergency response team *See* **CERT**.

Computer network A collection of computers that are physically and logically connected together to exchange information.[1]

Computer readable card A card capable of storing information in a form which can be read by a computer. Information may be written to the card on manufacture, or may be added during the use of the card. If the card contains a processor, the card is known as a 'smart card.'[4]

Computer security The protection of data and resources from accidental or malicious acts, usually by taking appropriate actions.[3]

Computer system An integrated arrangement of computer hardware and software operated by customers to perform prescribed tasks.[4]

Computer telephony integration *See* **CTI**.

Computer-aided instruction, computer-based training The development and use of computer technology to facilitate training or education on a topic. One of the most important advantages of using computer-based training is that the learner is provided with a self-paced training module. *See also* **CAL, CBL**.[6]

Computer-assisted learning *See* **CAL** and **CBL**.[4]

Computer-assisted medicine Use of computers directly in diagnostic or therapeutic interventions (e.g., computer-assisted surgery).

Computer-based learning *See* **CBL**.

Computer-based patient record *See* **EHR**.[4]

Computerized provider order entry *See* **CPOE**.

Computer-on-wheels *See* **COW**.

Computing environment The total environment in which an automated information system, network, or a component operates. The environment includes physical, administrative, and personnel procedures, as well as communication and networking relationships, with other information systems.[97]

COMSEC Measures and controls taken to deny unauthorized persons information derived from telecommunications and ensure the authenticity of such telecommunications. Communications security includes cryptosecurity, transmission security, emission security, and physical security of COMSEC material.[97]

Concentrator Network device where networked nodes are connected. Used to divide a data channel into two or more channels of lower bandwidth. *See also* **Hub**.[1]

Concept **1.** A concept is an abstraction or a general notation that may serve as a unit of thought or a theory. In terminology work, the distinction is made between a concept and the terms that reference the concept; the concept is identified as abstract from the language and the term is a symbol that is part of the language. **2.** A clinical idea to which a unique concept has been assigned. Each concept is represented by a row in the concepts table. Concept equivalence occurs when a post-coordinated expression has the same meaning as a pre-coordinated concept or another post-coordinated expression.[4,19] Note 1: Informally, the term 'concept' is often used when what is meant is 'concept representation.' However, this leads to confusion when precise meanings are required. Concepts arise out of human individual and social conceptualizations of the world around them. Concept representations are artifacts constructed of symbols.[96] Note 2: Concept representations are not necessarily bound to particular languages. However, they are influenced by the social or cultural context of use often leading to different categorizations.[96]

Concept harmonization Activity for reducing or eliminating minor differences between two or more concepts that are closely related to each other. Note: Concept harmonization is an integral part of standardization.[4]

Concept identifier Concept name, code, or symbol, which uniquely identifies a concept.[96]

Concept status A field in the concepts table that specifies whether a concept is in current use. Values include 'current,' 'duplicate,' 'erroneous,' 'ambiguous,' and 'limited.'[19]

Concept unique identifier *See* **CUI**.

Concepts table A data table consisting of rows, each of which represents a concept.[19]

Concurrent versioning system *See* **CVS**.

Conditional formatting *See* **CF**.

Confidentiality 1. Obligation of an entity that receives identifiable information about an individual as part of providing a service to that individual to protect that data or information; including not disclosing the identifiable information to unauthorized persons, or through unauthorized processes. **2.** A property by which information relating to an entity or party is not made available or disclosed to unauthorized individuals, entities, or processes.[48,3]

Configuration The components that make up a computer system, including the identity of the manufacturer, model, and various peripherals; the physical arrangement of those components (what is placed and where). The software settings that enable two computer components to communicate with each other.[1]

Configuration control Process of controlling modifications to an IT system's hardware, firmware, software, and documentation, to ensure the system is protected against improper modifications prior to, during, and after system implementation.[97]

Configuration management Management of security features and assurances through control of changes made to hardware, software, firmware, documentation, test, test fixtures, and test documentation, throughout the life-cycle of the IT.[97]

Configuration manager The individual or organization responsible for configuration control or configuration management.[97]

Configuration services This service is used to configure the EHRs. This includes configuration of the EHR data repository, the system, the metadata, the service components, EHR indexes, schema support, security, session and caching mechanism, etc.[8]

Conformance The precise set of conditions for the use of options which must be implemented in a standard. There are two types of conformance: dynamic and static. Dynamic conformance requirements of a standard are all those requirements (including options) which determine the possible behavior permitted by the standard. Static conformance is a statement of what conforming implementation should be capable of doing (i.e., what is implemented).[3]

Conformance assessment process The complete process of accomplishing all conformance testing activities necessary to enable the conformance of an implementation or system to one or more standards to be assessed.[4]

Conformance testing Testing to determine whether a system meets some specified standard. To aid in this, many test procedures and test setups have been developed, either by the standard's maintainers or external organizations, specifically for testing conformance to standards. Conformance testing is often performed by external organizations, or sometimes the standards body itself, to give greater guarantees of compliance. Products tested in such a manner are then advertised as being certified by that external organization as complying with the standard.[7]

Connectathon A testing event to which developers have registered their implementations for supervised interoperability testing with other implementations. Each participating system is tested for each registered combination of IHE actor and IHE integration or content profile.[93]

Connectivity The potential to establish links to, or interact with, another computer system or database.[1]

Consensus General agreement, characterized by the absence of sustained opposition to substantial issues by any important part of the concerned interests, and by a process that involves seeking to take into account the views of all parties concerned, and to reconcile any conflicting arguments.[4]

Consensus standards These are standards developed or adopted by consensus standards bodies, both domestic and international. Such work and the resultant standards are usually voluntary.[3]

Consent Under the Privacy Rule, consent is made by an individual for the covered entity to use or disclose identifiable health information for treatment, payment, and healthcare operations purposes only. This is different from consent for treatment, which many providers use and which should not be confused with the consent for use or disclosure of identifiable health information.

Consent for use and/or disclosure of identifiable health information is optional under the Privacy Rule, although it may be required by state law, and may be combined with consent for treatment unless prohibited by other law.[48]

Consent directive The record of a healthcare consumer's privacy policy that grants or withholds consent for: one or more principals (identified entity or role); performing one or more operations (e.g., collect, access, use, disclose, amend, or delete); purposes, such as treatment, payment, operations, research, public health, quality measures, health status evaluation by third parties, or marketing; certain conditions (e.g., when unconscious); specified time period (e.g., effective and expiry dates); and certain context (e.g., in an emergency).[48]

Consent informed *See* Informed consent.

Consenter An author of a consent directive; may be the healthcare consumer or patient, a delegate of the healthcare consumer (e.g., a representative with healthcare power of attorney), or a provider with legal authority to either override a healthcare consumer's consent directive, or create a directive that prevents a patient's access to personal health information until the provider has had an opportunity to review the PHI with the patient.[48]

Consistency The transaction takes the resources from one consistent state to another. *See also* **ACID**.[7]

Consistent presentation of images *See* **CPI**.

Consistent time *See* **CT**.

Consumer Empowerment Use Case This HITSP Interoperability Specification (IS-03) is designed to meet the specific requirements of the Consumer Empowerment Use Case, defined as the active involvement of consumers (i.e., individuals) in managing their healthcare and gaining the benefits of having their health information in a format easily accessible to them. This includes having a personal health record (PHR) to track patient information, insurance, family history, medications, and other special conditions.[48]

Contact An electrical connecting surface between an integrated circuit chip and its interfacing device that permits a flow of current.[1]

Content coverage The ability of a coding system to capture the meaning of a document.[1]

Content profile An IHE content profile specifies a coordinated set of standards-based information content, exchanged between the functional components of communicating healthcare IT systems and devices. An IHE content profile specifies a specific element of content (e.g., a document) that may be conveyed through the transactions of one or more associated integration profile(s).[93]

Continuity A performance dimension addressing the degree to which the care for a patient is coordinated among practitioners and organizations, and over time, without interruption, cessation, or unnecessary repetition of diagnosis or treatment.[123]

Continuity of care document *See* **CCD**.

Continuity of care record *See* **CCR**.

Continuous improvement 1. A management strategy to embed awareness of quality in all organizational processes. It has been widely used in healthcare (beginning in the 1990s), manufacturing, education, government, and service industries, as well as NASA space and science programs. It employs teamwork, statistical techniques, and motivational factors. 2. When applied to healthcare in the 1990s, the first generation of clinical decision support tools emerged, including casemix systems and rudimentary medical alerting systems.[7]

Control Means of managing risk, including policies, procedures, guidelines, practices, or organizational structures which can be of an administrative, technical, management, or legal nature.[124]

Control chart A graphic display of the results of a process over time and against established control limits. The dispersion of data points on the chart is used to determine whether the process is performing within prescribed limits, and whether variations taking place are random or systematic.[123]

Control rights The right of an individual to know where his/her data are stored, to authorize who can access his/her own data, to correct his/her own record, to make certain segments inaccessible via standard process, and to know that the data keeper observes the laws and professional ethical tenets.[1]

Control unit   *See* **CU**.

Controlled access   Authorized user access limited to specific data and resources, according to that user's authorization.[1]

Controlled resource   A resource to which an access control mechanism has been specifically applied.[1]

Conventional memory   The range of RAM used by MS-DOS to run real-mode applications.[1]

Convergence   The end-point of any algorithm that uses iteration or recursion to guide a series of data processing steps. An algorithm is usually said to have reached convergence when the difference between the computed and observed steps falls below a predefined threshold.[104]

Cookies   Chunks of information sent from Web sites to an individual's Internet browser, then saved on the system's hard drive. Helps the programs at the Web site keep track of what the user has been doing during the visit at the Web site.[1]

Coordination of benefits   *See* **COB**.

Coprocessor   A chip designed specifically to handle a particular task, such as math calculations or displaying graphics on screen; faster at its specialized function than the main processor; relieves the processor of some work.[1]

CORBA   **Common object request broker architecture.** A language-independent object model and specification for a distributed applications development environment.[1]

Core based statistical area.   *See* **CBSA**.

Core values   Guiding principles of an organization.

Cost containment   The process of planning in order to keep cost within certain constraints.[4]

Cost effectiveness   A system contributing to cost savings in healthcare by efficiently collecting, storing, and aggregating data and by providing decision support and augmented practices with appropriate and timely information.[6]

Cost-benefit analysis   A comparison of the costs of a proposed course of action with its benefits, considering tangible and intangible economic impacts, and the time value of money.[6]

Countermeasure Response Administration   *See* **CRA**.

Covered entity   Health plans, healthcare clearing houses, and healthcare providers who transmit any health information in electronic form, in connection with a transaction that is subject to federal Health Insurance Portability and Accountability Act (HIPAA) requirements, as those terms are defined and used in the HIPAA regulations, 45 CFR Parts 160 and 164.[118]

Covered function   Functions that make an entity a health plan, a healthcare provider, or a healthcare clearing house.[10]

COW   Computer-on-wheels.[16]

CP   **Certificate policy.** Named set of rules that indicates the applicability of a certificate to a particular community and/or class of application with common security requirements.[121]

CPI   **Consistent presentation of images.** Specifies a number of transactions that maintain the consistency of presentation for grayscale images and their presentation state information (including user annotations, shutters, flip/rotate, display area, and zoom). It also defines a standard contrast curve, the Grayscale Standard Display function, against which different types of display and hardcopy output devices can be calibrated. It thus supports hardcopy, softcopy, and mixed environments. *See also* Profile.[56]

CPM   **Control program for microcomputers.** Introduced in the late 1970s, this was the first standard microcomputer operating system, and generally used by the first generation of microcomputers. It relied on an 8-bit architecture, and was configured to run on a variety of microprocessors. Usage decreased after the advent of MS-DOS and the Apple operating system.[99]

CPOE   **Computerized practitioner order entry. 1.** An order entry application specifically designed to assist clinical practitioners in creating and managing medical orders for patient services and medications. This application has special electronic signature, workflow, and rules engine functions that reduce or eliminate medical errors associated with practitioner ordering processes. **2.** A computer application that accepts the provider's orders for diagnostic and treatment services electronically, instead of the clinician recording them on an orders sheet or prescription pad.[2] Also known as *computerized physician order entry, computerized patient order entry,* and *computerized provider order entry.*[45]

CPR **Computer-based patient record.** *See* **EHR.**[45]

CPRS **Computer-based patient record system.** *See* **EHR.**[45]

CPS **Certification practices statement.** Statement of the practices which a certification authority employs in issuing certificates.[121]

CPT **Current Procedural Terminology.** A medical code set, maintained and copyrighted by the AMA, that has been selected for use under HIPAA for noninstitutional and nondental professional transactions. The current version is the CPT-4.[9]

CPU **Central processing unit. 1.** The component in a digital computer that interprets and executes the instructions and data contained in software. Microprocessors are CPUs that are manufactured on integrated circuits, often as a single-chip package. **2.** Brain of the computer. Main system board (motherboard) integrated chip that directs computer operations. Performs the arithmetic, logic, and controls operations in the computer.[1]

CRA **Countermeasure Response Administration.** Systems that manage and track measures taken to contain an outbreak or event, and to provide protection against a possible outbreak or event. This public health information network (PHIN) functional area also includes multiple dose delivery of countermeasures: anthrax vaccine and antibiotics; adverse events monitoring; follow-up of patients; isolation and quarantine; and links to distribution vehicles (such as the Strategic National Stockpile).[46]

Crash A data system error condition leading to a total termination of all computing activities, requiring a restart procedure for recovering the normal operational status.[1]

Crawler A program that automatically fetches Web pages. Crawlers are used to feed pages to search engines. *See also* **Spider, Web crawler.**[1]

Credential Evidence attesting to one's right to credit or authority; in this standard, the data elements associated with an individual that authoritatively binds an identity (and, optionally, additional attributes) to that individual.[114]

Critical path A tool that supports collaborative, coordinated practices. It provides for multidisciplinary communication, treatment and care planning, and documentation of caregiver's evaluations and assessments.[6]

CRM **Customer relationship management.** The approach of establishing relationships with customers on an individual basis, then using collected information about the customer and their buying habits to treat different customers differently.[1]

Cross enterprise clinical document sharing *See* **XDS.**

Cross map A reference from one concept in one terminology to another in a different terminology. A concept may have a single, or a set of alternative cross maps.[19]

Cross-platform Refers to software or network functionality that will work on more than one platform or type of computer.[1]

Crosstalk Signal overflow from one wire to an adjacent wire, with the possibility of causing information distortion. UTP cable is the most susceptible transmission medium to crosstalk.[1]

Crosswalk *See* **Data mapping.**[5]

CRUD **Create, retrieve, update, and delete.**[1]

Cryptographic algorithm cipher Method for the transformation of data in order to hide its information content, prevent its undetected modification, and/or prevent its unauthorized use.[121]

Cryptography The art of keeping data secret, primarily through the use of mathematical or logical functions that transform intelligible data into seemingly unintelligible data and back again.[1]

CSMA/CD **Carrier sense multiple access with collision detection.** A network control protocol in which: a. carrier sensing scheme is used; and b. a transmitting data station that detects another signal while transmitting a frame, stops transmitting that frame, transmits a jam signal, and then waits for a random time interval (known as 'backoff delay' and determined using the truncated binary exponential backoff algorithm), before trying to send that frame again. Ethernet is the classic CSMA/CD protocol.[7]

CSO   Chief security officer. The person with the responsibility for the security of the paper-based and electronic health information, as well as the physical and electronic means of managing and storing that information.[1]

CSU/DSU   Channel sharing unit/data service unit. A unit that shapes digital signals for transmission. The CSU is a device that performs protective and diagnostic functions for a tele-communications line.[1]

CT   Computed tomography. A specialized x-ray imaging technique.[7]

CT   Consistent time. Mechanisms to synchronize the time base between multiple actors and computers. Various infrastructure, security, and acquisition profiles require use of a consistent time base on multiple computers. The consistent time profile provides a median synchronization error of less than one second.[56]

CTI   Computer telephony integration. Systems that enable a computer to act as a call center, accepting incoming calls, and routing them to the appropriate device or person.[1]

CTO   Chief technology officer. Has overall responsibility for managing technical vendor relationships and performance, as well as the physical and personnel technology infrastructure, including technology deployment, network and systems management, integration testing, and developing technical operations personnel.[1]

CTS   Common terminology services. Specification developed as an alternative to a common data structure.[16]

CU   Control unit. Portion of the CPU that coordinates all computer operations through the machine cycle: fetch, decode, execute, and store.[1]

CUI   Concept unique identifier. The class of names that uniquely identify an instance of entity. Some examples of unique identifiers are the keys of tables in database applications and the ISBN (International Standard Book Number).[1]

Culture   The mindset of an organization (e.g., a culture may be collaborative vs. regimented, favor open vs. proprietary solutions, or be internally vs. externally focused).[1]

Cure letter   A letter sent by one party to another, proposing or agreeing to actions that a party will take to correct legal errors or defects that have occurred under a contract between the parties or other legal requirement.[118]

Current procedural terminology   *See* **CPT**.

Cursor   The representation of the mouse location on the screen; may take many shapes.[1]

Custom, customized   Software that is designed or modified for a specific user or organization; may refer to all or part of a system. *See also* **Vanilla**.

Customer relationship management   *See* **CRM**.[1]

Customer-centric   Placing the customer at the center or focus of design or service.[7]

Customer-driven   Systems design focused on user acceptance; focused on customer requirements.[7]

Cut   To save information by highlighting the desired text or object from the page and placing it onto the clipboard.[1]

CVE   Common vulnerabilities and exposures. A list of standardized names for vulnerabilities and other information security exposures. CVE aims to standardize the names for all publicly known vulnerabilities and secure exposures.[125]

CVS   Concurrent versioning system. An open source version control and collaboration system.

CWE   Coded with exceptions. A data type coded with exceptions.[16]

CWE   Common weakness enumeration. A community-developed formal list of software weaknesses, idiosyncracies, faults, and flaws.[125]

Cyberspace The realm of communications and computation. A term used to refer to the electronic universe of information available through the Internet.[1]

Cyberspace shadow The model in cyberspace of a person or of an organization (e.g., a person's medical files).[1]

D

Dashboard User interface based on predetermined data fields that facilitate domain-specific data queries and are suited to regular use with minimal training.[94]

DAT Digital audio tape. The most common type of tape backup.[1]

Data 1. A sequence of symbols to which meaning may be assigned. 2. Raw facts consisting of numbers, letters, and characters.[1,6]

Data aggregation Combining protected health information by a business associate, on behalf of more covered entities than one, to permit data analysis related to the healthcare operations of the participating covered entities.[48]

Data category A significant attribute of a data element or data set that may be used by a trust engine to determine what type of element is under discussion, such as physical contact information.[57]

Data center A data center supports the information technology needs of a minimum of two medical/surgical hospitals and their associated subacute and ambulatory entities. Data centers can be located within a hospital or can be free-standing facilities. Information technology needs supported by data centers include server hosting, network support, desktop support, application support, help desk support, etc.[2]

Data circuit-terminating equipment See DCE.

Data classification The conscious decision to assign a level of sensitivity to data as it is being created, amended, enhanced, stored, or transmitted. The classification of the data then determines the extent to which the data needs to be controlled/secured, and is indicative of its value in terms of information assets.[118]

Data cleaning A process whereby automated or semi-automated algorithms are used to process experimental data, including noise, experimental errors, and other artifacts, in order to generate and store high-quality data for use in subsequent analyses. Data cleaning is typically required in high-throughput sequencing where compression or other experimental artifacts limit the amount of sequence data generated from each sequencing run or 'read.'[104]

Data collection The acquisition of healthcare information or facts based upon patient and consumer race, ethnicity and language. Data collection provides healthcare providers with the ability to perform benchmarking measures on healthcare systems to determine areas where improvement is needed in providing care.[138]

Data compression The process of eliminating gaps, empty fields, redundancies, and unnecessary data to shorten the length of records or blocks so they take up less space when stored or transmitted.[1]

Data condition A description of the circumstances in which certain data is required.[102]

Data content All the data elements and code sets inherent to a transaction, and not related to the format of the transaction.[10]

Data corruption A deliberate or accidental violation of data integrity.[1]

Data definition language See DDL.

Data dictionary 1. A document or system that characterizes the data content of a system. 2. In databases, a centralized repository of information about the stored data, providing details of the meaning, relationship to other data, origin, usage, and format. Data dictionary is a vital part of the database management system providing information on the nature and usage of stored data, thus giving the database administrator overall control of an evolving database. Information describing the specifications and location of all data contained in a system.[1]

Data diddling Unauthorized data alteration; a common form of computer crime.[1]

Data element The smallest named unit of information in a transaction or database.[10]

Data element, composite Groups of closely related data elements that can repeat as a group (i.e., procedure code, as defined in a composite data element).[32]

Data elements for emergency department systems *See* **DEEDS.**

Data encryption standard *See* **DES** and **DEA.**

Data entry Changing information from the original source into machine readable format.[1]

Data exchange Securing transmissions over communication channels.[1]

Data field Limited area for listing of data elements.[1]

Data fields An appendix, the data dictionary provides an alphabetical listing of data elements, listings of recommended coded values, and a cross reference from data elements to segments.[16]

Data flow diagram A special form of flow chart intended to help illustrate a process by showing events, or by tracing the paths of data through a process or operation.[6]

Data granularity *See* **Granularity.**

Data integrity **1.** Assurance of the accuracy, correctness, or validity of data, using a set of validation criteria against which data is compared or screened. **2.** Protection of data from compromise and alteration, accidental or deliberate.[6,1]

Data interchange The process of transferring data from an originating system to a receiving system.[4]

Data leakage The practically undetectable loss of control over, or possession of, information.[1]

Data link layer Second layer in the OSI model. Consists of upper logical link control (LLC) and lower media access control (MAC) portions. Handles data flow control, the packaging of raw data in its frames, or frames into raw data bits, and retransmits frames as needed.[1]

Data manipulation language *See* **DML.**

Data mapping **1.** The process of matching one set of data elements of individual code values to their closest equivalents in another set of them. **2.** Describes the process of creating data element mappings between two distinct data models.[10,7]

Data mark A derivation of a data warehouse that is focused on publishing data from a single subject area or departmental point of view.[1]

Data mart **1.** A well organized, user-centered, searchable database system. A data mart picks up where a data warehouse stops, by organizing the information according to the user's needs (usually by specific subjects), with ease of use in mind. **2.** A repository of data that serves a particular community of knowledge workers. The data may come from an enterprise-wide database or a data warehouse.[8]

Data messaging *See* **Messaging.**

Data migration Steps taken to enable legacy data to be accessible as part of a system that uses a specific type of semantic content. Options for data migration include actual conversion of the data, or provision of methods for accessing the data in its original form.[19]

Data mining A decision support approach of analyzing data, and then extracting actionable information in the form of new relationships, patterns, clusters, predictive models, and trends.[1]

Data model **1.** A conceptual model of the information needed to support a business function or process. **2.** Describes the organization of data in an automated system. The data model includes the subjects of interest in the system (or entities) and the attributes (data elements) of those entities. It defines how the entities are related to each other (cardinality) and establishes the identifiers needed to relate entities to each other. A data model can be expressed as a conceptual, logical, or physical model.[10,8]

Data modeling A method used to define and analyze data requirements needed to support the business functions of an enterprise. Data modeling defines the data elements, their relationships, and their physical structure in preparation for creating a database.[1]

Data object A collection of data that has a natural grouping and may be identified as a complete entity.[117]

Data origin authentication Corroboration that the source of data is received as is claimed.[1]

Data originator The person who generates data, such as the patient for symptoms, the physician for examination and decisions, the nurse for patient care, etc.[1]

Data processing Data processing is defined as the systematic performance of operations upon data, such as handling, merging, sorting, and computing. The semantic content of the original data should not be changed, but the semantic content of the processed data may be changed.[104]

Data quality A comprehensive view of the usefulness of data to support decision making. The measurements of data quality include completeness, correctness, comprehensibility, and consistency in support of intended use.[1]

Data repository *See* **Repository and Data warehouse.**

Data service unit *See* **DSU.**[1]

Data services Group of services that will hold metadata for operations that are carried out on repositories, and abstract data access services for specific database management systems.[8]

Data set ready *See* **DSR.**

Data sets A known grouping of data elements. *See also* **PNDS, NMDS, NMMDS.**[57]

Data standards Consensual specifications for the representation of data from different sources and settings; necessary for the sharing, portability, and reusability of data.[110]

Data structure A hierarchical description of a set of data elements. A data set can be described according to its data structure. P3P1.0 defines a set of basic data structures that are used to describe data sets.[57]

Data subject The person whose information is stored in the computer.[1]

Data synchronization The process of sending data between two or more computers so that each repository contains the identical information.[7]

Data tagging A formatted word that represents a wrapper for a stored value. The data tag is a small piece of scripting code, typically JavaScript, which transmits page-specific information via query string parameters. The process begins when a page containing a data tag is requested from the server. The tag is a piece of scripting code executed when the page is loaded into the browser. The data tag constructs the query string by scanning the document source for HTML, beginning with a specific identifier.[18]

Data terminal ready *See* **DTR.**

Data transformation Methods by which stored data or information is processed according to the needs of the end user.[6]

Data types The categories of data that will be persisted in the EHR. They include voice, waveforms, clinical notes and summaries, diagnostic imaging, lab, and pharmacy information.[8]

Data use agreement Confidentiality agreement between a covered entity and the recipient of health information in a limited data set.[48]

Data user The person or organization that has justified need for certain data in order to perform his or her legitimate tasks.[1]

Data validation A process used to determine if data are accurate, complete, or meet specified criteria. Data validation may include format checks, check key tests, reasonableness checks, and limit checks.[3]

Data visualization A decision support methodology for turning data into information by using the high capacity of the human brain to visually recognize patterns and trends, using a wide variety of data plotting, graphing, and exploration techniques.[1]

Data warehouse 1. A repository where all types of data (clinical, administrative, and financial) are stored together for later retrieval. Data mining and decision support systems are uses of a data warehouse. When the perspective of the strategy or user shifts from the enterprise view of aggregate data to the individual user or knowledge worker (who may need access to a specialized or local database), then the system is referred to, instead, as a data mart. **2.** A collection of clinical and/or financial data in a database designed to support management decision making.[1]

Database **1.** A file created by a database manager that contains a collection of information. The basic database contains fields, records, and files; a field is a single piece of information, a record is one complete set of fields, and a file is a collection of records. **2.** A collection of stored data, typically organized into fields, records, files, and associated descriptions (schema).[1,4]

Database administrator The person responsible for a database system, particularly for defining the rules by which data are accessed, modified, and stored.[1]

Database design The process of producing a detailed data model of a database. This model contains all the needed logical and physical design choices, and physical storage parameters needed to generate a design in a data definition language, which can then be used to create a database. Sometimes called *database life cycle*.

Database management system *See* **DBMS**.

DATUM Any single observation or fact. A medical datum generally can be regarded as the value of a specific parameter (e.g., a patient, at a specific time).[4]

Daughterboard A board that attaches to another board, such as the motherboard or an expansion card. A daughter card may contain additional memory to an accelerator card.[1]

DBMS Database management system. **1.** A program that lets one or more computer users create and access data in a database. On personal computers, Microsoft Access is a popular example of a single or small group user DBMS. Microsoft's SQL server is an example of a DBMS that serves database requests from multiple users. **2.** A set of programs used to define, administer, store, modify, process, and extract information from a database.[2,1]

DCE Data circuit-terminating equipment. Typically a modem or other type of communication device.[90]

DDL Data definition language. A set of commands designed to create and remove phases of a database project.[7]

DEA Data encryption algorithm. A method for encrypting information.[7] *See also* **DES**.

Debugging The process of discovering and eliminating errors and defects, or bugs, in program code.[1]

DEC **Digital Equipment Corporation.**

Decentralized Hospital Computer System *See* **DHCP**.

Decipherment decryption Process of obtaining, from a ciphertext, the original corresponding data.[121]

Decision support (analytic) The collection of analysis tools, systems, models, and processes applied to organized information in support of management decision making.[1]

Decision support (clinical) Software that taps into database resources and messages, presents data to assist users in making business decisions. A clinical decision support system gives physicians structured (rules-based) information to help make decisions on diagnoses, treatment plans, orders, and results. *See also* **Alerts**.[8]

Decision support system *See* **DSS** and **CDS**.

Decision tree A data mining predictive model-building algorithm that segregates data into factors with high association to the predicted variable. The resulting set of decision rules branch off each other and resemble a tree.[1]

Decompression The expansion of compressed image files. *See also* **Lossless compression, Lossy**.[1]

Decryption The process of decoding a message so that its meaning becomes obvious. The reverse process of encryption in which cipher text is transformed back into the original plain text using a second complex function and a decryption key.[1]

Dedicated line A telephone or data line that is always available. This line is not used by other computers or individuals, is available 24 hours a day, and is never disconnected.[1]

DEEDS Data elements for emergency department systems. The recommended data set for use in emergency departments; it is published by the Centers for Disease Control and Prevention (CDC).[46]

Default gateway TCP/IP configuration option that specifies a device or computer to send packets out of a local subnet. *See also* **Gateway**.[1]

Default route A routing table entry used to direct packets addressed to networks not explicitly listed in the routing table.[1]

Definition Statement which describes a concept and permits differentiation from other concepts within a system.[3]

Degaussing Exposure to high magnetic fields. One method of destroying data on a disk.[1]

De-identified health information Removal of individual identifiers so that it cannot be used to identify an individual. De-identified health information is not protected by HIPAA.[48]

Deliberate threat Threat of a person or persons to damage a computer system consciously and willingly.[1]

Deliverable Any tangible outcome that is produced by the project. These can be documents, plans, computer systems, buildings, aircraft, etc. Internal deliverables are produced as a consequence of executing the project and are usually only needed by the project team. External deliverables are those that are created for clients and stakeholders.[12]

DELOS WP5 Network on Excellence on Digital Libraries (EURO), Knowledge Extraction & Semantic Interoperability.[142]

Demodulation Reverse of modulation. The analog-to-digital signal conversion process occurring in a modem at a receiving site. Analog signals are used to transfer data over phone lines. Digital signals are used by the computer.[1]

Demographic information Information concerning population statistics, such as birth date, birth place, sex, residence, etc. Collected and used for healthcare evaluation and planning purposes.[4]

Denial-of-service attack An attack in which a user (or a program) takes up so much of a shared resource that none of the resource is left for other users or uses.[1]

Deployment process The part of the IHE process that builds upon profile specifications

produced by the development process. It starts with the testing of actual implementations of these profiles, demonstrates effective interoperability between independent implementations, and concludes with the means for developers of IT products to state their compliance to one or more profiles.[93]

Derivative Any re-use of information at the application level. Captures the notion of 'collect once, use many times.' For example, detailed data information from an accounting system can be used for financial planning. Loosely adapted from mathematics, investing.[32]

DES Data encryption standard. An algorithm implemented in electronic hardware devices and used to protect computer data through cryptography.[1]

Description logics Description logics are a family of knowledge representation languages which can be used to represent the terminological knowledge of an application domain in a structured and formally well-understood way. The name *description logic* refers, on the one hand, to concept descriptions used to describe a domain and, on the other hand, to the logic-based semantics which can be given by a translation into first-order predicate logic.[7]

Descriptor The text defining a code in a code set.[10]

Desiderata A list of things considered necessary or highly desirable (plural); a definitive list.[28]

Design **1.** Phase of software development following analysis, and concerned with how the problem is to be solved. **2.** The process and result of describing how a system or process is to be automated. Design must thoroughly describe the function of a component and its interaction with other components. Design usually also identifies areas of commonality in systems and optimizes reusability.[8]

Designated approving authority Official with the authority to formally assume the responsibility for operating a system or network at an acceptable level of risk.[97]

Designated code set Specified within the body of a rule.[10]

Designated record set Healthcare provider's medical records and billing records about individuals, a health plan's enrollment, payment, claims adjudication, and case or medical management records, and any other records used by a covered entity to make decisions about individuals.[48]

Development process The part of the IHE process that identifies and prioritizes use cases, selects interoperability standards, and documents these in the form of a profile.[93]

Device Any piece of equipment used in computer input/output operations.[1]

DHCP Decentralized Hospital Computer System. The earlier name of the Veterans Administration Clinical Information System, developed in the late 1970s and early 1980s by staff in local VA hospitals, over the objection of some of the Veterans Hospital Central (Washington, DC) administrators. Eventually, the DHCP system was ported into the Indian Health System and Department of Defense. In the late 1990s, the DHCP development was renamed the VistA system, as it acquired more graphical user interface (GUI) characteristics and deeper clinical content.[99]

DHCP Dynamic host configuration protocol. Standard protocol that allows a network device to obtain all network IP configuration information automatically from host-based pooled IP addresses. Alleviates manual static IP address assignment.[1]

DI Diagnostic imaging. The use of digital images and textual reports prepared as a result of performing diagnostic studies, such as x-rays, CT scans, MRIs, etc.[8]

Diagnosis related group Group of patients defined using a case-mix approach. Note: Originally the approach involved coding with ICD-9-CM or ICD-AM and grouping by homogeneous cost; used major diagnosis, length of stay, secondary diagnosis, surgical procedure, age, and type of services required.[4]

Diagnosis related groups *See* **DRGs**.

Diagnostic and statistical manual *See* **DSM-IV**.

Diagnostic procedure A procedure aimed at finding a diagnosis (the identification of diseases and other clinical conditions from the examination of signs and symptoms). A diagnostic procedure can involve an interview with a patient, physical examination, the use of laboratory tests.[4]

Dial-up line A communication connection from a computer to a host computer over standard phone lines. Unlike a dedicated line, user must dial the host computer to establish a connection.[1]

DICOM Digital imaging and communications in medicine. 1. DICOM is a standard for the electronic communication of medical images and associated information. DICOM relies on explicit and detailed models of how the patients, images, and reports involved in radiology operations are described and how they are related. The DICOM standards contain information object definitions, data structure, data dictionary, media storage, file format, communications formats, and print formats. **2.** These models are called entity-relationship models and are a way to be sure that manufacturers and users understand the basis for developing the data structures.[48]

Dictionary Structured collection of lexical units with linguistic information about each unit.[4]

Digital A digital system is one that uses numbers for input, processing, transmission, storage, or display, rather than a continuous spectrum of values (an analog system) or non-numeric symbols, such as letters or icons. The word 'digital' is commonly used in computing, especially where real-world information is converted to numeric form, as in digital audio and digital photography.[7]

Digital audio tape *See* **DAT**.

Digital certificate A digital document issued by a certification authority that contains the holder's name, serial number, public key, and the document's expiration date. Digital certificates are used in public key infrastructure to send and receive secure, encrypted messages.[8]

Digital envelope Data appended to a message that allow the intended recipient to verify the integrity of the content of the message.[3]

Digital Equipment Corporation *See* **DEC**.

Digital imaging and communications in medicine *See* **DICOM**.

Digital radiography Digital imaging technology applied to standard x-rays (such as chest x-rays). Because of the high resolution to approach analog file, digital radiology was the last modality to be automated.[8]

Digital signal Transmission signal that carries information in the discrete value form of 0 and 1. *See also* **DS-2-3**.[1]

Digital signature A means to guarantee the authenticity of a set of input data the same way a written signature verifies the authenticity of a paper document. A cryptographic transformation of data that allows a recipient of the data to prove the source and integrity of the data and protect against forgery. Specifically, an asymmetric cryptographic technique, in which each user is associated with a public key distributed to potential verifiers of the user's digital signature used to encrypt messages destined for other uses; and a private key, which is known only to the user, and is used to decrypt incoming messages. *See also* **Private key, Public key**.[1]

Digital signature standard Digital signatures provide a signature manifestation whereby signer identity, as well as document and signature attributes, are bound by a public key based cryptographic process. Public key, or asymmetric, cryptography involves two mathematically related keys. A 'signature' key is used to encrypt a one-way hash or 'digest' of the electronic data to obtain a digital signature of that data. The unique mathematical inverse of the signature key, also known as the 'verification' key, can be used to decrypt the digital signature. Verification of the digital signature follows from comparison of the decrypted hash with the verifier's application of the hashing function to the purportedly signed record. In digital signature applications, the signature key is uniquely associated with a particular signer by means of data structure, known as a 'verification certificate.' The certificate includes the verification key and provides a 'trusted' basis for associating a person with that key. The security of a digital signature depends upon the ability of the signer to maintain exclusive control over the use of the signature key. Typically, the assurance that the signer has this capability is provided by the process by which verification certificates are created and distributed.[3]

Digital subscriber line *See* **DSL**.

Digital subscriber line access multiplexer *See* **DSLAM**.

Digitize To convert an analog signal to a digital signal.[1]

Digitized signature An electronic image of an actual written signature. A digitized signature looks much the same as the original, but it does not provide the same protection as a digital signature, as it can be forged and copied.[1]

Dimension table A building block of a star schema data model; it contains the descriptive data regarding the data in a fact table that are used for column headings, query constraints, and OLAP dimensions.[1]

DIP switch Dual in-line package switch. A grouping of small on (1)/off (0) switches used in computers and associated devices to configure hardware options. DIP switches commonly allow a user to change the configuration of a circuit board to suit a particular computer.[1]

Direct connection A permanent communication connection between a computer system (either a single CPU or a LAN) and the Internet. This is also called a leased line connection because the telephone connection is leased from the phone company. A direct connection is in contrast to a dial-up connection.[1]

Direct memory access *See* **DMA**.

Direct sequence spread spectrum *See* **DSSS**.

Directory A system that the computer uses to organize files on the basis of specific information.[1]

Directory services markup language *See* **DSML**.

DIS Draft international standard. The fourth balloting stage for a draft international standard document. This most important phase of balloting lasts five months.[3]

Disclosure history Under the Health Insurance Portability and Accountability Act (HIPAA), this is a list of any entities that have received personally identifiable healthcare information for uses unrelated to treatment and payment.[10]

Disclosure/disclose The release, transfer, relay, provision of access to, or conveying client information to any individual or entity outside a specific healthcare system.[118]

Discovery Locating a resource on the enterprise, using a process (such as a search engine) to obtain knowledge of information content or services that exploit metadata descriptions of enterprise IT resources, stored directories, registries, and catalogs.[4]

Discrete data Data that can only take certain values.[143]

Disease episode An episode of care focused on the treatment of a specific disease.[141]

Disease management A system of coordinated healthcare interventions and communications for populations with conditions in which patient self-care efforts are significant.[101] *See also* **Chronic disease management**.

Disease registry A large collection or registry belonging to a healthcare system that contains information on different chronic health problems affecting patients within the system. A disease registry helps to manage and log data on chronic illnesses and diseases. All data contained within the disease registry are logged by healthcare providers and are available to providers to perform benchmarking measures on healthcare systems.[138]

Disease staging A type of severity system which maps progression through degrees of morbidity. *See* **Severity system**.[32]

Disk Rotating magnetic device used for file storage. Can be magnetic floppy disk (diskette), hard disk, or optical CD.[1]

Disk duplexing Fault-tolerant storage technique that mirrors the information from a primary drive to a secondary drive, while maintaining additional redundancy through the use of separate disk controllers. Mirrors data from a primary drive to a secondary drive to make files accessible in the event of a drive failure.[1]

Disk mirroring Fault-tolerant storage technique that mirrors data from a primary drive to a secondary drive to make files accessible in the event of a drive failure.[1]

Disk operating system *See* **DOS**.

Disk striping with parity Fault-tolerant storage technique that distributes data and parity across three or more physical disks. Storage technique that stripes data and parity in 64K blocks across all disks in the array. Striping provides fast data transfer and protection from a single disk failure by regenerating data for a failed disk through the stored parity. Minimum of three physical disks are required for disk striping with parity. Also known as *RAID 5*.[1]

Disk striping without parity Storage technique that distributes data across two or more physical disks in 64K blocks across all disks in the array. Striping provides fast data transfer. Minimum of two physical disks are required for disk striping without parity. Also known as *RAID 0*.[1]

Diskette Small, flexible, removable, magnetic storage media used for file storage.[1]

Display codes A parameter users can set that allows for the display of classification codes on the selection list during searches.

Distance learning Using communication technology to bring seminars and classes from distant locations into schools and homes. Distance learning technologies can range from one-way video to two-way video and audio transmission, with two or more PCs for the purpose of instruction. Distance learning provides virtual classroom, seminar, or meeting attendance without the expense and difficulty of travel.[1]

Distinguished name A set of data that identifies a real-world entity, such as a person in a computer-based context.[114]

Distributed computing environment (DCE) A client-server environment in which data are located in many servers that might be geographically dispersed, but connected by a wide area network (WAN).[1]

Distributed database A database that is stored in more than one physical location. Parts or copies of the database are physically stored in one location, and other parts are stored and maintained in other locations.[1]

Distributed processing The distribution of computer processing work among multiple computers, linked by a communications network.[1]

Dithering Within the context of the 216-color, browser-safe palette for Web engineering, the use of colors outside the selection of the 216 'safe' colors may bring distortion or dithering. This is caused by interpretation by another operating system, yielding a color not intended by the designer.[1]

DLC **Dynamic link control.** Protocol used for networked-enabled HP printers and for connectivity to IBM mainframe machines from Windows NT.[1]

DLL **Dynamic link library.** A file of code-containing functions that can be called from other executable code (either an application or another DLL). Programmers use DLLs to provide code that they can reuse and to parcel out distinct jobs. Unlike an executable file, a DLL cannot be directly run. DLLs must be called from other code that is already executing.[1]

DMA **Direct memory access.** Rapid data movement between computer subsystems. Accomplished through the use of the DMA controller without the use of the CPU.[1]

DMA controller **Direct memory access controller.** Integrated computer chip that handles direct memory operations without CPU intervention. Allows the CPU to concentrate on other computer operations.[1]

DML **Data manipulation language.** A language which enables users to access and manipulate data; includes retrieval, insertion, deletion, and modification.

DNS **Domain name server.** An online database that resolves human readable names to IP addresses. The DNS is a distributed database used by TCP/IP applications to map between host names and IP addresses and to provide electronic mail routing information. The DNS provides the protocol to allow clients and servers to communicate with each other.[1]

DNSSEC Secure Domain Name System for authentication and integrity.[1]

Document imaging The process by which print and film documents are fed into a scanner and converted into electronic documents.[2]

Document integrity To ensure the integrity of a document that is exchanged or shared.[48]

Document management Software systems allowing organizations to control the production, storage, management, and distribution of electronic documents, yielding greater efficiencies in the ability to reuse information and to control the flow of the documents, from creation to archiving.[2]

Document type definition *See* **DTD**.

Documentation and procedures test A testing event that evaluates the accuracy of user and operations documentation, and determines whether the manual procedure will work correctly as an integral part of the system.[6]

Domain The problem or subject to be addressed by a set of information technology messages or by a system ('application domain'). A particular area of interest in healthcare.[8]

Domain information model The model describing common concepts and relationships for a problem domain.[4]

Domain name server *See* **DNS**.

Domain specific data Information and knowledge specific to a given discipline (nursing, medicine, physical therapy, nutrition, etc.). Examples include data banks, online consultants, side effects of patients' medications, knowledge retrieval systems, etc.[6]

Domain synchronization Process in which a primary domain controller (PDC) updates all backup domain controllers (BDCs) with an updated copy of the accounts database through the replication service. Default PDF-to-BDC synchronization occurs every five minutes. BDCs can also be manually synchronized with the PDC through server manager.[1]

Domains Spheres of interest or concern, its constituent elements are called 'components.'[8]

DOS **Disk operating system.** The first widely installed operating system for personal computers.[42]

Dot bust Years of the 'Internet Bust' (early 2000 to October 2003), in which many '.com' companies went bankrupt and many investors lost money.[32]

Dot com   An Internet-based business, or '.com.'

Dot pitch   A measurement (in millimeters) of the distance between dots on a monitor. The lower the number, the higher the clarity of the display.[11]

Dots per square inch   *See* **DPI**.

Download   To retrieve a file from another computer.[1]

DPI   **Dots per square inch.** A measure of the resolution of a printer, scanner, or monitor. It refers to the number of dots per inch. The more dots per inch, the higher the resolution.[1]

Draft international standard   *See* **DIS**.

Draft standard for trial use   *See* **DSTU**.

Draft supplement for public comment   A specification candidate for addition to an IHE Domain Technical Framework (e.g., a new profile) that is issued for comment by any interested party.[93]

Draft technical report   *See* **DTR**.

DRAM   **Dynamic RAM.** RAM that must be continuously refreshed to maintain the current RAM value. Most RAM in microcomputers is dynamic RAM B, although there is a trend toward SDRAM.[1]

DRG   *See* **DRGs**.

DRGs   **Diagnosis related groups.** Groups of International Classification of Disease (ICD) coded diagnoses, procedures, and other information used to group patients for reimbursement by Medicare.[102]

Drilldown   Exploration of multidimensional data allows moving down from one level of detail to the next, depending on the granularity of data in the level.[94]

Driver   A piece of software that tells the computer how to operate an external device, such as a printer, hard disk, CD-ROM drive, or scanner.[1]

Drop   Wiring run made from a modular wall plate to a comm/wiring closet. UTP is the most common medium used in drops. Also identified as the connection between a computer and thicknet cabling.[1]

Drop-down list (or menu)   A menu of commands or options that appears when you select an item with a mouse. The item you select is generally at the top of the display screen, and the menu appears just below it, as if you had it dropped down or you had pulled it down.[32]

Drug information system   A computer-based system that maintains drug-related information, such as information concerning appropriate dosages and side effects, and may access a drug interaction database. A drug information system may provide, by way of a directed consultation, specific advice on the usage of various drugs.[4]

Drug interaction database   Database containing information on drug interactions.[4]

Drug therapy   The use of drugs to cure a medical problem, to improve a patient's condition, or to otherwise produce a therapeutic effect.[4]

DS-2-3   **Digital signal.** Digital Signal 2. 6.312-3.45 Mbps synchronous digital 1 transmission.[1]

DSA   **Digital signature algorithm.** *See* **Digital signature**.

DSG   **Document digital signature.** *See* **Digital signature**.

DSL   **Digital subscriber line.** DSL technologies use sophisticated modulation schemes to pack data onto copper wires.[1]

DSLAM   **Digital subscriber line access multiplexer.** A mechanism at a phone company's central location that links many customer DSL connections to a single high-speed ATM line. When the phone company receives a DSL signal, an ADSL modem with a POTS splitter detects voice calls and data.[1]

DSM-IV   **Diagnostic and Statistical Manual.** The Diagnostic and Statistical Manual of Mental Disorders, published by the American Psychiatric Association, is the handbook used most often in diagnosing mental disorders in the United States and internationally. The International Statistical Classification of Diseases and Related Health Problems (ICD) is sometimes used as an alternative.[7]

DSML   **Directory services markup language.** Bridges the world of directory services with the world of XML by continuing work on the DSML specification to add support for querying and modifying directories.

DSMO Designated standard maintenance organization. Designed to maintain ongoing updates to ISO standards. Responsible to ISO Central Secretariat and the Technical Committee secretariat.[3]

DSR Daily response message. Request and response messages may be exchanged between a client and server.[12]

DSR Data set ready. Modem control that indicates that the modem is attached to a communications line.[1]

DSS Decision support system. Any computer-based support of medical, managerial, administrative, and financial decisions in healthcare, using knowledge bases and/or reference material.[4]

DSSS Direct sequence spread spectrum. Also known as *direct sequence code division multiple access*. Allows a digital signal to resist interference, and also enables the original data to be recovered if data bits are damaged during transmission.[2]

DSTU Draft standard for trial use. An archaic term for any standard that has been approved.[10]

DSU Data service unit. Provides digital-to-digital communication.[1]

DSU/CSU Data service unit/channel service unit.[1]

DT Date data type (YYYYMMDD). International method of writing the date.

DTD Document type definition. Defines the legal building blocks of an XML document. It defines the document structure with a list of legal elements.[1]

DTR Data terminal ready. Modem control that indicates that a terminal is ready for transmission.[1]

DTR Draft technical report. Draft technical report containing only informative information that is ready for ballot.[3]

Dual-use technology Technology that has both civilian and military applications (e.g., cryptography).[1]

Dumb terminal Terminal with no localized processing, storage, or GUI capacity. VT-320s, VT-420s, and VT-510s are dumb terminals associated with Center for Healthcare Strategies. Mainly associated with mainframes and centralized computing.[1]

Durability Changes made by the committed transaction are permanent and must survive system failure. *See also* **ACID**.

Duration A field within a certificate that is composed of two subfields: 'date of issue' and 'date of next issue.'[114]

DVD Digital video disk or **digital versatile disk.** Backwardly compatible with CD-ROMs (i.e., they can read CD-ROMs). The DVD specification can support a disk with capacities from 4.7 gigabytes to 17 gigabytes.[11]

DXPlain A decision support system from Massachusetts General Hospital which uses a set of clinical findings (signs, symptoms, laboratory data) to produce a ranked list of diagnoses which might explain, or be associated with, clinical manifestations.[141]

Dynamic host configuration protocol *See* **DHCP.**

Dynamic link control *See* **DLC.**

Dynamic link library *See* **DLL.**

Dynamic RAM *See* **DRAM.**

E

e-[text] or e-text Electronic. Short for 'electronic,' 'e' or 'e-' is used as a prefix to indicate that something is Internet-based, not just electronic. The trend began with e-mail in the 1990s and now includes eCommerce, eHealth, e-GOV, etc.[32]

E-1-3 European digital signal. 2.048-3.139.254 Mbps digital transmission that is similar to ISDN.[1]

EAI Enterprise application integration. 1. The use of software and architectural principles to bring together (integrate) a set of enterprise computer applications. It is an area of computer systems architecture that gained wide recognition from about 2004 onwards.

EAI is related to middleware technologies, such as message-oriented middleware (MOM), and data representation technologies, such as XML. Newer EAI technologies involve using Web services as part of service-oriented architecture as a means of integration.[7] **2.** A presentation level integration technology that provides a single point of access to conduct business transactions that utilize data from multiple disparate applications.[1] *See also* **System integration**.

EAP Extensible authentication protocol. A general protocol for authentication that also supports multiple authentication methods, such as token cards, one-time passwords, certificate, public key authentication, and smart cards.[2]

Early event detection *See* **EED**.

EBB Eligibility-based billing. Process in which a payer bills a customer based on the eligibility. Clients are responsible for their own eligibility and data accuracy.

EBCDIC Extended binary coded decimal interchange code. A standard character-to-number encoding (like ASCII) used by some IBM computer systems.

EC Electronic commerce. Also known as *eCommerce*.[5]

ECG Retrieve ECG for display. Specifies a mechanism for broad access throughout the enterprise to electrocardiogram (ECG) documents for review purposes. The ECG documents may include 'diagnostic quality' waveforms, measurements, and interpretations. This integration profile allows the display of this information without requiring specialized cardiology software or workstations, but with general purpose computer applications, such as a Web browser. This integration profile is intended primarily for retrieving resting 12-lead ECGs, but may also retrieve ECG waveforms gathered during stress, Holter, and other diagnostic tests. This integration profile only addresses ECGs that are already stored in an information system. It does not address the process of ordering, acquiring, storing, or interpreting the ECGs. *See also* **Profile**.[56]

ECHO Describes the workflow associated with digital echocardiography, specifically that of transthoracic echo, transesophageal echo, and stress echo. As does the Cath Workflow integration profile, this profile deals with patient identifiers, orders, scheduling, status reporting, multi-stage exams (especially stress echo), and data storage. It also specifically addresses the issues of acquisition modality devices that are only intermittently connected to the network, such as portable echo machines, and addresses echo-specific data requirements. *See also* **Profile**.[56]

ECN Explicit congestion packet. A 2-bit IP packet header field that allows reduction of the number of TCP re-transmissions in the Internet.[1]

ED Encapsulated data type. The coupling or encapsulation of the data with a select group of functions that defines everything that can be done with the data.[7]

ED Evidence documents. Defines interoperable ways for observations, measurements, results, and other procedure details recorded in the course of carrying out a procedure step to be output by devices, such as acquisition systems and other workstations; to be stored and managed by archival systems; and to be retrieved and presented by display and reporting systems. This allows detailed non-image information, such as measurements, CAD results, procedure logs, etc., to be made available as input to the process of generating a diagnostic report. The evidence documents may be used either as additional evidence for the reporting physician or in some cases, for selected items in the evidence document to be included in the diagnostic report. *See also* **Profile**.[56]

EDDS Electronic document digital storage. Document management systems available online.[32] *See also* **Decision support clinical and analytic**, and **Decision support system**.

EDI Electronic data interchange. 1. Even before HIPAA, American National Standards Institute (ANSI) approved the process for developing a set of EDI standards known as the X12. EDI is a collection of standard message formats that allows businesses to exchange data via any electronic messaging service. **2.** The electronic transfer of data between companies using networks to include the Internet. Secure communications are needed in healthcare to exchange eligibility information, referrals, authorization, claims, encounter, and other payment data needed to manage contracts and remittance.[43] **3.** The sending, transmission, reception, and interchange of information and data relating to business transactions (typically an order or an invoice) via electronic means.[4]

EDI Electronic data interchange gateway. An electronic process to send data (claims, membership, and benefits) back and forth between providers and insurance companies.[15]

EDIT In CMS (Centers for Medicare & Medicaid Services), the logic within the Standard Claims Processing System (or PSC Supplemental Edit Software) that selects certain claims, evaluates, or compares information on the selected claims or other accessible source; and, depending on the evaluation, takes action on the claims, such as pay in full, pay in part, or suspend for manual review.[118]

EED Early event detection. This component of public health information network preparedness uses case and suspect case reporting, along with statistical surveillance of health-related data, to support the earliest possible detection of events that may signal a public health emergency.[46]

EEPROM Electronically erasable programmable read only memory. A reprogrammable memory chip that can be electronically erased and reprogrammed via a reader/writer device.[1]

Effective date Under the Health Insurance Portability and Accountability Act (HIPAA), this is the date that a final rule is effective, which is usually 60 days after it is published in the *Federal Register*.[10]

EGA Color display system providing 16 to 64 colors at a resolution of 640x480. Not supported by Windows 95 and Windows NT.[1]

E-GOV The 'E-Government Act of 2002' was signed into law by President George W. Bush in July 2002: "This legislation builds upon my Administration's expanding E-Government initiative by ensuring strong leadership of the information technology activities of Federal agencies, a comprehensive framework for information security standards and programs, and uniform safeguards to protect the confidentiality of information provided by the public for statistical purposes. The Act will also assist in expanding the use of the Internet and computer resources in order to deliver Government services, consistent with the reform principles I outlined on July 10, 2002, for a citizen-centered, results-oriented, and market-based Government."[44]

EGP Exterior gateway protocol. An old protocol that advertises the networks that can be reached within an autonomous system by advertising its IP addresses to a router in another autonomous system.[1]

eHealth eHealth (also written e-health) is a term for healthcare practice which is supported by electronic processes and communication; some people would argue the term is interchangeable with 'health informatics.' However, the term 'eHealth' encompasses a whole range of services that is at the edge of medicine/healthcare and information technology, including electronic medical records, telemedicine, and evidence-based medicine.[7]

EHR Electronic health record. A longitudinal electronic record of patient health information generated by one or more encounters in any care delivery setting. Included in this information are patient demographics, progress notes, problems, medications, vital signs, past medical history, immunizations, laboratory data, and radiology reports and images. The EHR automates and streamlines the clinician's workflow. The EHR has the ability to generate a complete record of a clinical patient encounter, as well as supporting other care-related activities directly or indirectly via interface; including evidence-based decision support, quality management, and outcomes reporting. *See also* **CPR, EMR,** and **Appendix A.**[45]

EHRS Electronic health record system.

EIDE Enhanced or extended integrated drive electronics. A standard interface for high-speed disk drives that operates at speeds faster than the standard IDE interface. It allows the connection of four IDE devices.[1]

EIN Employer identification number. 1. Employers, as sponsors of health insurance for their employees, often need to be identified in healthcare transactions, and a standard identifier for employers would be beneficial for transactions exchanged electronically. Healthcare providers may need to identify the employer of the participant on claims submitted to health plans electronically. **2.** The HIPAA standard is the EIN, the taxpayer identifying number for employers that is assigned by the Internal Revenue Service. This identifier has nine digits with the first two digits separated by a hyphen, as follows: 00-0000000.[1,10]

EIP Enterprise information portal. 1. Intranet portals are also known as enterprise information portals (EIP). The building blocks of portals are portlets, which contain portions of content published using markup languages, such as HTML and XML. **2.** An Internet-based approach to consolidate and present an organization's business intelligence and information resources through a single access point via an intranet.[7,1]

EIS Enterprise information system. A class of decision support systems that provide predefined and easy-to-use data presentation, and exploration functionality to top-level executives.[1]

EIS Executive information system. A computer-based system intended to facilitate and support the information and decision making needs of senior executives by providing easy access to both internal and external information relevant to meeting the strategic goals of the organization. It is commonly considered as a specialized form of decision support system. The emphasis of EIS is on graphical displays and easy-to-use user interfaces. They offer strong reporting and drill-down capabilities. In general, EIS are enterprise-wide DSS that help top-level executives analyze, compare, and highlight trends in important variables so that they can monitor performance and identify opportunities and problems. EIS and data warehousing technologies are converging in the marketplace.[7]

EISA Extended industry standard architecture. 32-bit internal bus. Introduced in 1988 to compete with the PS/2 (Micro Channel) line of computers.[1]

Electromagnetic interference *See* **EMI**.

Electronic *See* **e-[text] or e-text**.

Electronic attestation Verifies the identity of an individual by linking signature verification data to that person. The purpose of attestation is to show authorship and assign responsibility for an act, event, condition, opinion, or diagnosis.

Every entry in the health record must be identified with the author and should not be made or signed by someone other than the author. Attestation functionality must meet applicable legal, regulatory, and other applicable standards or requirements.[2]

Electronic certificate *See* **Digital certificate**.

Electronic claim 1. Electronic transactions sent to payers to receive payments for healthcare services covered by the payers. These are the HIPAA 837 transactions, responsible for remittance advice for claims payment made by payers. **2.** Any claim submitted for payment to the health plan by a central processing unit, tape diskette, direct data entry, direct wire, dial-in telephone, digital fax, or personal computer download or upload. *See* **EDI**.[2,1]

Electronic commerce Electronic commerce, or eCommerce, consists primarily of the distributing, buying, selling, marketing, and servicing of products or services over electronic systems, such as computer networks. HIPAA was intended, in large part, to facilitate eCommerce in healthcare. *See* **HIPAA**.

Electronic commerce *See* **EC**.

Electronic data Recorded or transmitted electronically, while non-electronic data would be everything else. Special cases would be data transmitted by fax and audio systems, which is, in principle, transmitted electronically, but which lacks the underlying structure usually needed to support automated interpretation of its contents.[10]

Electronic data interchange *See* **EDI**.

Electronic data interchange gateway *See* **EDI**.

Electronic forms management A software system that automatically generates forms and can be populated by importing data from another system and/or can export data that has been entered into another system.[2]

Electronic health record *See* **EHR** and **Appendix A**.

Electronic health record provider Entity in legitimate possession of electronic health record data, and in a position to communicate it to another appropriate entity.[116]

Electronic Health Records (EHR) Laboratory Results Reporting Use Case This HITSP Interoperability Specification (IS-01) is designed to meet the specific requirements of the Electronic Health Record (EHR) Use Case, defined as sending laboratory test results and laboratory interpretations in an electronic format to clinicians for patient care. Laboratory test results and interpretations are then available for integration into an electronic health record (EHR), local or remote, or other clinical systems.[48]

Electronic media **1.** Electronic storage media, including memory devices in computers (hard drives) and any removable/transportable digital memory media, such as magnetic tapes or disks, optical disks, or digital memory cards. **2.** Transmission media used to exchange information already in electronic storage media, including, for example, the Internet (wide open), extranet (using Internet technology to link a business with information accessible only to collaborating parties), leased lines, dial-up lines, private networks, and the physical movement of removable/transportable electronic storage media. Certain transmissions, including paper via facsimilie and voice via telephone, are not considered to be transmissions via electronic media because the information being exchanged did not exist in electronic form before the transmission.[118]

Electronic media claims *See* **EMC.**

Electronic medical record *See* **EMR.**

Electronic Medical Record Adoption Model *See* **EMRAM.**

Electronic medication administration record *See* **eMar.**

Electronic patient record *See* **EHR.**

Electronic personal health record *See* **ePHR** and **PHR.**

Electronic prescribing *See* **E-prescribing.**

Electronic protected health information. *See* **EPHI.**

Electronic purse A mechanism that allows end users to pay electronically for goods and services. The function of the electronic purse is to maintain a pool of value that is incrementally reduced as transactions are performed.[114]

Electronic remittance advice *See* **ERA.**

Electronic signature **1.** An electronic signature creates the logical manifestation of a signature, including the possibility for multiple parties to sign a document and have the order of application recognized and proven and supply additional information, such as time stamp and signature purpose, specific to that user. **2.** Verifying a signature on a document verifies the integrity of the document and associated attributes and verifies the identity of the signer. Several technologies are available for use authentication, including passwords, cryptography, and biometrics.[1]

Electronically erasable programmable read only memory *See* **EEPROM.**

Eligibility-based billing *See* **EBB.**

E-mail **Electronic mail.** Electronic messages sent via networks between users on other computer systems. A service that permits a message or response to be created on one computer and sent over a network to another machine, another person, a group, or a computer program.[1]

eMar **Electronic medication administration record.** An electronic record-keeping system that documents every drug taken by a patient during a hospital stay. This application supports the five rights of medication administration (right patient, right medication, right dose, right time, and right route of administration) by utilizing bar coding functionality with pharmacy medication dispensing and nursing medication administration services. This functionality is implemented to reduce medication errors. This functionality requires tightly coupled data flows between the CPOE, pharmacy, automated dispensing machines, robotic devices, and nursing medication administration applications. Medical errors are reduced, drug inventory costs are reduced, and billing is more accurate.[2]

EMC **Electronic media claims.** This term usually refers to a flat file format used to transmit or transport claims.[10]

Emergency Sudden demand for action; a condition that poses an immediate threat to the health of the patient. This definition is further clarified to mean "any potential denial of critical health services, or information, that could reasonably result in personal injury or death to an individual or the public."[39,48]

Emergency access Granting of user rights and authorizations to permit access to protected health information and applications in emergency conditions outside of normal workflows. (Emergency room access is considered to be a normal workflow.)[48]

Emergency care system An application that assists emergency department clinicians and staff in the critical task of managing patients quickly and efficiently; directs each step of the patient management/patient flow and patient documentation process, including triage, tracking, nursing and physician charting, disposition, charge capture, and management reporting.[2]

Emergency permission Permission granted to certain caregivers in advance that allows self-declaration of an emergency and assumption of an emergency role. Emergency permissions defined in standard ways, compliant with appropriate ANSI standards and Health Level Seven (HL7) healthcare permission definitions, are suitable for federated circumstances, where the person declaring the emergency is not a member of the organization possessing the requested information.[48]

Emergency repair disk *See* **ERD**.

EMI Electromagnetic interference. Any disruption caused by electromagnetic waves.[1]

Emissions security *See* **EMSEC**.

Emoticons A combination word for 'emotional icon,' it is a small 'picture' created with the normal keys on a keyboard meant to denote the writer's mood in an e-mail message.[11]

EMPI Enterprise Master Person Index. A system that coordinates client identification across multiple systems, namely by collecting and sorting IDs and person-identifying demographic information from source system (track new persons; track changes to existing persons). These systems also take on several other tasks and responsibilities associated with client management.[2]

Employee Retirement Income and Security Act *See* **ERISA**.

Employee welfare benefit plan A plan, fund, or a program maintained by an employer, or an employee organization, that provides medical, surgical, or hospital care.[48]

Employer identification number *See* **EIN**.

EMR An application environment that is composed of the clinical data repository, clinical decision support, controlled medical vocabulary, order entry, computerized practitioner order entry, and clinical documentation applications. This environment supports the patient's electronic medical record across inpatient and outpatient environments, and is used by healthcare practitioners to document, monitor, and manage healthcare delivery.[2]

EMRAM Electronic Medical Record Adoption Model. A tool developed by HIMSS Analytics guiding hospitals to improved clinical outcomes.[2]

EMSEC Measures taken to deny unauthorized persons information derived from intercept and analysis of compromising emanations from crypto-equipment of an IT system.[97]

Emulation A software program that allows a computer to imitate another computer with a differing operating system.[1]

Encapsulated data type *See* **ED**.

Encipherment encryption Cryptographic transformation of data to produce ciphertext.[121]

Encoded data Data represented by some identification of classification scheme, such as a provider identifier or a procedure code.[5]

Encoder This application enables health information management personnel to find and use complete and accurate codes and code modifiers for procedures and diagnoses to optimize billing and reimbursement. For example, 1234 is bronchitis, whereas 1235 is bronchitis with asthma, and 1236 is bronchitis with stomach flu.[2]

Encoding-decoding services This service will encode and/or decode messages from and to different coding formats, such as Unicode, UTF-8, Base64, etc.[8]

Encounter Clinical encounter is: **1.** An instance of direct provider/practitioner to patient interaction, regardless of the setting, between a patient and practitioner vested with primary responsibility for diagnosing, evaluating, or treating the patient's condition, or both, or providing social worker services. **2.** A contact between a patient and practitioner who has primary responsibility for assessing and treating the patient at a given contact, exercising independent judgment. Encounter serves as a focal point linking clinical, administrative and financial information. Encounters occur in many different settings—ambulatory care, inpatient care, emergency care, home health care, field and virtual (telemedicine).[39]

Encounter data Detailed data about individual services provided by a capitated managed care entity. The level of detail about each service reported is similar to that of a standard claim form. Encounter data are also sometimes referred to as 'shadow claims.'[102]

Encryption 1. An application/technology that provides the translation of data into a secret code. Encryption is the most effective way to achieve data security. To read an encrypted file, you must have access to a secret key or password that enables you to decrypt it. Unencrypted data is called plain text; encrypted data is referred to as cipher text. **2.** Means of securing data by transforming/generating them into apparently meaningless random characters between source and destination. A process by which a message is encoded so that its meaning is not obvious. It is transformed into a second message using a complex function and a special encryption key.[2,1]

Encryption-decryption services This encrypts and decrypts messages. It could use X.509 certificates and other cryptography mechanisms.[8]

Enhanced or extended integrated drive electronics *See* **EIDE**.

Enhanced small device interface *See* **ESDI**.

ENP® **European Nursing care Pathways.** Provides nursing knowledge for nursing professionals in terms of a nursing language implemented in a classification system for the illustration of the nursing process. The nursing classification ENP consists of the vertical level of the classes nursing diagnoses, characteristics, resources, nursing objectives and nursing interventions, and intervention guiding specifications. Within the individual classes, the organizing principle is either hierarchical or coordinate. In the ENP system, every single ENP nursing diagnosis, supported by nursing

literature, relates horizontally and class-spanning to other objects (characteristics, etiologies, resources, nursing objectives, and nursing interventions). According to the ENP developers, these nursing diagnosis-related pathways represent up-to-date nursing knowledge and can be understood as a knowledge management system for nursing due to semantic networks. ENP is among the pre-combined nursing classifications and is conceived for front-end use.[113]

Enterprise A business organization.[32]

Enterprise application integration *See* **EAI**.

Enterprise architecture A business-focused framework developed in accordance with the Clinger-Cohen Act of 1996 that identifies the business processes, systems that support processes, and guidelines and standards by which systems must operate.[23]

Enterprise architecture integration Tools and techniques that promote, enable, and manage the exchange of information and distribution of business processes across multiple application systems, typically within a sizeable electronic landscape, such as large corporations, collaborating companies, and administrative regions.[8]

Enterprise electronic health record An application environment that is composed of the clinical data repository, clinical decision support, controlled medical vocabulary, order entry, computerized physician order entry, and clinical documentation applications. This environment supports the patient's electronic medical record across the continuum of care (e.g., across inpatient and outpatient environments) and is used by healthcare professionals to document, monitor, and manage healthcare delivery. *See also* **EHR**.[2]

Enterprise information portal *See* **EIP**.

Enterprise information system *See* **EIS**.

Enterprise Master Patient Index A system which coordinates client identification across multiple systems, namely by collecting and storing IDs and person-identifying demographic information from source systems (track new persons, track changes to existing persons). These systems also take on several other tasks and responsibilities associated with client ID management.[8]

Enterprise Master Person Index *See* **EMPI**.

Enterprise network A network consisting of multiple servers and domains over a small or large geographical area.[1]

Enterprise network services Examples are security, messaging, administration, host connectivity, wide area network (WAN) communication.[1]

Enterprise resource planning *See* **ERP**.

Enterprise scheduling The ability to schedule procedures, exams, and appointments across multiple systems and/or locations spanning an entire jurisdiction.[8]

Enterprise user authentication *See* **EUA**.

Entity Something that has a distinct, separate existence, though it need not be a material existence.[7]

Entity identity assertion Ensure that an entity is the person or application that claims the identity provided.[48]

Entity-relationship diagram The entity-relationship model or entity-relationship diagram (ERD) is a data model or diagram for high-level descriptions of conceptual data models, and it provides a graphical notation for representing such data models in the form of entity-relationship diagrams. Such data models are typically used in the first stage of information-system design; they are used, for example, to describe information needs and/or the type of information that is to be stored in the database during the requirements analysis.[7]

Entries Health record data in general (clinical observations, statements, reasoning, intentions, plans, or actions) without particular specification of their formal representation, hierarchical organization, or of the particular record component class(es) that might be used to represent them.[116]

EOB Explanation of benefits. A document detailing how a claim was processed according to the insured's benefits.[15]

EOP Explanation of payment. Generated to the provider in reply to a claim submission.[15]

EPHI Electronic protected health information. Any protected health information (PHI) which is created, stored, transmitted, or received electronically.[48]

ePHR Electronic Personal Health Record. A universally accessible, layperson comprehensible, lifelong tool for managing relevant health information, promoting health maintenance, and assisting with chronic disease management via an interactive, common data set of electronic health information and eHealth tools. The ePHR is owned, managed, and shared by the individual or his or her legal proxy(s), and must be secure to protect the privacy and confidentiality of the health information it contains. It is not a legal record unless so defined, and is subject to various legal limitations.[45] *See also* **PHR**.

Episode of care An encounter, or series of encounters, related to the detection and subsequent care for a particular patient.

E-prescribing Electronic prescribing. The use of computing devices to enter, modify, review, and output or communicate drug prescriptions.[1]

EPROM Erasable programmable memory. Reusable firmware that can be programmed. Previous contents are erased by applying ultraviolet light through the window in the chip.[1]

ERA Electronic remittance advice. Any of several electronic formats for explaining the payments of healthcare claims.[10]

Erasable programmable memory *See* **EPROM**.

ERD Emergency repair disk. Disk that contains machine-specific repair process information on registry (system, software, security, SAM) and system files for use when failures occur.[1]

ERD Entity relationship diagram (or model). A diagram showing entities and their relationships. Relates to business data analysis and database design.

ERISA Employee Retirement Income and Security Act of 1975. Most group health plans covered by ERISA are also health plans under the Health Insurance Portability and Accountability Act (HIPAA).[48]

ERP   Enterprise resource planning. Management information systems that integrate and automate many of the business functions associated with the operations or production aspects of an enterprise, such as general ledger, budgeting, materials management, purchasing, payroll, and human resources.[7,1]

Error   An act of commission (doing something wrong) or omission (failing to do the right thing) that leads to an undesirable outcome or significant potential for such an outcome. For instance, ordering a medication for a patient with a documented allergy to that medication would be an act of commission. Failing to prescribe a proven medication with major benefits for an eligible patient (e.g., low-dose unfractionated heparin as venous thromboembolism prophylaxis for a patient after hip replacement surgery) would represent an error of omission. Errors of omission are more difficult to recognize than errors of commission but likely represent a larger problem. In other words, there are likely many more instances in which the provision of additional diagnostic, therapeutic, or preventive modalities would have improved care than there are instances in which the care provided quite literally should not have been provided. In many ways, this point echoes the generally agreed-upon view in the healthcare quality literature that underuse far exceeds overuse, even though the latter historically received greater attention. *See also* **Underuse, Overuse, Misuse**.[14]

Error chain   Generally refers to the series of events that led to a disastrous outcome, typically uncovered by a root cause analysis. Sometimes the chain metaphor carries the added sense of inexorability, as many of the causes are tightly coupled, such that one problem begets the next. A more specific meaning of error chain, especially when used in the phrase "break the error chain," relates to the common themes or categories of causes that emerge from root cause analyses. These categories go by different names in different settings, but they generally include (1) failure to follow standard operating procedures; (2) poor leadership; (3) breakdowns in communication or teamwork; (4) overlooking or ignoring individual fallibility; and (5) losing track of objectives. Used in this way, "break the error chain" is shorthand for an approach in which team members continually address these links as a crisis or routine situation unfolds. The

checklists that are included in teamwork training programs have categories corresponding to these common links in the error chain (e.g., establish team leader, assign roles and responsibilities, monitor your teammates).[14]

ESDI   Enhanced small device interface. Short-lived hard disk drive interface standard introduced by Compaq. Step in technology after MFM, but before IDE.[1]

ESL   *See* **Extensible style sheet language**.

Ethernet   A frame-based computer networking technology for local area networks (LANs). The name comes from the physical concept of ether. It defines wiring and signaling for the physical layer, and frame formats and protocols for the media access control (MAC)/data link layer of the OSI model. Ethernet is mostly standardized as IEEEs 802.3. It has become the most widespread LAN technology in use during the 1990s to the present.[7]

ETL   Extraction transformation loading. A data warehousing term. The collection of methods, processes, and technology that perform the acquisition, cleansing, transformation, integration, and loading of raw data sources into a data warehouse.[1]

EUA   Enterprise user authentication. A means to establish one name per user that can then be used on all of the devices and software that participate in this integration profile, greatly facilitating centralized user authentication management and providing users with the convenience and speed of a single sign-on. This profile leverages Kerberos (RFC 1510) and the HL7 CCOW standard (user subject).[56]

European digital signal   *See* **E-1-3**.

European Nursing care Pathways®   *See* **ENP®**.

Event   Action or activity that occurs within a system and/or network scope, inclusive of its boundaries.[48]

Event aggregation   Consolidation of similar log entries into a single entry, containing a count of the number of occurrences of the event.[48]

Event correlation   Relationships between two or more log entries.[48]

Event filtering Suppression of log entries from analysis, reporting, or long-term storage, because their characteristics indicate that they are unlikely to contain information of interest.[48]

Event reduction Removal of unneeded data fields from all log entries to create a new log that is smaller.[48]

Evidence documents *See* **ED**.

Evidence-based medicine Evidence-based medicine asks questions, finds and appraises the relevant data, and harnesses that information for everyday clinical practice. Evidence-based medicine follows four steps: formulate a clear clinical question from a patient's problem; search the literature for relevant clinical articles; evaluate (critically appraise) the evidence for its validity and usefulness; and implement useful findings in clinical practice. The term 'evidence-based medicine' was coined at McMaster Medical School in Canada in the 1980s to label this clinical learning strategy, which people at the school had been developing for over a decade.[5] *See* **Best practices**.

Evidence-based practice *See* **Evidence-based medicine**.

Exception A transaction that does not receive authorization by the accepted rules and procedures.[1]

Exchange format The representation of the data elements and the structure of a message, while in transfer between systems.[4]

Exclusive branching Splits a process in several branches, only one of which can be selected, based on the fulfillment of a condition associated with a given branch.[111]

Exclusive choice The divergence of a branch into two or more branches, such that when the incoming branch is enabled, the thread of control is immediately passed to precisely one of the outgoing branches, based on a mechanism that can select one of the outgoing branches.[112] *See* **Simple merge**.

Executive information system *See* **EIS**.

EXL Commercial grade Internet access with your choice of managed routers, managed firewalls, managed virtual private network, managed anti-spam and anti-virus.

Expert system A software system with two basic components: a knowledge base and an inference engine.[7]

Explanation of benefits *See* **EOB**.

Explanation of payment *See* **EOP**.

Explicit congestion notification *See* **ECN**.

Expression The textual means to convey a concept to the user. It can be a major concept, a synonym, or a lexical variant.[32]

Extended ASCII **Extended American Standard Code for Information Interchange.** Extensively used 8-bit standard information processing code with 256 characters.[1]

Extended binary coded decimal interchange code *See* **EBCDIC**.

Extended industry standard architecture *See* **EISA**.

Extended memory Additional area of memory beyond 1MB associated with DOS machines.[1]

Extensibility The ability to economically modify or add functionality.[8]

Extensible authentication protocol *See* **EAP**.

Extensible markup language *See* **XML**.

Extensible style sheet language *See* **XSL**.

Exterior gateway protocol *See* **EGP**.

Extraction transformation loading *See* **ETL**.

Extranet An internal network or intranet opened to selected business partners to allow access to internal information in support of essential information for a business relationship, such as supply-chain management information.[1]

F

Facility directory Listing or reference document maintained by a healthcare provider, such as (but not limited to) a hospital, nursing home, or treatment center, of persons receiving care or treatment from that provider, and containing information about each individual patient or resident receiving care or treatment.[48]

Fact table   A table, typically in a data warehouse, that contains the measures and facts (the primary data).

Failsafe   Pertaining to avoidance of compromise in the event of a failure.[3]

False acceptance rate   *See* **FAR**.

Family set   Group of backup tapes consisting of a single run of backup information.[1]

FAQ   Frequently asked questions. A collection of information on any subject for which questions are typically asked. FAQ postings provide quick answers without the need or expense of a staff person answering the question on the phone or in writing, and are viewed as a time-saving feature of Web sites which provides a return on investment.[1]

FAR   False acceptance rate. Refers to the rate at which an unauthorized individual is accepted by the system as a valid user.[114]

Fast SCSI   Fast small computer system interface. 10 Mbps high-speed 8-bit bus interface for connecting devices to the computer bus.[1]

Fast small computer system interface   *See* **Fast SCSI**.

FAT   File allocation table. 16-bit file cluster system technique used by MS-DOS and Windows operating systems to manage disk space. Can also be used with Windows NT.[1]

Fat client   In a client/server system, a client that performs most of the necessary data processing itself, rather than relying on the server.[107]

FAT32   File allocation table 32-bit. 32-bit file system technique used by the Windows 95 operating system to manage disk space. Cannot be used with Windows NT.[1]

FDDI   Fiber distributed data interface. Fiber optic dual token-ring network within the 802.8 standard. Provides 1000MHz of bandwidth at a distance of 200km.[1]

Federal Health Architecture   *See* **FHA**.

Federal Privacy Act of 1974   HIPAA. U.S.C. Section 552a. The Federal Privacy Act established a framework within which the government collects and uses information about individuals. Medicare recipients are protected because Medicare contractors are prohibited from releasing personal information, such as a person's health insurance claim number, claim data, diagnoses, etc., without written or verbal permission from the beneficiary or their official representative. Privacy rights of individuals were further strengthened in various revisions and through HIPAA.[1]

Fee for service   *See* **FFS**.

Feeder systems   Operational systems that will feed patient/person data to the EHR in the form of real-time single, multiple messages or batch file uploads. *See also* **Source systems**.[8]

FFS   Fee for service. Contract method to pay a contracted fee for services performed by providers.[32]

FHA   Federal Health Architecture. The FHA is one of five Lines of Business (LoB) supporting the President Bush's Management Agenda goal to expand electronic government. The FHA will create a consistent federal framework to facilitate communication and collaboration among all healthcare entities to improve citizen access to health-related information and high-quality services. It will link health business processes to their enabling technology solutions and standards to demonstrate how these solutions achieve improved health performance outcomes. It will also provide the ability to identify cross-functional processes, redundant systems, areas for collaboration, and opportunities to enhance interoperability in critical information systems and infrastructure.[144]

Fiber   distributed   data   interface   *See* **FDDI**.

Fiber optic cable   A pure glass cable used for the transmission of digital signals. It generates no radiation of its own and is resistant to electromagnetic interference. It is used in areas where security is of prime importance because tapping into the cable is detectable. Can be used over longer distances than copper cable.[1]

Fiber optics   Extremely fast communications technology that uses glass or plastic medium to transmit light pulses produced by LEDs or ILDs to represent data. Immune to electronic magnetic interference, but susceptible to chromatic dispersion. Information is transmitted through the fiber as pulsating light. The light pulses represent bits of information. Fiber optics give users of telecommunications added capacity, better transmission quality, and increased clarity.[1]

Fiber transceiver Device that converts fiber optic signals to digital signals and vice versa. Usually used to make a connection from a fiber run to an Ethernet segment.[1]

Field When a unit of data can be subdivided, the individual subdivisions are known as fields or data elements.[1]

Field components A field entry may also have discernable parts or components. For example, the patient's name is recorded as last name, first name, and middle initial, each of which is a distinct entity separated by a component delimiter.[16]

Field level security Data protection and/or authorization of specified fields or data elements within files, rather than of entire files.[1]

FIFO First in first out.

File Electronic data collected in related records. Files have unique names and entities that allow for them to be stored, moved, and edited. Often, a file's suffix describes its type, such as a Microsoft document file (.doc) or an executable file (.exe).[1]

File allocation table *See* **FAT**.

File allocation table 32-bit *See* **FAT32**.

File extension A group of characters appended to the end of a disk file name. File extensions usually consist of a full stop (dot) and one to three characters.[4]

File server A networked computer that provides file handling and storage for users with network access. A computer that each computer on a network can use to access and retrieve files that can be shared among the attached computers. Access to a file is usually controlled by the file server software, rather than by the operating system of the computer that accesses the file.[1]

File transfer protocol *See* **FTP**.

Filmless radiology Use of devices that replace film by acquiring digital images and related patient information, and transmit, store, retrieve, and display them electronically.[106]

Filter The purpose of a filter is to limit the responses displayed on a selection list during searches to specific categories of terminology.

FIPS **Federal Information Processing Standards.** A standard for adoption and use by federal departments and agencies that has been developed within the Information Technology Laboratory and published by NIST, a part of the U.S. Department of Commerce. A FIPS covers some topics in information technology to achieve a common level of quality or some level of interoperability.[114]

Firewall **1.** Used to prevent unauthorized access by blocking and checking all incoming network traffic. A firewall permits only authorized users to access and transmit privileged information, and denies access to unauthorized users. **2.** A system designed to prevent unauthorized access to or from a private network. Firewalls can be implemented in both hardware and software, or in combination of both. Firewalls are frequently used to prevent unauthorized Internet users from accessing private networks connected to the Internet, especially intranets. All messages entering or leaving the Intranet pass through the firewall, which examines each message, and blocks those that do not meet the specified security criteria.[1,2]

Firmware Computer instructions written to a read-only ROM, PROM, or EPROM chip.[1]

First in first out *See* **FIFO**.

Fishbone diagram The fishbone diagram, or cause-and-effect diagram, is a tool for capturing, displaying, and classifying the various theories about the causes of a problem.[120]

Five rights of medication administration The "Five Rights"—administering the Right Medication, in the Right Dose, at the Right Time, by the Right Route, to the Right Patient—are the cornerstone of traditional nursing teaching about safe medication practice.[14]

Fixed wireless Refers to wireless devices or systems that are situated in fixed locations, such as an office or home, as opposed to devices that are mobile, such as cell phones and PDAs. The point-to-point signal transmissions occur through the air over a terrestrial microwave platform rather than through copper or fiber cables; therefore, fixed wireless does not require satellite feeds or local phone service. The advantages of fixed wireless over traditional cabling infrastructure include the ability to connect with users in remote areas without the need for laying new cables, and the capacity for broad bandwidth that is not impeded by fiber or cable capacities. *See also* **PDA.**[1]

Flash drive Portable memory in a space the size of a key. Also called memory key, jump drive, thumb drive, stick drive, removable drive, and other names.[7]

Flash memory Non-volatile memory that provides read-only operations for computer boot-up. Contents can be updated. Smart card memory technology that emulates a hard disk, except that the data are stored electronically, and there are no moving parts.[1]

Flat files **1.** Files in which each record has the same length, whether or not all the space is used. Empty parts of the record are padded with a blank, or zero, depending on the data type of each field. **2.** Refers to a file that consists of a series of fixed-length records that include some sort of record type code.[1,10]

Flat table One data element per field, tables are in the simplest form.[6]

Flexibility The ability to support architectural and hardware configuration changes.[8]

Flexible spending account *See* **FSA.**

Flip-flop Digital signal circuit that can store one bit of information or be in a cleared state. 1-bit memory.[1]

Flow chart A diagram that combines symbols and abbreviated narratives to describe a sequence of operations and/or a process.[6]

Flow sheet A tabular summary of information that is arranged to display the values of variables as changed over time.[4]

Foreground Application or task that is executing and accepting user input and subsequent output on a multi-tasking machine.[1]

Foreign key A primary key of one data table that is placed into another data table to represent a relationship among those tables. Foreign keys resolve relationships and support navigation among data structures. *See also* **Primary key.**[1]

Formal system In a concept representation, a set of machine processable definitions in a subject field.[90]

Format Specifications of how data or files are to be characterized.[5]

Fortezza card A credit card-sized electronic module that stores digital information that can be recognized by a network or system. It is used to provide data encryption and authentication services.[1]

Frame A packet that can be 64 to 1,518 bytes long and contains header/data/trailer information, in addition to a preamble to mark the start of a frame.[1]

Frame relay A packet-oriented communication switching method used for local area network (LAN) interconnections and wide area network (WAN) connections. Used in both private and public networks. Frame relay networks in the U.S. support data transfer rates at T-1 (1.544 Mbps) and T-3 (45 Mbps) speeds. *See also* **ATM, SONET.**[1]

Framework **1.** A structured description of a topic of interest, including a detailed statement of the problem(s) to be solved and the goals to be achieved. An annotated outline of all the issues that must be addressed while developing acceptable solutions to the problem(s). A description and analysis of the constraints that must be satisfied by an acceptable solution, and detailed specifications of acceptable approaches to solving the problem(s)[114] **2.** Provides a unified view of the needs and functionality of a particular service or application, thus allowing a coherent approach to the specification of protocols and protocol elements as needed to realize the implementation of the service or application.[4]

Free text Unstructured, uncoded representations of information in text format (e.g., sentences describing the results of a patient's physical condition).[4]

Frequently asked questions *See* **FAQ.**

FSA **Flexible spending account.** A method of setting aside pre-tax dollars for healthcare reimbursement.[15]

FTF **Face to face.**

FTP **File transfer protocol. 1.** A standard high-level protocol for transferring files of different types between computers over a TCP/IP network. FTP can be used with a command line interface or graphical user interface. **2.** The name of a utility program available on several operating systems, which makes use of this protocol to access and transfer files on remote computers.[1]

Full duplex Communication channel/circuit that allows simultaneous two-way data transmission.[1]

Fully specified name A phrase that describes a concept uniquely and in a manner that is intended to be unambiguous.[19]

Functional health status Refers to a patient's ability to perform typical daily physical and social/role functions, plus other measures of self-perceived health status, such as well-being, vitality, and mental health.[120]

Functional requirements A statement of the system behavior needed to enforce a given policy. Requirements are used to derive the technical specifications of a system. Describes the performance expectations for a system.[1]

Functional role Role an individual is acting under when executing a function.[122]

Functional specifications A precise description of a computer system's functional requirements containing an overall picture of the proposed system's conditions, prerequisites, and restraints.[6]

G

Gantt chart A type of bar chart used in process or project planning, and control to display planned work targets for completion of work in relation to time. Typically, a Gantt chart shows the week, month, or quarter in which each activity will be completed, and the person or persons responsible for carrying out each activity.[123]

Gap analysis Evaluation of results of a security inventory against requirements.[48]

Garbage in garbage out See **GIGO**.

Gateway **1.** A computer or a network that allows access to another computer or network. **2.** A phrase used by Webmasters and search engine optimizers to describe a Web page designed to attract visitors and search engines to a particular Web site. A typical gateway page is small, simple, and highly optimized. **3.** A technical term for the software interface between a Web-based shopping cart (or order form) and a merchant account. See also **Electronic commerce**.[7]

GB Gigabyte.[1]

Gbps Gigabytes per second. Transmission of a billion bits per second.[1]

GELLO An object-oriented query and expression language for clinical decision support.[92]

General order message ORM. The function of this message is to initiate the transmission of information about an order. This includes placing new orders, cancellation of existing orders, discontinuation, holding, etc. ORM messages can originate also with a placer, filler, or interested third party.[16]

GIF Graphics interchange format. Standard for encoding, transmitting, decoding, and providing photo quality images. Introduced by CompuServe in 1987 to allow network transmission of photo-quality graphics images.[1]

GIFanim An animated picture created by including two or more .gif images in one file.[1]

GIG Global information grid. A globally interconnected, end-to-end set of information capabilities, associated processes, and personnel for collecting, processing, storing, disseminating, and managing information on demand.[23]

Gigabit A measure of computer storage that is approximately equal to one billion bits, most commonly used to describe telecommunications transfer speeds. For example, gigabit Ethernet allows local area network (LAN) transfer of about one billion bits, or discrete signal pulses, per second.[1]

Gigabyte Approximately one billion (1,024 megabytes) bytes. Unit of computer storage capacity.[1]

Gigahertz One billion cycles per second.[1]

GIGO Garbage in garbage out. Synonymous with the entry of inaccurate or useless data and processed output of worthless/useless information.[1]

Global information grid See **GIG**.

Global system for mobile communications *See* **GSM**.

Glossary A list of terms (usually alphabetically sorted) with explanations pertaining to a particular field (glossary is synonymous with vocabulary).[4]

Gnutella A file sharing network.[42] *See* **P2P**.

Google™ Popular Internet search engine.[32]

Gopher Text-based menu-driven document retrieval information service used on the Internet. Has virtually been made obsolete by the introduction of graphical-based Web browsers. A tool for finding data on the Internet that enables the user to locate essentially all textual information stored on Internet servers through a series of easy-to-use, hierarchical menus.[1]

Graduated security A security system that provides several levels of protection based on threats, risks, available technology, support services, time, human concerns, and economics.[114]

Granularity An expression of the relative size of a unit. The smallest discrete information that can be directly retrieved. In security, it is the degree of protection. Protection at the file level is considered coarse granularity, whereas protection at the field level is finer granularity.[1]

Graphical user interface *See* **GUI**.

Graphics interchange format *See* **GIF**.

Greenscreen **Monochrome computer monitors. 1.** Named for the green phosphor commonly used in monitors in the 1970s and 1980s. **2.** Refers to a computer application based on a character-cell terminal, which typically displayed about 80 characters wide by 24–25 lines tall, vs. the graphic user interfaces (GUI) commonly used in 2000 and later.[7]

Grid computing Uses the resources of many separate computers connected by a network (usually the Internet) to solve large-scale computation problems.[7]

Group health plan Under the Health Insurance Portability and Accountability Act (HIPAA), this is an employee welfare benefit plan that provides for medical care that either has 50 or more participants, or is administered by another business entity.[10]

GroupWare Network software that defines applications used by a group of people. Allows users on different systems to collaborate and interact. Electronic mail is an example.[1]

GSM **Global system for mobile communications. 1.** A worldwide digital standard used in nearly all countries in the world except Japan and the U.S. GSM is a pure digital service that can transmit Internet packets (IP) to the Internet, and uses an array of fixed antennas in geographical cells that connect various mobile devices to the network. **2.** GSM uses 1,900 MHz in the U.S., and 800 to 900 MHz in Europe and Asia. GSM providers also offer wireless application protocol (WAP) services, such as connection of a GSM phone to a laptop with a PC card or cable at a data rate of 9.6 Kbps.[1]

GSNW **Gateway services for NetWare.** Provides the ability to connect to and make NetWare server resources available to a Windows NT server.[1]

GUI **Graphical user interface. 1.** User interface that employs graphical images for the execution of resources as opposed to command line entry. Employs windows, icons, and menus in lieu of text to run programs and give commands to the computer. It is usually a window system accessed through a pointing device, such as a mouse. **2.** Options on how the mouse interacts with the objects on the screen allows a point-and-click interface to identify or activate an icon, or a drag-and-drop interface to move an item to another location. **3.** A type of display format that enables the user to choose commands and initiate programs and other options by selecting pictorial representation (icons) via a mouse or a keyboard.[1]

Guideline **1.** A recommended approach, parameter, etc. for conducting an activity or task or utilizing a product. **2.** A description that clarifies what should be done and how, to achieve the objectives set out in policies.[123] *See* **Clinical practice guideline**.

H

Hacker A person who gains unauthorized access to a computer network for profit, criminal mischief, or personal pleasure.[1]

Half duplex Communication channel/circuit that allows data transmission in one direction at a time, but not in both directions simultaneously.[1]

HAN Health alert network. To ensure that each community has rapid and timely access to emergent health information; a cadre of highly-trained professional personnel; and evidence-based practices and procedures for effective public health preparedness, response, and service on a 24/7 basis.[46]

Handheld A portable computer that is small enough to hold in one's hand. Used to refer to a variety of devices ranging from personal data assistants, such as the BlackBerry, to more powerful devices that offer many of the capabilities of desktop or laptop computers. Handhelds are used in clinical practice for such tasks as ordering prescriptions, accessing patients' medical records, and documenting patient encounters.[107]

Hard copy File printed to a paper document.[1]

Hard disk A hard disk is part of a unit, often called a 'disk drive' or 'hard disk drive,' that stores and provides relatively quick access to large amounts of data on an electromagnetically charged surface or set of surfaces.[1]

Hardware The physical equipment of a computer system, including the central processing unit, data-storage devices, terminals, and printers.[4]

Hardware address Unique low-level address burned into each piece of network hardware.[1]

Harm Physical injury or damage to the health of people, or damage to property or the environment.[68]

Harmonization Harmonization of national standards is the prevention or elimination of differences in the technical content of standards having the same scope, particularly differences that may cause hindrances to trade. Processes to achieve harmonization include convergence, modeling mapping, translation, and other technical specifications.[4]

Hashing Iterative process that computes a value (referred to as a hashword) from a particular data unit in such a manner that, when the hashword is protected, manipulation of the data is detectable.[1]

Hazard Potential source of harm.[68]

Hazardous situation Circumstance in which people, property, or the environment are exposed to one or more hazards.[68]

HCO Healthcare organization. Coordinates the delivery of healthcare. The organization should equip healthcare personnel with the knowledge, tools and expertise that they need to deliver care and act as a link to community resources. One approach to addressing healthcare systems is to divide them into the micro level (patient interaction), meso level (healthcare organization and community) and the macro level (policy). This section focuses on the role of the meso level of the healthcare system in delivering the best possible healthcare.[25]

HCPCS A set of healthcare procedure codes based on the American Medical Association's Current Procedural Terminology.[102]

HDSL High bit-rate digital subscriber line. One of the earliest forms of DSL, used for wideband digital transmission within a corporate site and between the telephone company and a customer. The main characteristic of HDSL is that it is symmetrical: an equal amount of bandwidth is available in both directions.[1]

Heads-up An electronically generated display of flight, navigational, attack, or other data superimposed upon a military pilot's forward field of view; more recently, being adapted to medicine. 'Heads up' is also used as a metaphor for an alert or forewarning.[35]

Health alert network *See* **HAN**.

Healthcare A broad term that directly refers to different activities and means used to prevent or cure different processes of morbidity.[4]

Healthcare clearing house Organization that processes health information received from another entity in a nonstandard format or containing nonstandard data content, into standard data elements or a standard transaction, or vice versa.[48]

Healthcare Common Procedure Coding System *See* **HCPCS**.

Heathcare data card A machine-readable card conformant to ISO 7810, intended for use within the healthcare domain.[117]

Healthcare enterprise Healthcare business organization (e.g., Hospital Corporation of America).[32]

Healthcare evaluation Methods for determining the success of healthcare delivery.[4]

Healthcare information framework High-level logical model of healthcare system.[4]

Healthcare Information Technology Standards Panel *See* **HITSP**.

Healthcare operations Operations, including quality assessment and improvement, peer review, underwriting, medical review audits, and business planning, management, and development.[48]

Healthcare organization *See* **HCO**.

Healthcare practitioner Person entrusted with the provision of healthcare services.[4]

Healthcare provider Person or organization that furnishes, bills, or is paid for healthcare in the normal course of business.[48]

Health indicator Measure that reflects the state of health of a group of patients that have common characteristics.[94]

Health information Information, whether oral or recorded in any form or medium, that (1) is created or received by a healthcare provider, health plan, public health authority, employer, life insurer, school or university, or healthcare clearinghouse; and (2) relates to the past, present, or future physical or mental health or condition of an individual; the provision of healthcare to an individual; or the past, present, or future payment for the provision of healthcare to an individual.[48]

Health information exchange *See* **HIE**.

Health information organization *See* **HIO**.

Health information privacy An individual's right to control the acquisition, uses, or disclosures of his or her identifiable health data.[48]

Health information security Refers to physical, technological, or administrative safeguards or tools used to protect identifiable health data from unwarranted access or disclosure.[48]

Health information system A health information system is an information system (i.e., a system of computer equipment, programs, procedures, and personnel designed, constructed, operated, and maintained to collect, record, process, retrieve, and display information) specific to the healthcare domain.[4]

Health insurance Insurance to cover the cost of healthcare. Health insurance can be privately managed or can be part of a government managed scheme.[4]

Health Insurance Portability and Accountability Act of 1996 *See* **HIPAA**.

Health maintenance organization *See* **HMO**.

Health outcome *See* **Outcome**.

Health Plan Employer Data Information Set *See* **HEDIS**.

Health services research The integration of epidemiologic, sociological, economic, and other analytic sciences in the study of health services. Health services research is usually concerned with relationships between need, demand, supply, use, and outcome of health services. The aim of the research is evaluation, particularly in terms of structure, process, output, and outcome.[1]

HEDIS Health Plan Employer Data Information Set. Set of standards for employers to use as a guide to compare health plans. *See also* **MPI**.[1]

Hercules graphics card *See* **HGC**.

Hexadecimal Base 16 numbering system where 4 bits are used to represent each digit. Uses the 0–9 digits and A–F letters for the representations of the 10–15 digits.[1]

HGC Hercules graphics card. Monochrome graphics display at a resolution of 720x348. Display type used before CGA and EGA.[1]

HIE Health information exchange. **1.** The sharing action between any two or more organizations with an executed business/legal arrangement that have deployed commonly agreed-upon technology with applied standards, for the purpose of electronically exchanging health related data between the organizations. **2.** A catch-all phrase for all health information exchanges, including RHIOs, QIOs, AHRQ funded communities, and private exchanges.[45,15] *See also* **Appendix D**.

Hijacking The ability of a hacker to misuse a system by gaining entry through the computer of a user who failed to logoff from a previous use.[1]

HIO Health information organization. An organization that oversees and governs the exchange of health-related information among organizations according to nationally recognized standards. The purpose of an HIO is to perform oversight and governance functions for health information exchanges (HIEs).[84] *See also* **Appendix D**.

HIPAA Health Insurance Portability and Accountability Act of 1996. According to the Centers for Medicare & Medicaid Services (CMS) Web site, Title I of HIPAA protects health insurance coverage for workers and their families when they change or lose their jobs. Title II of HIPAA, the Administrative Simplification (AS) provisions, requires the establishment of national standards for electronic healthcare transactions and national identifiers for providers, health insurance plans, and employers. The AS provisions also address the security and privacy of health data. The standards are meant to improve the efficiency and effectiveness of the nation's healthcare system by encouraging the widespread use of electronic data interchange in healthcare. Also known as the *Kennedy-Kassebaum Bill, K2,* or *Public Law 104-191.*[7]

HIPAA administrative code sets Code sets that characterize a general business situation, rather than a medical condition or service. Also called *non-medical code sets.*[1]

HIPAA administrative simplification HIPAA, Title II, Subtitle F, gives the Department of Health and Human Services the authority to mandate the use of standards for the electronic exchange of healthcare data; specify what medical and administrative code sets should be used within those standards; require the use of national identification systems for healthcare patients, providers, payers (or plans), and employers (or sponsors); and specify the types of measures required to protect the security and privacy of personally identifiable healthcare information.[1]

HIPAA chain of trust A term used in the HIPAA Security Notice of Proposed Rulemaking (NPRM) for a pattern of agreements that extend protection of healthcare data by requiring that each covered entity sharing healthcare data provide comparable protections offered by the original covered entity.[1]

HIPAA clearinghouse (or healthcare clearinghouse) Under HIPAA, this is a public or private entity that reformats health information, especially billing transactions, from a nonstandard format into a standard and approved format.[1]

HIPAA data dictionary A data dictionary that defines and cross-references the contents of all X12 transactions included in the HIPAA mandate. The dictionary is maintained by the X12N/TG3.[1]

HIPAA standard Any data element or transaction that meets each of the standards and implementation specifications adopted or established by the Secretary of the Department of Health and Human Services.[1]

HIPAA standard setting organization An organization accredited by the American National Standards Institute (ANSI) to develop information transactions or data elements for health plans, clearinghouses, and/or providers.[1]

HIPAA unique identifier A standard unique health identifier for each individual, employer, health plan, and healthcare provider, for use in the healthcare system.[1]

HIS Health information system. The National Committee on Vital and Health Statistics describes HIS as 'a comprehensive, knowledge-based system, capable of providing information to all who need it to make sound decisions about health.'[103]

Histogram A graphic display used to plot the frequency with which different values of a given variable occur. Histograms are used to examine existing patterns, identify the range of variables, and suggest a central tendency in variables.[123]

HIT Health information technology. A 'marriage' between the clinical healthcare activities and computer science for the benefit of patients and those who provide healthcare services.[138]

Hit analysis An analysis that uses the collected detail transactions of an organization's Web site to determine how, when, why, and what visitors did during their Web site visits. Within the analysis, the number of clicks, or hits, is shown from various perspectives—including which search engine may have referred them to the site, how long they stayed, and how many different pages were viewed.[1]

HITSP   Healthcare Information Technology Standards Panel. A multi-stakeholder coordinating body, based on a contract by the Department of Health and Human Services (DHHS), Office of National Coordinator for Health Information Technology (ONC), and the American Health Information Community (AHIC), designed to provide the process within which affected parties can identify, select, and harmonize standards for communicating healthcare information throughout a National Healthcare Information Network (NHIN).[48]

HMO   Health maintenance organization. An entity that provides, offers, or arranges for coverage of designated health services needed by plan members for a fixed, prepaid premium.[15]

Home page   The first and main view of a World Wide Web document, under which a series of pages may be placed. A top-level document of an organization, or a document that a user frequently visits.[1]

Host   An end user computer that is connected to at least one network.[1]

Host file   Text file that maps remote host names to IP addresses. Acts as a local DNS equivalent to provide a static type of DNS service.[1]

HTML   Hypertext markup language. 1. ASCII-based language used for creating files to display documents or Web pages to Web browsers. 2. Hypertext markup language is the standard provided by W3G (World Wide Web Group) used for Web pages on the Internet.[1,4]

HTTP   Hypertext transfer protocol. 1. Communication link protocol used by World Wide Web servers and browsers to transfer/exchange HTML documents or files (text, graphic images, sound, video, and other multimedia files) over the Internet. 2. Protocol with lightness and speed necessary for a distributed collaborative hypermedia information system. It is a generic, stateless, object-oriented protocol, which may be used for many similar tasks, such as name servers, and distributed object-oriented systems, by extending the commands or 'methods' used. *See also* **S-HTTP**.[1,16]

HTTP over SSL/HTTPS   HTTPS is a secure way of using HTTP. It supplements HTTP's transport layer, the insecure TCP, with Secure Socket Layer (SSL), a secure transport layer. HTTPS is a Web protocol developed by Netscape and built into its and other browsers that encrypts and decrypts user page requests, as well as the pages that are returned by the Web server.[8]

Hub   Electronic network device to which multiple networked computers are attached. Divides a data channel into two or more channels of lower bandwidth. Hubs function at the physical layer (first layer) of the OSI model. *See also* **Concentrator**.[1]

Hybrid network   Type of LAN topology in which networked nodes are connected to a hub, where star and ring topologies are combined into one overall topology.[1]

Hybrid smart card   A card that combines both optical and smart card technologies.[1]

Hype cycle   Hype Cycle of Emerging Technology (Gartner Group), a five-stage progression concerning 'the visibility' of an emerging technology (e.g., in the popular press): **1.** technology trigger; **2.** peak of inflated expectations; **3.** trough of disillusionment; **4.** slope of enlightenment; and **5.** plateau of productivity. Relative values on a 0–10 scale: 0, 9, 2, 3, 4. Used to convey the sense that new technologies are always oversold at first. Though they eventually are useful, they seldom live up to initial expectations.[47]

Hypertext markup language   *See* **HTML**.

Hypertext transfer protocol   *See* **0**.

Hz   Hertz. One cycle per second. Processing speeds for CPUs are measured in MHz.[1]

I

I/O   Input/output device. Allows computer to communicate with external devices, such as printers.[4]

IAM   Identity access management. Set of services to include authentication, user provisioning (UP), password management, role matrix management, enterprise single sign-on, enterprise access management, federation, virtual and metadirectory services, and auditing.[48]

IAP   Internet access provider. Company that provides basic Internet connection access. No additional services are provided, such as e-mail hosting.[1]

ICC   Integrated circuit chip. Another name for a chip, an integrated circuit is a small electronic device made out of a semiconductor material. Integrated circuits are used for a variety of devices, including microprocessors, audio and video equipment, and automobiles. Integrated circuits are often classified by the number of transistors and other electronic components they contain.[1]

ICD   The International Statistical Classification of Diseases and Related Health Problems (commonly known by the abbreviation ICD) is a detailed description of known diseases and injuries. It is published by the World Health Organization and is used worldwide for morbidity and mortality statistics. It is revised periodically and is currently in its tenth edition, known as the ICD-10. Every disease (or group of related diseases) is described with its diagnosis and given a unique code, up to five letters long.[25]

ICIDH   International Classification of Functioning and Disability. Classification system issued by the World Health Organization for common language for clinical use, data collection and research.[145]

ICON   A picture or symbol that graphically represents an object or a concept.[32]

ICON   An informational tool to describe nursing practice, it provides data representing nursing practice in comprehensive health information systems. A combinatorial terminology for nursing practice that includes nursing phenomena, nursing actions, and nursing outcomes, and facilitates cross-mapping of local terms and existing vocabularies and classifications.[49]

ICR   Intelligent call routing. Capability that automatically routes each call, based on caller profile, to the best available agent to handle the need, anywhere in the network. *See also* **PING**.[1]

ICR   Intelligent character recognition. The computer translation of manually entered text characters into machine-readable characters.[1]

ICR   Internet relay chat. A program that allows 'live' conversations between people all over the world by typing messages back and forth across the Internet.[1]

ICU   Intensive care unit. A specialized section of a hospital containing the equipment, medical and nursing staff, and monitoring devices necessary to provide intensive care. Also called critical care unit, or may have a specialty name such as cardiac care unit. [32]

IDCOP   Idealized design of the clinical office practice. A collaborative initiative, sponsored by the Institute for Healthcare Improvement, aimed at comprehensive redesign of the office system. IDCOP designs, tests, and deploys new models of office-based practices, including e-communication practices, to improve performance.[107]

IDE   Integrated device electronics. A standard ISA 16-bit bus interface for high-speed disk drives that operates a 5 Mbps with two attached devices (master and slave). Invented in 1986 and introduced in microcomputers in 1989/1990.[1]

Idealized design of the clinical office practice   *See* **IDCOP**.

Identification   The process of discovering the true identity of a person or item from the entire collection of similar persons or items.[114]

Identification authentication   1. The process of determining the identity of a user that is attempting to access a physical location or computer resource. Authentication can occur through a variety of mechanisms, including challenge/response, time-based code sequences, biometric comparison, or other techniques. **2.** Use of a password, or some other form of identification, to screen users and to check their authorization.[114,1]

Identifier   Unique data used to represent a person's identity and associated attributes. A name or a card number are examples of identifiers.[114]

Identity   The set of physical and behavioral characteristics by which an individual is uniquely recognizable.[114]

Identity access management *See* **IAM**.

Identity digital management *See* **IDM**.

Identity proofing The process of providing sufficient information (e.g., identity history, credentials, documents) to a personal identity verification (PIV) registrar when attempting to establish an identity.[114]

Identity verification The process of confirming or denying that a claimed identity is correct by comparing the credentials of a person requesting access with those previously proven and stored in the personal identity verification (PIV) card/system, and associated with the identity being claimed.[114]

IDM Identity digital management. Comprised of the set of business processes, and a supporting infrastructure, for the creation, maintenance, and use of digital identities within a legal and policy context.[48]

IDMS Identity management system. Comprised of one or more systems or applications that manages identity verification, validation, and issuance process.[114]

IDN Integrated delivery network. Commonly used to refer to an integrated delivery system, but may also be used when referring more to the network of providers vs. the system as a whole.[1]

IDR Intelligent document recognition. Based on intelligent character recognition, the IT system automatically identifies structural features of a document to allow for a more rapid creation of the document text.[17]

IDS Integrated delivery system. A healthcare organization (HCO) that owns at least two hospitals.[2]

IGP Interior gateway protocol. Used to advertise routing information within an autonomous system.[1]

IHE Integrating the Healthcare Enterprise. An initiative by healthcare professionals and industry to improve the way computer systems in healthcare share information. IHE promotes the coordinated use of established standards such as DICOM and HL7 to address specific clinical needs in support of optimal patient care. Physicians, medical specialists, nurses, administrators, and other care providers envision a day when vital information can be passed seamlessly from system to system within and across departments and made readily available at the point of care.[56] *See also* listing in Organizations and Associations section.

IHE profile Provides a common language for purchasers and vendors to discuss the integration needs of healthcare sites and the integration capabilities of healthcare IT products. They offer developers a clear implementation path for communication standards supported by industry partners that are carefully documented, reviewed and tested. They give purchasers a tool that reduces the complexity, cost and anxiety of implementing operating systems.[56]

IIF Information in identifiable form. Any representation of information that permits the identity of an individual to whom the information applies to be reasonably inferred by either direct or indirect means.[114]

IIS Internet information server. Server that provides HTTP and FTP services to Web browsers.[1]

IKE Internet key exchange. A key management protocol standard which is used in conjunction with the IPSec standard. IPSec is an IP security feature that provides robust authentication and encryption of IP packets.[1]

ILD Injection laser diode. Laser diode that provides the light pulses used with single-mode fiber to convey data transmission information.[1]

Image compression Used to reduce the amount of memory required to store an image (e.g., an image that has a resolution of 640x480 and is in the RGB color space at 8 bits per color requires 900 Kbytes of storage). If this image can be compressed at a compression ratio of 20:1, the amount of storage required is only 45 Kbytes. There are several methods of image compression, including iVEX, JPEG, MPEG, H.261, H.263, and Wavelet.[1]

Image exchange format The logical data format used for image exchange and storage.[4]

Imaging The process of capturing, storing, displaying and printing graphical information, such as the capturing of paper documents for archival purposes. Can be used to store and call up documents from centralized image storage systems.[1]

IMP Internet control message protocol. An extension to the Internet protocol, or IP, that supports packets containing error, control, and information messages. The PING command uses IMP to test an Internet connection.[1]

Impact A change in the status (e.g., health, standard of living) of individuals, families, or communities as a result of a program, project, or activity. For example, the impact of an immunization program might be the reduction in infant mortality by 15 percent.[123]

Implementation The carrying out, execution, or practice of a plan; a method, or any design for doing something. Implementation is the action that must follow any preliminary thinking in order for something to actually happen.[8]

Implementation guide A document explaining the proper use of a standard for a specific purpose.[10]

Implementation specification Specific instructions for implementing a standard.[10]

In-band Communications that occur together in a common communications method or channel. For example, a privacy label that applies to a clinical document will be sent in-band with the document.[48]

Indicator A measurable variable (or characteristic) that can be used to determine the degree of adherence to a standard or the level of quality achieved.[123]

Individual Person who is the subject of information collected, used, or disclosed by the entity holding the information.[48]

Individual practice association See **IPA**.

Individually identifiable data Data that can be readily associated with a specific individual. Examples would be a name, a personal identifier, or a full street address.[5]

Individually identifiable health information That which relates to an individual's physical or mental health; the provision of healthcare to an individual; or the payment for healthcare provided to an individual that identifies the individual or could be used to identify the individual.[48]

Individually identifying information Single item or compilation of information or data that indicates or reveals the identity of an individual specifically (such as the individual's name or Social Security number), or that does not specifically identify the individual, but from which the individual's identity can reasonably be ascertained.[48]

Industry standard architecture See **ISA**.

Infiltration Entry into the system via the communication lines of an inactive user that is still connected to the computer. Canceling a user's sign-off signal and then continuing to operate his password and authorization. See also **Piggyback**.[1]

Infobutton A simple alerting system which provides information on request. The information may be keyed to topic and/or user. May or may not be linked to decision support system.[146]

Informatics 1. The discipline concerned with the study of information and manipulation of information via computer-based tools. 2. Information science or informatics is the science of information. It is often, though not exclusively, studied as a branch of computer science and information technology and is related to database, ontology, and software engineering.[4,7]

Information 1. Knowledge derived from study, experience, or instruction; a collection of facts or data; the act of informing or the condition of being informed. 2. Data to which meaning is assigned, according to context and assumed conventions.[60,1]

Information access model Depicts access to key processes and organization information for reporting and/or security purposes.[127]

Information asset Refers to any information in any form (e.g., written, verbal, oral, or electronic) upon which the organization places a measurable value. This includes information created by the entity holding the information, gathered for the entity, or stored by the entity for external parties.[48]

Information compromise An intentional or accidental disclosure or surrender of clinical data to an unauthorized receiver.[1]

Information exchange initiative Attempts by two or more independent healthcare organizations (HCOs) in a geographic area to collaborate to share common patient information for the improvement in community health status, patient care, or viability of the HCOs. A common variety of information exchange initiatives is regional healthcare information networks (RHINs).[2]

Information flow model Visually depicts information flows in the business-to-business functions, business organizations, and applications.[127]

Information highway The Internet. *See also* **Information superhighway.**

Information infrastructure The combination of computers and an information system.[1]

Information in identifiable form *See* **IIF.**

Information Interchange Information Interchange (American Standard Code) is a code for information exchange between computers made by different companies; a string of seven binary digits represents each character; used in most microcomputers.[147]

Information model A conceptual model of the information needed to support a business function or process.[5]

Information modeling The building of abstract models for the purpose of developing an abstract system.[4]

Information privacy The contractual right of a person to know that his/her recorded personal medical information is accurate, pertinent, complete, up to date, and that effective steps have been taken to restrict access to mutually agreed-upon purposes by authorized data users.[1]

Information resource department *See* **IRD.**

Information resource management *See* **IRM.**

Information security The result of effective protection measures that safeguard data or information from undesired occurrences and exposure to accidental or intentional disclosure to unauthorized persons, accidental or malicious alteration, unauthorized copying, loss by theft and/or destruction by hardware failures, software deficiencies, operating mistakes, or physical damage by fire, water, smoke, excessive temperature, electrical failure, or sabotage.[1]

Information superhighway The Internet. The information highway is a term used, especially in the 1990s, to describe the Internet. The official project was dubbed the National Information Infrastructure (NII) and went beyond the interconnectivity of just computers; the scope broadened to include all types of data transmissions between a plethora of places, people, and devices. *See also* **Internet.**[7]

Information system A system that takes input data (data keyed in, transferred from other systems, etc.), processes it, and provides information as output (reports, screens, displays, etc.).[6]

Information system architecture A framework from which applications, system software, and hardware can be developed in a coherent manner, and in which every part fits together without containing a mass of design details.[4]

Information systems A general description that may include any combination of hardware, software, and network components that comprise the ability to store, process, and retrieve information.[1]

Information technology The hardware, firmware, and software used as part of the information system to perform information functions. This definition includes computers, telecommunications, automated information systems, and automatic data processing equipment. IT includes any assembly of computer hardware, software, and/or firmware configured to collect, create, communicate, compute, disseminate, process, store, and/or control data or information.[97]

Information Technology Management Reform Act of 1996 *See* **ITMRA.**

Information Technology Security *See* **ITSEC.**

Information warfare Deliberate attacks on data confidentiality and possession, integrity and authenticity, and availability and utility.[1]

Informed consent Refers to the requirement that all researchers explain the purposes, risks, benefits, confidentiality protections, and other relevant aspects of a research study to potential human subjects so that they may make an informed decision regarding their participation in the research. Institutional Review Boards

(IRBs) review informed consent processes and forms documenting the consent to ensure compliance with research regulations and policies.[48]

Infrared Data Association   *See* **IrDa**.

Infrastructure-centric   A security management approach that considers information systems and their computing environment as a single entity.[97]

Initiator   An (authenticated) entity (e.g., human user or computer-based entity) that attempts to access other entities. Also known as *claimant* or *principal*.[125]

Injection laser diode   *See* **ILD**.

Inpatient   Patient who is admitted to a healthcare facility in order to receive healthcare.[4]

Inpatient record   Healthcare record of a hospitalized patient.[4]

Inputs   The resources needed to carry out a process or provide a service. Inputs required in healthcare are usually financial, physical structures, such as buildings, supplies and equipment, personnel and clients.[123]

Institutional review board   *See* **IRB**.

Integrated call management   An important strategy to improve speed and efficiency in many healthcare applications through the use of multiple automated system components for telecommunications support or medical information systems design.[1]

Integrated circuit chip   *See* **ICC**.

Integrated client   Existing applications in hospitals and other medical facilities that will provide EHR functionality by integrating with the EHR using specified HL7 v3 messages.[8]

Integrated delivery network   *See* **IDN**.

Integrated delivery system   *See* **IDS**.

Integrated device electronics   *See* **IDE**.

Integrated networks   Propose to provide seamless access to unified data across multiple-care delivery sites to support patient care.[6]

Integrated service digital network   *See* **ISDN**.

Integrating the Healthcare Enterprise   *See* **IHE**.

Integration   **1.** The process of bringing together related parts into a single system. To make various components function as a connected system. **2.** Combining separately developed parts into a whole so that they work together. The means of integration may vary, from simply mating the parts together at an interface to radically altering the parts or providing something to mediate between them.[8]

Integration layer   Software component that presents a single, consolidated point of access to several systems and/or services.[8]

Integration profile   A precise description of how standards are to be implemented to address a specific clinical integration need. Each integration profile includes the definition of the clinical use case, the clinical information and workflow involved, and the set of actors and transactions that address that need. Integration profiles reference the fully detailed integration specifications defined in the IHE technical framework in a form that is convenient to use in requests for proposals and product descriptions.[56]

Integration services   This group of services is made up of services that manage the integration, message brokering, and service catalog functions.[8]

Integration testing   A testing event that seeks to uncover errors in the interactions and interfaces among application software components when they are combined to form larger parts of a system.[6]

Integrity   **1.** Quality of an IT system reflecting the logical correctness and reliability of the operating system; the logical completeness of the hardware and software implementing the protection mechanisms; and the consistency of the data structures and occurrence of the stored data. It is composed of data integrity and system integrity. **2.** Knowledge that a message has not been modified while in transit. May be done with digitally signed message digest codes. Data integrity, the accuracy and completeness of the data, program integrity, system integrity, and network integrity are all components of computer and system security.[97,1]

Intelligent agent A program that can learn from its owner and complete a task according to the owner's personal preferences. These programs incorporate artificial intelligence technology, which allows them to be able to offer intuitive suggestions and make judgments.[1]

Intelligent call routing *See* **ICR**.

Intelligent character recognition *See* **ICR**.

Intelligent document recognition *See* **IDR**.

Intended use/intended purpose Use for which a product, process, or service is intended according to the specifications, instructions, and information provided by the manufacturer.[68]

Intensive care unit *See* **ICU**.

Intentionally unsafe acts Any events that result from a criminal act, a purposefully unsafe act, an act related to alcohol or substance abuse by an impaired provider and/or staff, or events involving alleged or suspected patient abuse of any kind.[96]

Interaction model Logical diagram or narrative describing the exchange of data and sequence of method invocation between objects to perform a specific task within a use case.[8]

Interactive services Services that allow the customer to decide which information they will be presented with next, such as requesting a search or conducting business-to-business or electronic commerce.[1]

Interactive video disc *See* **IVD**.

Interactive voice response *See* **IVR**.

Interface **1.** A common boundary between two associated systems across which information may flow. **2.** The juncture at which two computer components (hardware and/or software) meet and interact with each other. A specific interface program may be necessary to enable this interaction.[4,2]

Interface engine An interface engine is an interface tool that translates functions from different systems and protocols into a common format to facilitate information sharing. It is a translator for data for files to pass between systems.[2]

Interface terminology Support interactions between healthcare providers and computer-based applications. They aid practitioners in converting clinical 'free text' thoughts into the structured, formal data representations used internally by application programs.[108]

Interior gateway protocol *See* **IGP**.

Internal protocol An Internet working protocol that executes in hosts and routers to interconnect a number of packet networks.[1]

International standard Standard that is adopted by an international standardizing/standards organization and made available to the public.[4]

Internet A global network interconnecting thousands of dissimilar computer networks and millions of computers worldwide.[1]

Internet access provider *See* **IAP**.

Internet control message protocol *See* **ICMP**.

Internet Explorer™ A graphical Web browser developed and distributed by Microsoft to allow Web pages to incorporate sound, graphics, movies, and Java applets along with text.[1]

Internet information server *See* **IIS**.

Internet key exchange *See* **IKE**.

Internet network information center *See* **InterNIC**.

Internet protocol *See* **IP**.

Internet protocol address *See* **IP address**.

Internet protocol datagram *See* **IP datagram**.

Internet protocol security *See* **IPsec**.

Internet relay chat *See* **IRC**.

Internet service provider *See* **ISP**.

Internet work packet exchange/sequence A network of computer networks.[1]

InterNIC Internet Network Information Center. Agency that provides and coordinates Internet services, such as IP addresses. In addition, the center also handles registration of IP addresses and domain names. Also called *NIC*.[1]

Interoperability Interoperability means the ability of health information systems to work together within and across organizational boundaries in order to advance the effective delivery of healthcare for individuals and communities.[45] *See also* Appendix B.

Interpreted language Code that is not compiled. A line-by-line interpretation of code takes place each and every time an interpreted language program is run. Tends to run slowly.[1]

Interrupt A request for service from an external device seeking attention. The external device requests service by asserting an interrupt request line connected to the processor.[1]

Interrupt request *See* **IRQ**.

Intranet Private computer network that uses Internet protocols and Internet derived technologies, including World Wide Web browsers, Web servers and Web languages, to facilitate collaborative data sharing within an enterprise.[2]

Intrusion detection Tools to detect unauthorized system break-ins.[1]

IP **Internet protocol.** Basic Internet transmission protocol based on a connectionless best-effort packet delivery.[1]

IP address **Internet protocol address.** The equivalent of an Internet mailing address, which identifies the network, the subnet and the host, such as 168.100.209.246. A specific 32-bit (4 octet) unique address assigned to each networked device.[1]

IP datagram **Internet protocol datagram.** Basic unit of information that passes across the Internet. Contains data and source and destination address information.[1]

IPA **Individual practice association.** HMO model that contracts with an entity, which in turn contracts with physicians to provide healthcare services in return for a negotiated fee. Physicians continue in their existing individual or group practices and are compensated on a per capita fee schedule or fee-for-service basis.[15]

IPsec **Internet protocol security.** A developing low-level protocol for encrypting the Internet protocol (IP) packet layer of a transmission instead of the application layer to provide improved confidentiality, authentication, and integrity. IPsec can be handled without requiring changes to individual user computers.[1]

IRB **Institutional Review Board.** A specially constituted review body established or designated by an entity, in accordance with 45 CFR Part 46, to protect the welfare of human subjects recruited to participate in biomedical or behavioral research.[118]

IRD **Information resource department.** Department within a facility that provides data automation, hardware, software, and user support. Usually associated with U.S. Army facilities.[1]

IrDA **Infrared Data Association.** A group of device manufacturers that worked on the development of a standard for transmitting data via infrared light waves, the IrDA port.[143]

IRM **Information resource management.** Department within a facility that provides data automation, hardware, software, and user support. Usually associated with U.S. Air Force and Marine Corps facilities.[1]

IRQ **Interrupt request.** Standard interrupt assignment for the system timer.[1]

ISA **Industry standard architecture.** 8- and 16-bit internal bus, or used to identify an Internet server application.[1]

ISDN **Integrated service digital network.** A data transfer technology that can transfer data significantly faster than a dial-up modem. ISDN enables wide-bandwidth digital transmission over the public telephone network, which means more data can be sent at one time. A typical ISDN connection can support transfer rates of 64K or 128K of data per second. While these speeds are faster than what you can get with a dial-up modem, the newer DSL technology can support even faster transfer rates, and is less costly to set up and maintain.[2]

ISO/TC 215 International Standards Organization (ISO) technical committee for health informatics.[3]

Isolation A transaction's effect is not visible to other transactions until the transaction is committed. *See also* **ACID**.

ISP **Internet service provider.** Company that provides Internet connectivity and Internet-related services, online computer access, Web site hosting, and domain name registration for an added fee beyond their costs with the Inter-NIC or other registration retailers.[1]

ITMRA   Information Technology Management Reform Act of 1996. Former name of the Clinger-Cohen Act of 1996.[1]

ITSEC   Information Technology Security. Protection of information technology against unauthorized access to or modification of information, whether in storage, processing, or transit, and against the denial of service to authorized users, including those measures necessary to detect, document, and counter such threats. Protection and maintenance of confidentiality, integrity, availability, and accountability.[97]

IVD   Interactive video disc. A combination of computer and laser disc technology, which can be rapidly accessed through instructions on the computer disc to hold still and motion pictures; useful for providing simulation experiences.[6]

IVR   Interactive voice response. Ability to access information over the phone (claim payments, claim status, and a patient's eligibility).[15]

J

Java   A language for adding interactivity to Web pages.[1]

JavaScript   1. JavaScript is used in Web site development to do such things as automatically change a formatted date on a Web page, cause a linked-to page to appear in a popup window, or cause text or graphic images to change during a mouse rollover. **2.** JavaScript is an interpreted programming or script language.[8]

J-codes   A subset of the HCPCS level II code set with a high-order value of 'J' that has been used to identify certain drugs and other items. The final HIPAA transactions and code sets rule states that these J-codes will be dropped from the HCPCS, and that NDC codes will be used to identify the associated pharmaceuticals and supplies.[10]

Joins   A data query operation performed on data tables in a relational DBMS, in which the data from two or more tables are combined using common data elements into a single table.

Typically performed using Structured Query Language (SQL).[1]

Joint Photographic Experts Group   *See* **JPEG**.

Journaling   Recording of all computer system activities and uses of a computer system. Used to identify access violations and the individual accountable for them, determine security exposures, track the activities of selected users, and adjust access control measures to changing conditions.[1]

JPEG   Joint Photographic Experts Group. Standard for encoding, transmitting, and decoding full-color and gray-scale still images. JPEG is a graphic file format that has a sophisticated technique for compressing full-color bitmapped graphics, such as photographs.[1]

JPEG compression   A generic algorithm to compress still images.[1]

JTC   Joint technical committee.

JWG   Joint working group.

K

KB   Kilobyte. Equal to 1,024 bytes of digital data.[1]

Kbps   Kilobits per second. Transmission of a thousand bits per second.[1]

Kennedy-Kassebaum Bill   Original name for the Health Insurance Portability and Accountability Act of 1996 (HIPAA).[1]

Kerberos   Network security service for securing higher-level applications and providing confidentiality and authentication. Kerberos was developed in the Athena Project at the Massachusetts Institute of Technology. The name is taken from Greek mythology; Kerberos was a three-headed dog who guarded the gates of Hades.[1]

Kernel   The core components of most operating systems. It is the part of the system that manages files, peripherals, memory, and system resources. It runs the processes and provides communication between the processes.[1]

Key   1. A value that particularizes the use of a cryptographic system. **2.** An input that controls the transformation of data by an encryption algorithm.[114,1]

Key image notes *See* **KIN**.

Key management services As data is brought in from various sources, there will be cases where certain primary source identity keys are not unique across source systems. The key management service will generate and manage keys during insert and update operations in the EHR repository.[8]

Keystroke verification The determination of the accuracy of data entry by the reentry of the same data through a keyboard.[3]

Keyword Specified words used in text search engines. Through the use of multiple keywords, an organization increases its chances that search engines will locate its Web page and serve it up to the requesting user.[1]

KHz **Kilohertz.** One thousand cycles per second.[1]

Kill UNIX command to stop a process.[1]

KIN **Key image notes.** Specifies transactions that allow a user to mark one or more images in a study as significant by attaching to them a note managed together with the study. This note includes a title stating the purpose of marking the images and a user comment field. Physicians may attach key image notes to images for a variety of purposes: referring physician access, teaching files selection, consultation with other departments, image quality issues, etc. *See also* **Profile**.[56]

Klugey Clunkey, inefficient, inelegant. "It's kind of a klugey solution, but we don't have the cycles to clean it up." Also used in noun form as 'kluge' or 'kludge.'[148]

Knowledge Considered to be the distillation of information that has been collected, classified, organized, integrated, abstracted, and value-added. Knowledge is at the level of abstraction higher than the data and information on which it is based, and can be used to deduce new information and new knowledge.[4]

Knowledge acquisition The process of eliciting, analyzing, transforming, classifying, organizing, and integrating knowledge; and representing that knowledge in a form that can be used in a computer system.[4]

Knowledge engineering Converting knowledge, rules, relationships, heuristics, and decision-making strategies into a form understandable to the artificial software upon which an expert system is built.[6]

Knowledge representation The process and results of formalization of knowledge in such a way that the knowledge can be used automatically for problem solving.[4]

L

Laboratory information system An application to streamline the process management of the laboratory for basic clinical services, such as hematology and chemistry. This application may provide general functional support for microbiology reporting but does not generally support blood bank functions. Provides an automatic interface to laboratory analytical instruments to transfer verified results to nurse stations, chart carts, and remote physician offices. The module allows the user to receive orders from any designated location, process the order and report results, and maintain technical, statistical, and account information. It eliminates tedious paperwork, calculations, and written documentation, while allowing for easy retrieval of data and statistics.[2]

Laboratory scheduled workflow *See* **LWF**.

LAN **Local area network.** A single network of physically interconnected computers that is localized within a small geographical area. Operates in a span of short distances (office, building, or complex of buildings). *See also* **MAN, WAN**.[1]

LAN adapter Allows access to a network, usually a wireless network.[100]

Laser printer Desktop printers that use the dry toner and Xerographic printing process.[1]

Laserdisc A 12-inch disk that is similar to an audio CD but holds visual images (such as high-quality movies), as well as music. Also called a *videodisc*.[1]

Last in first out *See* **LIFO**.

LAT **Local-area transport.** Non-routable but bridgeable protocol used by DEC to support terminal servers.[1]

LCD **Liquid crystal display.** The display screen of an electronic device.[1]

LEAP **Lightweight and efficient application protocol.** One of several protocols used with the International Electric and Electronic Engineers (IEEE) 802.1 standard for local area network (LAN) port access control. In the IEEE framework, a LAN station cannot pass traffic through an Ethernet hub or wide local area network (WLAN) access point until it successfully authenticates itself. The station must identify itself and prove that it is an authorized user before it is actually allowed to use the LAN.[2]

Leased line Permanent communications link owned by the telephone companies, leased for dedicated customer use.[1]

Legacy systems **1.** Usually refers to mainframe computers that have been in use for a long period of time that contain many years of data and have been used over many years of software development. **2.** Data that were collected and maintained using a 'previous' system, but are now preserved on a 'current' system.[1,116]

Level Seven Level Seven refers to the highest level of the International Standards Organization's (ISO) communications model for Open Systems Interconnection (OSI)—the application level. Issues within the application level include definition of the data to be exchanged, the timing of the interchange, and communication of certain errors to the application.[16]

Lexicon A group of related terms used in a particular profession, subject, or style.[32]

Lexicon query service *See* **LQS**.

License Authorization to use a software product.[1]

Licensure A process by which a governmental authority grants permission to individual practitioners or healthcare organizations to operate or to engage in an occupation or profession.[123]

Lifecycle All phases in the life of a medical device, from the initial conception to final decommissioning and disposal.[68]

LIFO **Last in first out.** A queue that executes last-in requests before previously queued requests. Also called a *stack*.[1]

Lightweight and efficient application protocol *See* **LEAP**.

Limited data set Specifies health information from which identifiers have been removed. Information in a limited data set is protected, but may be used for research, healthcare operations, and public health activities without the individual's authorization.[48]

Line-of-sight Propagation along an unobstructed path.[1]

Link A connection between two network devices. Also called *anchors, hotlinks,* and *hyperlinks*.[1]

Liquid crystal display *See* **LCD**.

LISTSERV A distribution list management package whose primary function is to operate mailing lists. An e-mail program that allows multiple computer users to connect onto a single system, thus creating an online discussion.[1]

LLC **Logical link control.** Upper part of the second layer of the OSI model. Oversees and controls the exchange of data between two network nodes.[1]

LMHOSTS Text file that maps IP addresses to Windows computer names (NetBIOS names) to network computers outside the local subnet. Acts as a local WINS equivalent to provide a static type of WINS service.[1]

Local area network *See* **LAN**.

Local area transport *See* **LAT**.

Local codes Generic term for code values that are defined for specific payers, providers, or political jurisdictions.[15]

Local talk Networking cabling standard used by Macintosh computers. Transmits 230kb per second over STP at distances up to 300 feet. Supports only 32 computers per segment.[1]

Log Record that is created by an event(s).[48]

Log analysis Studying log entries to identify events of interest or suppress log entries for insignificant events.[48]

Log archival Retaining logs for an extended period of time, typically on removable media, a storage area network (SAN), or a specialized log archival appliance or server.[48]

Log clearing Removal of all entries from a log that precede a certain date and time.[48]

Log compression Storing a log file in a way that reduces the amount of storage space needed for the file without altering the meaning of its contents.[48]

Log conversion Parsing a log in one format and storing its entries in a second format.[48]

Log entry Individual record within a log.[48]

Log management Process for generating, transmitting, storing, analyzing, and disposing of log data.[48]

Logging Activities involved in creating logs.[48]

Logic bomb A program deliberately written or modified to produce unexpected results when certain conditions are met.[1]

Logical access control An automated system that controls an individual's ability to access one or more computer system resources, such as a workstation, network, application, or database.[114]

Logical drive Subdivision of a large physical drive into numerous smaller drives.[1]

Logical link control See **LLC**.

Logical observation identifiers, names, and codes See **LOINC**.

Logical threat A threat of the possibility of destruction or alteration of software or data. Would be realized by logical manipulation within the system, rather than by physical attack.[1]

Logical unit See **LU**.

Login To enter and identify yourself as a proper customer of the computer.[4]

Login controls Specific conditions users must meet for gaining access to a computer system.[1]

Login/Logging into Action performed by an end user, when authenticating in to a computer system.[48]

Logoff Process of closing an open server session.[1]

Logon Process of opening a server session through authentication.[1]

Logon process The interaction between a user and the clinical computer system that enables the user to utilize the computer system.[1]

Logout To formally exit from the computer's environment.[4]

LOINC Logical observation identifiers, names, and codes. Universal identifiers for laboratory and clinical observations, including such things as vital signs, hemodynamic measures, intake/output, EKG, obstetric ultrasound, cardiac echo, urologic imaging, gastroendoscopic procedures, pulmonary ventilator management, selected survey instruments, and other clinical observations.[50]

Longitudinal lifetime patient record The concept of access to health information across an individual's lifetime. See also **EHR**.[1]

Long-term care See **LTC**.

Loop 1. A repeating structure or process. 2. A collection of segments that can repeat.[5,59]

Loophole An incompleteness or error in a computer program, or in the hardware that permits circumventing the access control mechanism.[1]

Loosely coupled Loosely coupled application roles do not assume that common information about the subject classes participating in a message is available to system components outside of the specific message.[8]

Lossless compression Method of data compression that permits reconstruction of the original data exactly, bit-for-bit. The graphics interchange file (GIF) is an image format used on the Web that provides lossless compression.[57]

Lossy compression Method of data compression that permits reconstruction of the original data approximately, rather than exactly.[57]

LQS Lexicon query service. Standardizes a set of read-only interfaces able to access medical terminology system definitions, ranging from sets of codes, to complex hierarchical classification and categorization schemes.[124]

LTC Long-term care. The segment of the healthcare continuum that consists of maintenance, custodial, and health services for the chronically ill or disabled; may be provided on an inpatient (rehabilitation facility, nursing home, mental hospital) or outpatient basis, or at home.[1]

LU   Logical unit. Portion of the ALU within the CPU that coordinates logical operations.[1]

Luminance   Brightness; the amount of light, in lumens, that is emitted by a pixel or an area of the computer screen.[57]

LWF   Laboratory   scheduled   workflow. Establishes the continuity and integrity of clinical laboratory testing and observation data throughout the healthcare enterprise. It involves a set of transactions to maintain the consistency of ordering and patient information, to control the conformity of specimens, and to deliver the results at various steps of validation. *See also* **Profile.**[56]

M

MAC   Mandatory access control. A system of access control that assigns security labels or classifications to system resources and allows access only to entities (people, processes, devices) with distinct levels of authorization or clearance.[1]

MAC   Media access control. Lower portion of the second layer of the OSI model. Identifies the actual physical link between two nodes.[1]

MAC   Message authentication code. A digital code generated using a cryptographic algorithm, defined in an ISO (International Organization for Standardization) standard that establishes that the contents of a message have not been altered or generated by an unauthorized party.[3]

MAC address   Media   access   control address. Synonym for unique hardware physical address of a network device identified at the media access control layer and stored in ROM.[1]

Machine code   The elemental language of computers, consisting of a stream of 0s and 1s. Ultimately, the output of any programming language analysis and processing is machine code.[1]

Machine language   The lowest-level programming language (except for computers that utilize programmable microcode), machine languages are the only languages understood by computers. While easily understood by computers, machine languages are almost impossible for humans to use because they consist entirely of numbers. Programmers, therefore, use either a high-level programming language or an assembly language. An assembly language contains the same instructions as a machine language, but the instructions and variables have names instead of being just numbers.[7]

Macro   Small program that automates a function for an application program. Although many of these are supplied with the purchase of a program, in many applications, users can create their own by either recording keystrokes or writing the commands using the language that the application program provides. (This process is usually very similar to the Basic language.)[11]

Magnetic resonance imaging   *See* **MRI.**

Magnetic stripe card   A smart card containing a magnetic stripe that can store about 800 bits (100 bytes) of information. Largely used as banking cards and for security access applications.[1]

Mail merge   The merging of database information, such as names and addresses, with a letter template in a word processor to create personalized letters.[1]

Mailing list   A list of e-mail users who are members of a group. A mailing list can be an informal group of people who share e-mail with one another, or it can be a more formal LIST-SERV group that discusses a specific topic.[1]

Mailslots   Connection-oriented interprocess messaging interface between clients and servers in a Windows NT environment.[1]

Mainframe computer server   Industry term for a large computer, typically manufactured for commercial applications and other large-scale computing purposes. Historically, a mainframe is associated with centralized, rather than distributed, computing.[2]

Mainframe computer system   A computing environment in which the main processing is done by a mainframe, and information is accessed via terminals or PCs linked to the host mainframe. Because the terminals do not actually do any processing, this is sometimes referred to as a master/slave environment. Operating systems for this hardware environment include Multiple Virtual Storage and Customer Information Control System.[2]

Malicious software Software, e.g., a virus, designed to damage or disrupt a system.[118]

MAN Metropolitan-area network. 1. Provides high-speed data transfer regional connectivity through multiple physical networks. Operates over distances sufficient for a metropolitan area. An IEEE 802.6 standard. **2.** A backbone network that covers a metropolitan area and is regulated by state or local utility commissions. Suppliers that provide MAN services are telephone companies and cable services. *See also* **LAN, WAN.**[1]

Manage consent directives Ensure that protected health information is only accessed with a consumer's consent.[48]

Managed care Use of a planned and coordinated approach to providing healthcare with the goal of quality care at a lower cost. Usually emphasizes preventive care, and often associated with a health management organization.[6]

Management information department *See* **MID.**

Management information systems (or services) *See* **MIS.**

Management service organization *See* **MSO.**

Mandatory access control *See* **MAC.**

Manufacturer Natural or legal person with responsibility for the design, manufacture, packaging, or labeling of a medical device, assembling a system, or adapting a medical device before it is placed on the market or put into service, regardless of whether these operations are carried out by that person, or on that person's behalf by a third party.[68]

Manufacturing automation protocol *See* **MAP.**

MAP Manufacturing automation protocol.

Map A relationship between a concept in a terminology and a concept in the same or another terminology, according to a mapping scheme or rules.[98]

Mapping 1. Assigning an element in one set to an element in another set through semantic correspondence. **2.** A rule of correspondence established between data sets that associates each element of a set with an element in the same or another set. *See also* **Data mapping, Crosswalk.**[126,32]

Mapping services The mapping service helps create a map file that translates a source document format to the destination format. This service can be used to map from XML to flat file and other formats, and vice versa.[8]

Marketing Communications that encourage the purchase or use of a product or service. This does not include a covered entity's communications about its own products, services or benefits, or communications for treatment, case management, care coordination, or referral for care.[48]

Masquerading Obtaining proper identification through improper means (such as wiretapping), and then accessing the system as a legitimate user.[1]

Massachusetts Utility Multi-Programming System *See* **MUMPS.**

Massively parallel processing *See* **MPP.**

Master browser Computer on a network that maintains a list of all computers and services available on the network.[1]

Master patient index *See* **MPI.**

Match/matching The process of comparing biometric information against a previously stored biometric data, and scoring the level of similarity.[114]

Math co-processor Accompanying integrated chip to the CPU that performs arithmetic functions, which allows the CPU to perform system functions.[1]

MAU Media access unit. A token-ring network hub.[1]

Maximum defined data set All of the required data elements for a particular standard based on a specific implementation specification. An entity creating a transaction is free to include whatever data any receiver might want or need. The recipient is free to ignore any portion of the data that is not needed to conduct his or her part of the associated business transaction, unless the inessential data is needed for coordination of benefits.[10]

Mb Megabit. 1,048,576 bits or 1,024kb.[1]

MBDS Minimum basic data set. A set of data that is the minimum required for a healthcare record to conform to a given standard.[4]

Mbps Megabits per second. Transmission of a million bits per second.[1]

MDA Model driven architecture. A platform independent model providing for separate business and application functionality from the technology-specific code, while enabling interoperability within and across platform boundaries.[111]

MDI-X port Hub port that can be configured to provide a crossover function that reverses the transmit and receive wire pairs. Used to connect hubs together with a standard drop cable. Alleviates creating a crossover cable to perform the same function.[1]

MDM Medical document management message.

MDS Minimum data set. A core of elements to use in performing comprehensive assessments in long-term care facilities.[102]

Mean time between failure *See* **MTBF.**

Mean time to diagnose *See* **MTTD.**

Mean time to repair *See* **MTTR.**

Measure A number assigned to an object or an event. Measures can be expressed as counts (45 visits), rates (10 visits/day), proportions (45 primary healthcare visits/380 total visits = .118), percentages (12 percent of the visits made), or ratios (45 visits 4 health workers = 11.25).[123]

MedDRA Medical Dictionary for Regulatory Activities. Used by regulatory agencies and drug manufacturers.[14]

Media access control *See* **MAC.**

Media access control address *See* **MAC address**.

Medical code sets Codes that characterize a medical condition to treatment. These code sets are usually maintained by professional societies and public health organizations.[10]

Medical device Any instrument, apparatus, implement, machine, appliance, implant, in vitro reagent or calibrator, software, material, or other similar or related article, intended by the manufacturer to be used, alone or in combination, for human beings for one or more of the specific purposes(s) of diagnosis, prevention, monitoring, treatment, or alleviation of disease; diagnosis, monitoring, treatment, alleviation of, or compensation for an injury; investigation, replacement, modification, or support of the anatomy or of a physiological process; supporting or sustaining life; control of conception; disinfection of medical devices; providing information for medical purposes by means of in vitro examination of specimens derived from the human body; and which does not achieve its primary intended action in or on the human body by pharmacological, immunological, or metabolic means, but which may be assisted in its function by such means.[68]

Medical error **1.** The failure of a planned action to be completed as intended, or the use of a wrong plan to achieve an aim in the healthcare delivery process. **2.** A mistake that harms a patient. Adverse drug events, hospital-acquired infections and wrong-site surgeries are examples of preventable medical errors.[107,138]

Medical informatics Scientific discipline concerned with the cognitive, information processing and communication task of healthcare practice, education, and research, including the information science and technology to support healthcare tasks.[4]

Medical information bus *See* **MIB.**

Medical logic model *See* **MLM.**

Medical home **1.** A model of delivering primary care that is accessible, continuous, comprehensive, family-centered, coordinated, compassionate, and culturally effective. **2.** In a medical home model, primary care clinicians and allied professionals provide conventional diagnostic and therapeutic services, as well as coordination of care for patients who require services not available in primary care settings. The goal is to provide a patient with a broad spectrum of care, both preventive and curative, over a period of time and to coordinate all of the care the patient receives.[134,135]

Medical record *See* **EHR, EMR.**[4]

Medical subject heading *See* **MeSH.**

Medical terminology/controlled medical vocabulary A vocabulary server application that normalizes various medication vocabularies used by system applications in a healthcare delivery environment.[2]

Medication error Mishaps that occur during prescribing, transcribing, dispensing, administering, adherence, or monitoring a drug.[96]

MEDIX A terminology developed for use in monitoring medical products throughout all phases of their regulatory cycle.[111]

MEDS Minimum emergency data set. A standardized view of the critical components of a patient's past medical history.[1]

Megabyte One million bytes of data used as a measure of computer processor storage and real and virtual memory. A megabyte is actually 2 to the 20th power of 1,048,576 bytes.[1]

Memorandum of understanding *See* **MOU.**

Memory **1.** The part of a system which holds program instructions and information being processed. Sometimes referred to as RAM (random access memory). **2.** Area of a computer used to store data. Can be RAM or ROM. Another word for dynamic RAM, the chips where the computers store system software, programs, and data currently being used. *See also* **RAM, ROM.**[1]

Menu A list of options listed on the screen from which to choose. Usually labeled; customer is asked to press the key corresponding to a choice.[4]

Merchant status Term used to indicate a business is authorized to accept credit cards in payment for goods and services.[1]

MeSH Medical subject heading. A thesaurus of concepts and terms used for the indexing of biomedical literature.[4]

Message An organized set of data exchanged between people or computer processes.[4]

Message authentication Ensuring that a message is genuine, has arrived exactly as was sent, and comes from the stated source.[4]

Message authentication code *See* **MAC.**

Message syntax System of rules and definitions specifying the basic component types of messages, interrelationships, and arrangement.[4]

Message type An identified, named, and structured set of functionally related information which fulfils a specific business purpose.[4]

Message, instant A package of information communicated from one application to another.[8]

Messaging Creating, storing, exchanging, and managing data messages across a communications network. The two main messaging architectures are publish-subscribe and point-to-point.[57]

Messaging services A group of services that handle messages. Services in this group include parsing, serialization, encryption and decryption, encoding and decoding, transformation, and routing.[8]

Meta tag A special HTML command that provides information about a Web page. Unlike normal HTML tags, meta tags do not affect how the page is displayed.[1]

Metadata Machine understandable information for the Web. Metadata describes the content, quality, condition, and other characteristics of the data. Fundamentally, metadata describes who, what, when, where, why, and how about a data set. Without proper documentation, a data set is incomplete. Metadata is critical to preserving the usefulness of data over time. Metadata captures important information on how data was collected and/or processed so that future users of that data understand these details.[18]

Metadata customer Individuals who need to access metadata (e.g., information system designers and survey form developers who ensure products meet national reporting requirements, analysts who need information to interpret data, and information managers who advise clinicians on how to report data).[18]

Metadata developers Individuals responsible for developing and proposing new metadata content and revising existing metadata.[18]

Metadata registry A metadata registry is a system that contains information that describes the structure, format, and definitions of data.[18]

Metadata stewards Organizations that have the responsibility for the ongoing maintenance of a metadata item.[18]

Metathesaurus An integration of several different thesauri to produce a new large thesaurus. A metathesaurus includes cross-references between the different thesauri from which it is composed (e.g., Meta-1). *See also* **UMLS**.[4]

Metropolitan-area network *See* **MAN**.

MFM **Modified frequency modulation.** A line code used by most floppy disk formats, notably by most CP/M machines, as well as PCs running DOS.[7]

MHz **Megahertz.** One million times, cycles, occurrences, alterations, or pulses per second. Used to describe a measurement of CPU or processor speed.[1]

MIB **Medical information bus. 1.** The backbone of information exchange, allowing data to be moved from one point to another. **2.** International Electronic Electric Engineers P1073 (standard designation) standard proposed for data exchange in a medical environment.[51]

Micro channel Micro channel architecture. IBM 32-bit multi-processing system and interface hardware bus standard for PS/2 computers.[1]

Micro channel architecture *See* **Micro channel**.

Microcomputer Desktop or laptop/notebook computer employing a microprocessor.[1]

Microprocessor Central processing unit. A microprocessor is a computer processor on a microchip. It is the 'engine' that goes into motion when you turn your computer on. Designed to perform arithmetic and logic operations that make use of small number-holding areas, called registers. *See* **CPU**.[1]

Microsecond One millionth of a second.[1]

Microsoft disk operating system *See* **MS-DOS**.

MID **Management information department.** Department within a facility that provides data automation, hardware, software, and user support.[1]

Middleware Software systems that facilitate the interaction of disparate components through a set of commonly defined protocols. The purpose is to limit the number of interfaces required for interoperability by allowing all components to interact with the middleware using a common interface.[8]

Midrange A computer platform or system that typically has less processing power than mainframe systems, but more power than workstations or microcomputers. A midrange is sometimes referred to as a *minicomputer*.[2]

Migration tool for NetWare Utility included in Windows NT to migrate NetWare user accounts, group accounts, files, and directories from a NetWare server environment to a Windows NT server environment. GSNW and NWLink must be installed before a migration can take place.[1]

Millions of instructions per second *See* **MIPS**.

Millisecond One thousandth of a second.[1]

MIME **Multipurpose Internet mail extensions.** A format originally developed for attaching sounds, images, and other media files to electronic mail, but now also used with World Wide Web applications.[1]

Minicomputer Small- to medium-scale computer that often uses dumb terminals.[1]

Minimum basic data set *See* **MBDS**.

Minimum emergency data set *See* **MEDS**.

Minimum necessary Minimum amount of protected health information necessary to accomplish permitted use or disclosure for payment or healthcare operations.[48]

Minimum scope of disclosure The principle that, to the extent practical, individually identifiable health information should only be disclosed to the extent needed to support the purpose of the disclosure.[10]

MIPS **Millions of instructions per second.** Rate that a processor executes instructions. Used as a measurement of processing power and computer speed.[1]

Mirror set RAID Level 1. Two-disk array where one disk shadows the contents of the original disk to maintain instant redundancy.[1]

Mirror site An FTP site that is created after the contents of an original FTP archive server are copied to it. Usually, mirror sites use larger and faster systems than the original, so it is easier to obtain material from the mirror.[1]

MIS **Management information systems (or services).** MIS refers to either a class of software that provides management with tools for organizing and evaluating their department, or the staff that supports information systems.[1]

Mission critical Activities, processing, etc., which are deemed vital to the organization's business success, and possibly, its very existence.[48]

Misuse Occurs when an appropriate process of care has been selected, but a preventable complication or medical error occurs and the patient does not receive the full potential benefit of the service. Avoidable complications of surgery or medication use are misuse problems. A patient who suffers a rash after receiving penicillin for strep throat, despite having a known allergy to that antibiotic, is an example of misuse. A patient who develops a pneumothorax after an inexperienced operator attempted to insert a subclavian line would represent another example of misuse.[138]

MLM **Medical Logic Model.** Arden Syntax for Medical Logic Systems Version 1.0 was adopted by ASTM in 1992.[39]

Mobile devices A portable device that uses wireless technologies to transmit and exchange data.[2]

Model A very detailed description or scaled representation of one component of a larger system that can be created, operated, and analyzed to predict actual operational characteristics of the final produced component.[114]

Model driven architecture *See* **MDA**.

Modeling The process of defining concepts to reflect their unique definition and meaning. *See also* **Data modeling**.[19]

Modem **Modulator/demodular.** Device that converts digital data to analog signals for trans-

mission over a telephone line, and performs analog-to-digital signals conversion for the receiving node.[1]

Modified frequency modulation *See* **MFM**.

Modify/modification Under the Health Insurance Portability and Accountability Act (HIPAA), this is a change adopted by the Secretary, through regulation, to a standard or an implementation specification.[10]

Modularity The design goal of separating code into self-sufficient, highly cohesive, low coupling pieces.[1]

MOLAP **Multidimensional online analytical processing (OLAP).** A technical OLAP approach in which data are pre-summarized using specialized multidimensional DBMS technology in a very structured manner within predetermined dimensions, allowing for very high performance.[1]

Moore's Law The empirical observation that at our rate of technological development, the complexity of an integrated circuit, with respect to minimum component cost, will double in about 18 months. It is attributed to Gordon E. Moore, a cofounder of Intel.[7]

Motherboard Main system board of the computer that consists of the CPU, I/O bus, and built-in peripherals. Also called the logic board. *See also* **Daughterboard**.[1]

Motion Picture Expert Group *See* **MPEG**.

MOU **Memorandum of understanding.** A document providing a general description of the responsibilities that are to be assumed by two or more parties in their pursuit of some goals. More specific information may be provided in an associated statement of work (SOW).

Mouse Desktop input device used with GUI systems providing cursor control and program execution features.[1]

Mousing-around The nonproductive activity required by many graphic user interface software designs where the hands must leave the keyboard many times during entry of a page of information.[99]

MOV   A file extension found on the World Wide Web that denotes that the file is a movie or video in QuickTime format.[1]

MPEG   Motion Picture Expert Group. Standard for digital encoding, transmitting, decoding, and presentation of video recorder quality motion video.[1]

MPI   Master patient index. 1. The unique numerical index identity of a patient that may contain the patient's Social Security number or any other locally derived or system-generated unique number. **2.** The MPI is important because it serves as the centerpiece for all subsequent functionality and software applications, such as links to the patient clinical record, the patient schedule for appointments, reporting results of lab, x-ray, pharmacy, patient-related images, etc. **3.** As part of HIPAA's unique identifier codes, a mandated standard was controversial due to patient concern about these numbers being accidentally made available providing potential means for, and thereby identifying, the confidential records to other persons.[1]

MPP   Massively parallel processing. A computing platform technology that clusters multiple independent servers, each managed by its own operating system.[1]

MRI   Magnetic resonance imaging. Magnetic fields and radio waves to construct 2-D images or 3-D models of internal body structures.[2]

MSAU   Multiple station access unit, also called a media access unit. A device to attach multiple network stations in a star topology in a token-ring network, internally wired to connect the stations into a logical ring. The MAU contains relays to short out nonoperating stations. Multiple MAUs can be connected into a larger ring through their ring in/ring out connectors.[7]

MS-DOS   Microsoft disk operating system. Set of 16-bit software programs that direct system-level computer operation. Developed by Microsoft in the early 1980s for the 8086 CPU.[1]

MSO   Management service organization. A corporation owned by the system or network, or a physician's system or network joint venture, which provides management services to one or more medical group practices. As part of a full-service management agreement, the MSO purchases the tangible assets of the practices and leases them back, employs all nonphysician staff, and provides all supplies, IT services, and administrative services for a fee.[2]

MTBF   Mean time between failure. The average device operating time, as measured between the last failure until the next failure occurs.[1]

MTTD   Mean time to diagnose. The time it takes to diagnose a problem.[1]

MTTR   Mean time to repair. The time it takes to restore a device to service from a failure.[1]

Multi-axial taxonomy   Taxonomy that requires terms on more than one axis to create a term describing the phenomenon.[11]

Multicast   Network transmission meant for multiple, but not all, network nodes. Technique that allows copies of a single packet to be passed to a select number of nodes within a subnet.[1]

Multidimensional online analytical processing (OLAP)   *See* **MOLAP**.

Multi-homed host   Computer that is physically connected to two networks. Has two IP addressees assigned to it, one for each network interface.[1]

Multimedia   Communications that combine voice, video, and graphics that require large amounts of disk space for storage and large amounts of bandwidth for transmission.[1]

Multiple station access unit   *See* **SMAU**.

Multiplex   The division of a single transmission medium into multiple logical channels, supporting many apparently simultaneous sessions.[1]

Multiplexer, multipleXer, or multipleXor   *See* **MUX**.

Multiplicity   In mathematics, the multiplicity of a member of a multiset is how many memberships in the multiset it has. For example, the term is used to refer to the value of the totient valence function, or the number of times a given polynomial equation has a root at a given point. The common reason to consider notions of multiplicity is to count right, without specifying exceptions (e.g., double roots counted twice). Hence the expression "counted with (sometimes implicit) multiplicity."[16]

Multipurpose Internet mail extensions *See* **MIME.**

Multi-site testing A testing event that determines the ability of the application or its subsystems to function in multiple geographical settings.[6]

Multitasking Ability of an operating system to run multiple tasks concurrently. Windows NT and OS/2 are multitasking operating systems.[1]

MUMPS **Massachusetts Utility Multi-Programming System.** A procedural, interpreted general-purpose programming language oriented toward database applications, with built-in multi-user/multi-tasking support.[1]

Murphy's Law "If anything can go wrong, it will."[32]

Mutual authentication Occurs when parties at both ends of a communication activity authenticate each other.[48]

MUX **Multiplexer, multipleXer, or multipleXor.** A network device in which multiple streams of information are combined from different sources onto a common medium for transmission.[1]

N

NAHDO **National Association of Health Data Organizations.** A group that promotes the development and improvement of state and national health information systems.[9]

Name Designation of an object by a linguistic expression.[4]

Name resolution The process of mapping a name into a corresponding address. The domain name system provides a mechanism for naming computers in which programs use remote name servers to resolve a machine name into an IP address.[1]

Named pipes One- or two-way pipe used for connectionless interprocess messaging interface between clients and servers.[1]

NANDA taxonomy II A taxonomy of nursing diagnostic concepts that identify and code a patient's responses to health problems or life processes.[52]

Narrowband A telecommunications medium that uses (relatively) low-frequency signals, exceeding 1.544 Mbps.[106]

NAS **Network attached storage.** A hard disk storage system that has its own network address rather than being attached to the department computer that is serving applications to a network's workstation users. By removing storage access and its management from the department server, both application programming and files can be served faster because they are not competing for the same processor resources.[2]

NAT **Network address translation.** Involves rewriting the source and/or destination addresses of IP packets as they pass through a router or firewall. Most systems using NAT do so in order to enable multiple hosts on a private network to access the Internet using a single public IP address. According to specifications, routers should not act in this way, but many network administrators find NAT a convenient technique and use it widely. Nonetheless, NAT can introduce complications in communication between hosts. Also known as *network masquerading* or *IP-masquerading.*[7]

National drug codes *See* **NDC.**

National employer ID A system for uniquely identifying all sponsors of healthcare benefits.[9]

National Health Information Infrastructure *See* **NHII.**

National member body *See* **NMB.**

National patient identification or ID A system for uniquely identifying all recipients of healthcare services. Sometimes referred to as the National Individual Identifier, or as the Healthcare ID. *See also* **MPI.**[1]

National payer ID A system for uniquely identifying all organizations that pay for healthcare services.[10]

National provider file *See* **NPF.**

National provider identifier *See* **NPI.**

National provider registry The organization envisioned for assigning national provider IDs.[10]

National standard format *See* **NSF.**

National standardization Standardization that takes place at the level of a specific country.[4]

National standards body Standards body recognized at the national level that is eligible to be the national member of the corresponding international and regional standards organization.[4]

National standards system network *See* NSSN.

Native format The native format is generally readable only by that application, but other programs can sometimes translate it using filters.[1]

Natural language Spoken or written language in contrast to a formal language.[4]

Natural language processing *See* NLP.

NAV Notification of document availability. A mechanism allowing notifications to be sent point-to-point to systems and users within an affinity domain, eliminating the need for manual steps or polling mechanisms.[56]

Navigation tools Allows users to find their way around a Web site or multi-media presentation. They can be hypertext links, clickable buttons, icons, or image maps.[1]

NCPDP Batch Standard National Council for Prescription Drug Programs (NCPDP). An NCPDP standard designed for use by low-volume dispensers of pharmaceuticals, such as nursing homes. Use of Version 1 of this standard has been mandated under the Health Insurance Portability and Accountability Act (HIPAA).[10]

NCPDP Telecommunication Standard National Council for Prescription Drug Programs (NCPDP). An NCPDP standard designed for use by high-volume dispensers of pharmaceuticals, such as retail pharmacies. Use of Version 5.1 of this standard has been mandated under the Health Insurance Portability and Accountability Act (HIPAA).[10]

NDC National Drug Code. The Drug Listing Act of 1972 requires registered drug establishments to provide the Food and Drug Administration (FDA) with a current list of all drugs manufactured, prepared, propagated, compounded, or processed by it for commercial distribution. (*See* Section 510 of the Federal Food, Drug, and Cosmetic Act [Act] [21 U.S.C.

§ 360]). Drug products are identified and reported using a unique, three-segment number, called the National Drug Code (NDC), which is a universal product identifier for human drugs.[1]

NDIS Network driver interface specification. For writing device drivers for network interface cards. Using the NDIS specification, multiple protocols can be bound to a single network adapter.[1]

Near miss An event or situation that could have resulted in an adverse drug event or an adverse event, but did not, either by change or through timely intervention.[96]

NEDSS National Electronic Disease Surveillance System. An initiative that promotes the use of data and information system standards to advance the development of efficient, integrated, and interoperable surveillance systems at federal, state, and local levels. It is a major component of the Public Health Information Network (PHIN).[48]

Needs assessment The identification, definition, and description of the problems to be addressed for selected system.[6]

Need-to-know The explicit specification of the kind of data to be made available to a qualified, authorized user or an authorized computer system.[1]

Nesting Placing documents within other documents. Nesting allows a user to access material in a nonlinear fashion. This is the primary factor needed for developing hypertext.[1]

NetBEUI NetBIOS extended user interface. Fast, easy to install, nonconfigurable, nonroutable network protocol for use with up to 200 network nodes. Resides at the OSI transport layer.[1]

NetBIOS Network basic input output system. Standard interface to networks employing IBM and compatible PCs. Implemented at the application layer. NetBIOS names cannot exceed 15 characters.[1]

NetBIOS extended user interface *See* NetBEUI.

Net-centric The realization of a robust, globally interconnected, networked environment, in which data is shared timely and seamlessly among users, applications, and platforms.[18]

Network A collection of hardware, such as printers, modems, servers, and terminals/personal computers that enables users to store and retrieve information, share devices, and exchange information.[2]

Network adapter card Computer hardware adapter card that provides an interface between the computer and the network.[1]

Network address translation *See* **NAT**.

Network architecture Specifies the function and data transmission needed to convey information across a network.[4]

Network attached storage *See* **NAS**.

Network basic input output system *See* **NetBIOS**.

Network computer A computer with minimal memory, disk storage, and processor power designed to connect to a network, especially the Internet. The idea behind network computers is that many users who are connected to a network do not need all the computer power they get from a typical personal computer. Instead, they can rely on the power of the network servers.

Network drive A shared disk drive available to network users.[1]

Network driver interface specification *See* **NDIS**.

Network file system *See* **NFS**.

Network information center *See* **NIC**.

Network layer Third layer of the OSI model. Routes data from source to destination across networks, and handles addressing and switching. Also known as the *Internet layer*.[1]

Network operating system *See* **NOS**.

Network operation center *See* **NOC**.

Network printer Shared printer available to network users. Can be connected to a print server, directly connected to the network, or shared from a workstation.[1]

Network protocol services The network protocol service will provide communication capabilities over the physical network. The primary network protocol that will be supported is TCP/IP.[8]

Network redirector Operating system feature that intercepts requests from the computer and directs them to the local or remote machine for processing. Resides at the OSI presentation layer.[1]

Network server A network server supports the sharing of peripheral devices among the workstations in the network. Network servers provide printing, file sharing, and messaging services to end users' personal computers.[2]

Network service provider *See* **NSP**.

Network topology The pattern of links connecting pairs of nodes of a network. A given node has one or more links butt to others, and the links can appear in a variety of different shapes. The simplest connection is a one-way link between two devices. A second return link can be added for two-way communication. Modern communications cables usually include more than one wire in order to facilitate this, although very simple bus-based networks have two-way communication on a single wire. Network topology is determined only by the configuration of connections between nodes; it is, therefore, a part of graph theory. Distances between nodes, physical interconnections, transmission rates, and/or signal types are not a matter of network topology, although they may be affected by it in an actual physical network.[7]

Network traffic Data transmitted on a network for the purpose of sending information from one node to another, or from one network to another.[1]

Network weaving A penetration technique in which different communication networks are used to gain access to a data processing system to avoid detection and trace-back.[3]

Networking application Type of networking application (i.e., browser, database management system, interface engine, network operating systems, or Web development tools).[2]

Neural network A data mining predictive model-building algorithm that is composed of connected logical nodes with inputs, outputs, and processing at each node. The neural network is particularly useful for pattern recognition.[1]

New work item proposal *See* **NWIP**.

Newsgroups Public message or discussion areas on the Internet are called newsgroups or 'news' for short, and sometimes 'Usenet News' for the network that originated discussion groups.[1]

Newsreader A program that allows user to access, read, and post to Usenet newsgroups.[1]

NFS Network file system. A protocol developed by Sun Microsystems that allows a computer system to access files over a network as if they were on its local disks.[1]

NHII National Health Information Infrastructure. This is a healthcare-specific lane on the information superhighway, as described in the National Information Infrastructure (NII), or as in the Healthcare ID.[10]

Nibble First or last half of an 8-bit byte. A half byte.[1]

NIC Nursing intervention classification. A comprehensive, research-based, standardized classification of interventions that nurses perform. NIC is useful for clinical documentation, communication of care across settings, integration of data across systems and settings, effectiveness research, productivity measurement, competency evaluation, reimbursement, and curricular design.[26]

NIC Network information center. 1. An organization that provides information, assistance, and services to network users. 2. A computer circuit board or card that is installed in a computer so that it can be connected to a network.[1]

NIC Network interface card. A card that allows one to access a network. *See also* **LAN adapter**.

NLP Natural language processing. A subfield of artificial intelligence and linguistics. It studies the problems inherent in the processing and manipulation of natural language, and natural language understanding devoted to making computers 'understand' statements written in human languages.[7]

NM Nuclear medicine image integration. Specifies how nuclear medicine images should be stored by acquisition modalities and workstations, and how image displays should retrieve and make use of them. It defines the basic display capabilities that image displays are expected to provide, and also how result screens, both static and dynamic, such as those created by NM cardiac processing packages, should be stored using DICOM objects that can be displayed on general purpose image display systems. *See also* **Profile**.[56]

NMB National member body. The standards institute in each country that is a member of International Organization for Standardization (ISO).[3]

NMDS Nursing minimum data set. 1. The foundation for nursing languages development that identified nursing diagnosis, nursing intervention, nursing outcomes, and intensity of nursing care as unique nursing components of the Uniform Hospital Discharge Data Set (UHDDS). 2. Essential set of information items that has uniform definitions and categories concerned with nursing. It is designed to be an abstraction tool or system for collecting uniform, standard, compatible, minimum nursing data.[52,6]

NMMDS Nursing management minimum data set. A data set used to describe environment at unit level of service related to nursing delivery (unit/service, patient/client population, care delivery method), as well as nursing care resources and financial resources.[52]

NOC Nursing outcome classification. A comprehensive, standardized classification of patient/client outcomes developed to evaluate the effects of nursing interventions. Standardized outcomes are necessary for documentation in electronic records, for use in clinical information systems, for the development of nursing knowledge, and the education of professional nurses.[26]

NOC Network operation center. A location from which the operation of a network or Internet is monitored. Additionally, this center usually serves as a clearinghouse for connectivity problems and efforts to resolve those problems.[1]

Node 1. Originating or terminating point of information or signal flow in a telecommunications network. 2. Computer or device connected to a network, which is also called a *host*.[48,1]

NOI Notice of Intent. A document that describes a subject area for which the federal government is considering developing regulations. It may describe the presumably relevant considerations and invite comments from interested parties. These comments can then be used in developing a notice of proposed rulemaking (NPRM) or a final regulation.[10]

Nomenclature A consistent method for assigning names to elements of a system.[6]

Non-overwriting virus A computer virus that appends the virus code to the physical end of a program, or moves the original code to another location.[1]

Nonrepudiation Cryptographic receipts created so that an author of a message cannot falsely deny sending a message. Proof to a third party that only the signer could have created a signature. A basis of legal recognition of electronic signatures.[1]

Non-uniform memory architecture *See* **NUMA**.

Nonvolatile memory Memory that retains its content when power is removed.[1]

Normalization The process of creating a uniform and agreed-upon set of standards, policies, definitions, and technical procedures to allow for interoperability.[8]

Normalization services This service will take various concepts from different sources, normalize, and store them in the EHR's internal form. This service could be extended to include normal values based on incoming and outgoing profiles.[8]

Normative document Document that provides rules, guidelines, or characteristics for activities or results.[4]

NOS Network operating system. Operating system used on network servers to provide file, print, and other services to clients. Includes Windows NT Server, Novell NetWare, Banyan VINES (on top of UNIX), IBM OS/2 LAN Server, and OpenVMS.[1]

Notice of Intent *See* **NOI**.

Notice of proposed rulemaking *See* **NPRM**.

Notification of document availability *See* **NAV**.

NPF National provider file. The database envisioned for use in maintaining a national provider registry.[10]

NPI National provider identifier. A system for uniquely identifying all providers of healthcare services, supplies, and equipment.[10]

NPRM Notice of proposed rulemaking. A document that describes and explains regulations that the federal government proposes to adopt at some future date, and invites interested parties to submit comments related to them. These comments can then be used in developing a final regulation.[10]

NSF National standard format. Generically, this applies to any nationally standardized data format, but it is often used in a more limited way to designate the professional flat file record format used to submit professional claims.[10]

NSP Network service provider. A company providing consolidated service for some combination of e-mail, voice mail, phone, and fax configurations on broadband or wireless handheld devices. Also called *unified messaging solutions* or *universal messaging*.[1]

NSSN National standards system network. A National Resource for Global Standards is a search engine that provides users with standards-related information from a wide range of developers, including organizations accredited by the American National Standards Institute (ANSI), other U.S. private sector standards bodies, government agencies, and international organizations.[43]

Nuclear medicine image integration *See* **NM**.

Null modem cable Serial cable with transmit and receive pins crossed to simulate a modem for a direct connection between computers.[1]

NUMA Non-uniform memory architecture. A computing platform technology that clusters multiple symmetrical multi-processing (SMP) nodes together, similar to massively parallel processing (MPP) technology. *See also* **SMP, MPP**.[1]

Nursing informatics (from ANA Scope) The specialty that integrates nursing science, computer science, and information science in identifying, collecting, processing, and managing data and information to support nursing practice, administration, education, and research, and to expand the knowledge of nursing.[52]

Nursing information system Part of the healthcare information system that deals with nursing aspects, particularly the maintenance of the nursing record.[4]

Nursing intervention classification *See* **NIC**.

Nursing management minimum data set *See* **NMMDS**.

Nursing minimum data set *See* **NMDS**.

Nursing outcome classification *See* **NOC**.

Nursing procedure Systematic activity directed at, or performed on, an individual patient, with the object of providing nursing care or treatment.[4]

NWIP New work item proposal. First balloting phase for draft standards and draft technical specifications. During this phase, at least five experts from five participating ISO Technical Committee countries are chosen to work on the document.[3]

O

OASIS Outcome and Assessment Information Set. A group of data elements that represent core items of a comprehensive assessment for an adult home care patient, and form the basis for measuring patient outcomes for purposes of outcome-based quality improvement. This assessment is performed on every patient receiving services of home health agencies that are approved to participate in the Medicare and/or Medicaid programs.[102]

Object A block of information that is self-contained and has additional information that describes the data, the application that created it, how to format it, and the location of related information stored in a separate disk file.[1]

Object identifier *See* **OID**.

Object linking and embedding *See* **OLE**.

Object model Conceptual representation, typically in the form of a diagram, which describes a set of objects and their relationship.[8]

Object request broker The common interface that permits object-to-object communication.[1]

Object reuse Securing resources for the use of multiple users.[1]

Objective evidence Data supporting the existence or verity of something.[92]

Object-oriented **1.** An image, icon, illustration, or font file that is created by engineering code and mathematical equations, which provide functionality within a Windows programming environment. **2.** Applied to analysis, design and programming. The basic concept in this approach is that of objects, which consist of data structures encapsulated with a set of routines, often called 'methods,' which operate on the data. Operations on the data must be performed via these methods, which are common to all instances of objects of a particular class. Thus, the interface to objects is well defined, and allows the code implementing the methods to be changed, so long as the interface remains the same.[18]

Object-oriented **programming** **1.** An approach to software development that combines data and procedures into a single object. **2.** The idea behind object-oriented programming is that a computer program is composed of a collection of individual units, or objects, as opposed to a traditional view in which a program is a list of instructions to the computer. Each object is capable of receiving messages, processing data, and sending messages to other objects. Object-oriented programming is claimed to give more flexibility, easing changes to programs, and is widely popular in large scale software engineering. Furthermore, proponents of object-oriented programming claim that it is easier to learn for those new to computer programming than previous approaches, and that this approach is often simpler to develop and to maintain, lending itself to more direct analysis, coding, and understanding of complex situations and procedures than other programming methods. *See also* **SOA**.[1]

Obligation Operations specified in a policy, or policy set, that should be performed by the policy enforcement point (PEP) in conjunction with the enforcement of an authorization decision.[48]

OCR **Optical character recognition.** A technology that scans a printed page and converts it into a text document that can be edited in a word processor.[1]

OCSP **Online certificate status protocol.** A common scheme for maintaining the security of a server and other network resources.[42]

Octal Base eight numbering system where three bits are used to represent each digit. Uses the 0-7 digits for representations.[1]

Octet 8-bit or 1 byte unit of data. Four octets are used in an IP address.[1]

ODA **Open document architecture.** A standard document file format created by the International Telecommunications Union-Telecommunication Standardization (ITU-T) to replace all proprietary document file formats. It should not be confused with the OASIS Open Document Format for Office Applications, also known as Open Document.[7]

Odd parity A technique of checking whether data has been lost or written over during transmission.[1]

ODS **The operational data store.** A subject-oriented, integrated, real-time, volatile store of detailed data, in support of operational and tactical decision making.[1]

OEM **Original equipment manufacturer.**[1]

Off-line Device not available to be connected to or controlled by a computer.[1]

OID **Object identifier.** An identifier used to name an object, usually strings of numbers. In computer programming, an object identifier generally takes the form of an implementation-specific integer or pointer that uniquely identifies an object.[7]

OLAP **Online analytical processing.** A class of business intelligence tools that summarizes and allows efficient navigation of information along predetermined dimensions in an interactive manner.[1]

OLE **Object linking and embedding.** A document standard developed by Microsoft that allows for the creation of objects within one application, and linking them into a second application.[1]

OLTP **Online transaction processing.** A DBMS approach and technology that is optimized for defined, predictable, key-based transactions, in support of sub-second query response times. *See also* **Star schema.**[1]

OM **Outbreak management.** The capture and management of information associated with the investigation and containment of a disease outbreak or public health emergencies are primary functions of public health.[46]

Omaha nursing diagnosis/intervention *See* **Omaha System.**

Omaha System Omaha Nursing Diagnosis/Intervention. A research-based, comprehensive and standardized taxonomy designed to enhance practice, documentation, and information management. It consists of three relational, reliable, and valid components: the Problem Classification Scheme, the Intervention Scheme, and the Problem Rating Scale for Outcomes. The components provide a structure to document client needs and strengths, describe multidisciplinary practitioner interventions, and measure client outcomes in a simple, yet comprehensive, manner.[29]

On-chip applications Applications that reside on the integrated circuit chip.[1]

One-to-many Synonym for 'identification.'[114]

Online Device available to be connected to, or controlled by, a computer. Actively connected to other computers or devices. A device is online when it is logged on to a network or service.[1]

Online analytical processing *See* **OLAP.**

Online certificate status protocol *See* **OCSP.**

Online service provider An entity which provides a service online. It can include Internet service providers and Web sites, such as message board operators. In its original, more limited definition, it referred only to a commercial computer communication service, in which paid members could dial via a computer modem the service's private computer network, and access various services and information resources, such as bulletin boards, downloadable files and programs, news articles, chat rooms, and electronic mail services. The term 'online service' was also used in references to these dial-up services.[7]

Online transaction processing *See* **OLTP**.

On-site concurrent review A process to evaluate inpatient hospital services at delivery to determine that the member's clinical care is being provided in the appropriate hospital setting and facilitates timely discharge.[15]

Ontology A specification of a conceptualization of a knowledge domain. An ontology is a controlled vocabulary that describes objects and the relations between them in a formal way, and has a grammar for using the vocabulary terms to express something meaningful within a specified domain of interest. The vocabulary is used to make queries and assertions. Ontological commitments are agreements to use the vocabulary in a consistent way for knowledge sharing. Ontologies can include glossaries, taxonomies, and thesauri, but normally have greater expressivity and stricter rules than these tools. A formal ontology is a controlled vocabulary expressed in an ontology representation language.[1]

OOA **Out of area.** Not within the market geographic bounds.[15]

OON **Out of network.** In the geographic bounds, but not contracted.[7]

OOP **Out of pocket.** An amount patient pays at time of service.[8]

OpArc **Operational architecture.** *See also* Architecture.[20]

Open access A type of network that allows a member to self-refer.[15]

Open card system The open system model envisions that consumers will obtain from an independent third-party a single certificate which certifies that consumer's identity. Consumers will then use that certificate to facilitate transactions with potentially numerous merchants.[1]

Open source Software in which the source code is available free to users, who can read and modify the code.[107]

Open systems architecture In telecommunications, the term 'open systems architecture' means the layered hierarchical structure, config-

uration, or model of a communications or distributed data processing system that (1) enables system description, design, development, installation, operation, improvement, and maintenance to be performed at a given layer or layers in the hierarchical structure; (2) allows each layer to provide a set of accessible functions that can be controlled and used by the functions in the layer above it; (3) enables each layer to be implemented without affecting the implementation of other layers; and (4) allows the alteration of system performance by the modification of one or more layers without altering the existing equipment, procedures, and protocols at the remaining layers.[7]

Open systems environment Software systems that can operate on different hardware platforms because they use components that follow the same standards for user interfaces, applications, and network protocols.[1]

Open systems interconnection *See* **OSI**.

Operating system *See* **OS**.

Operating system (O/S) interface layer The layer that allows for the interconnection and interrelationship among the various operating systems in the form of two or more devices, applications, and the user interfacing with an application or device.[1]

Operating system 2 *See* **OS/2**.

Operation system certification A guarantee based on an objective and closed process or assessment that no design and/or implementation flaw is present, and that the occurrence of a random hardware and/or software error is below a specified value.[1]

Operational architecture Describes the mission, functions, information requirements, and business rules (operational requirements) for healthcare delivery. *See also* **Architecture, Enterprise architecture**.[20]

Operational data store Repository of clinical data used by client applications to create, update, and process encounter-specific information at the points of service.[8]

Optical card An optical memory card with laser-recorded and laser-read information that can be edited or updated, and has a storage capacity of 800 printed pages.[1]

Optical character recognition *See* **OCR**.

Optical disc An electronic data storage medium that is read or recorded using a low-powered laser beam. There has been a constant succession of optical disc formats, first in CD formats, followed by a number of DVD formats. Optical disc offers a number of advantages over magnetic storage media. An optical disc holds much more data.[2]

Optical resolution In scanning, this refers to the number of truly separate readings taken from an original image within a given distance, as opposed to the subsequent increase in resolution (but no detail) created by software interpolation.[1]

Optical video disk Compact discs that use lights to read information.[1]

Opt-in Mechanism that states data collection and/or use methods, and provides user choice to accept such collection and/or use.[36]

Opt-out Mechanism that states data collection and/or use methods, and provides user choice to decline such collection and/or use.[36]

OR Logical gating operation that provides a high output if any input is high.[1]

Order Request for a certain procedure to be performed.[4]

Order communications The interface from order entry applications to departmental systems that communicates the service needs for the department.[2]

Order entry system System for recording and processing orders.[4] *See also* **CPOE**.

Organized healthcare arrangement Organized system of healthcare in which more than one covered entity participates, and in which the participating covered entities hold themselves out to the public as participating in a joint arrangement; and participate in joint utilization review, quality assurance, or financial risk for healthcare services.[48]

ORM *See* **General order message**.

OS Operating system. Software that manages basic computer operations, and supervises and controls tasks, such as Windows 95, 98, NT, Windows 2000, Me, CE, Linus, Palm OS, MAC OS X, OS/2, and UNIX.[1]

OS/2 Operating system 2. IBM's 32-bit GUI multi-tasking operating system with the ability to run DOS, Win16, Win 32, OS/2 16, and OS/2 32 applications, for 80286 and 80386 computers.[1]

OSI Open systems interconnection. A reference model to the protocols in the seven-layer data communications networking standards model and services performed at each level. The OSI standard is defined by the International Standards Organization (ISO). The seven layers from the bottom are physical, data link, network, transport, session, presentation, and application.[1]

Otology A data model that represents a set of concepts within a domain and the relationships between those concepts. It is used to reason about the objects within that domain.[48]

Out of area *See* **OOA**.

Out of network *See* **OON**.

Out of pocket *See* **OOP**.

Outbreak management *See* **OM**.

Outcome The valued results of care as experienced primarily by the patient, but also by physicians, and all other participants in the processes contributing to the outcomes.[120]

Outcome and Assessment Information Set *See* **OASIS**.

Outcome assessment Research aimed at assessing the quality and effectiveness of healthcare as measured by the attainment of a specified end result or outcome. Measures include parameters, such as improved health, lowered morbidity or mortality, and improvement of abnormal states (such as elevated blood pressure).[5]

Outcome data Data that measure the health status of patients resulting from specific medical and health interventions.[102]

Outcome indicator An indicator that assesses what happens or does not happen to a patient following a process; agreed-upon desired patient characteristics to be achieved; undesired patient conditions to be avoided.[102]

Outcome measure A parameter for evaluating the success of a system; the parameter reflects the top-level of goals of the system.[4]

Outcomes-based practice Multidisciplinary clinical practice, based on evidence that specific treatments will improve patient outcomes.[120]

Out-of-band Communications which occur outside of a communications method or channel (e.g., the communication of security policies that will be applied to data in the future are communicated out-of-band; they communicated prior to, not at the same time as, the data).[48]

Outpatient Patient who does not reside in a healthcare facility.[4]

Outpatient record Healthcare record of an outpatient.[4]

Output The direct result of the interaction of inputs and processes in the system; the types and qualities of goods and services produced by an activity, project, or program.[123]

Overuse Providing a process of care in circumstances where the potential for harm exceeds the potential for benefit. Prescribing an antibiotic for a viral infection like a cold, for which antibiotics are ineffective, constitutes overuse. The potential for harm includes adverse reactions to the antibiotics and increases in antibiotic resistance among bacteria in the community. Overuse can also apply to diagnostic tests and surgical procedures.[14]

Overwriting virus A virus that reproduces by overwriting the first parts of the program with itself. Because important parts of the program are effectively destroyed, it will not ever run, but the virus code will. These viruses are dangerous and can damage a computer.[35]

OWL Web ontology language.

P

P2P Peer-to-peer. **1.** A network structure in which the computers share processing and storage tasks as equivalent members of the network. Different from a client/server network, in which computers are assigned specific roles. **2.** A general term for popular file-sharing systems like gnutella, in which there is no central repository of files. Instead, files can be stored on, and retrieved from, any user's computer.[107]

P4P **Pay for performance.** Refers to the general strategy of promoting quality improvement by rewarding providers (meaning individual clinicians or, more commonly, clinics or hospitals) who meet certain performance expectations with respect to healthcare quality or efficiency. Performance can be defined in terms of patient outcomes but is more commonly defined in terms of processes of care (e.g., the percentage of eligible diabetics who have been referred for annual retinal examinations, the percentage of children who have received immunizations appropriate for their age, patients admitted to the hospital with pneumonia who receive antibiotics within 6 hours). Pay-for-performance initiatives reflect the efforts of purchasers of healthcare—from the federal government to private insurers—to use their purchasing power to encourage providers to develop whatever specific quality improvement initiatives are required to achieve the specified targets. Thus, rather than committing to a specific quality improvement strategy, such as a new information system or a disease management program, which may have variable success in different institutions, pay for performance creates a climate in which provider groups will be strongly incentivized to find whatever solutions will work for them.[14]

Packet The unit of data that is routed between an origin and a destination on the Internet or any other packet-switched network. Packets have no set size; they can range from one character to hundreds of characters.[1]

Packet format Contains three sections: header, data, and trailer.[1]

Packet header First three octets of an X.25 packet that specifies packet destination, source, and contains an alert.[1]

Packet Internet groper *See* **PING.**

Packet sniffing A technique in which attackers surreptitiously insert a software program at remote network switches or host computers. The program monitors information packets as they are sent through networks, and sends a copy of the information retrieved to the hacker.[1]

Packet switched Transmission technique in which data are broken up into packets and sent along multiple destination paths using store and forward techniques. Once all the packets forming a message arrive at the destination, they are recompiled into the original message. *See also* **Circuit switched**.[1]

Packet switched telephone network *See* **PSTN**.

Packet switching Data are coded into small units and sent over an electronic communication network. Most traffic over the Internet uses packet switching, and the Internet is basically a connectionless network.[1]

Packet-filtering firewall A computer that decides packet-by-packet whether a packet should be copied from one network to another.[1]

PACS Picture archiving and communication systems. A system that begins by converting the standard storage of x-ray films into digitized electronic media that can later be retrieved by radiologists, clinicians, and other staff to view exam data and medical images. Computers or networks dedicated to the storage, retrieval, distribution, and presentation of images. Full PACS handle images from various modalities, such as ultrasonography, magnetic resonance imaging, positron emission tomography, computed tomography, and radiography (plain x-rays). Small-scale systems that handle images from a single modality (usually connected to a single acquisition device) are sometimes called *mini-PACS*.[1]

Palm operating system *See* **Palm OS**.

Palm OS Palm operating system. Handheld computer operating system from Palm, Inc., which provides a basic set of calendar, address book, and wireless access functions. Typing is done by either a mini-keyboard and stylus, or a graffiti style of handwritten shorthand.[1]

PAP Password authentication protocol. Allows the use of clear text passwords at its lowest level.[1]

Parallel branching Specifies that two or more tasks are executed independently of each other.[111] *See* **Exclusive branching**.

Parallel cable A cable used to connect peripheral devices through a computer's parallel port.[1]

Parallel port A type of port that transmits data in parallel, with several bits side by side.[1]

Parallel split The divergence of a branch into two or more parallel branches, each of which execute concurrently.[112]

Parameter A word, number, or symbol that is typed after a command to further specify how the command should function.[1]

Parameter RAM *See* **PRAM**.

Pareto chart A graphic representation of the frequency with which certain events occur. It is a rank-order bar chart that displays the relative importance of variables in data sets and may be used to set priorities regarding opportunities for improvement.[123]

Pareto Principle The so-called Pareto Principle (also known as the 80-20 rule, the law of the vital few and the principle of factor sparsity) states that for many phenomena, 80% of consequences stem from 20% of the causes. The idea has rule-of-thumb application in many places, but it is commonly misused.[7]

Parity Parity is used to check a unit of data for errors during transmission through phone lines or modem cables.[1]

Parser 1. A function that recognizes valid sentences of a language by analyzing the syntax structure of a set of tokens passed to it from a lexical analyzer. 2. A software tool that parses programs or other text, often as the first step of assembly, compilation, interpretation, or analysis.[8]

Parser services This service will parse the messages that come in through the protocol layer. The parser will provide support for input formats such as XML, flat files positional, flat file fixed field length, etc.[8]

Passive threat A potential breach of security, the occurrence of which would not change the state of the system. Such threat could arise from unauthorized reading of files, or use of the computer system for an unauthorized application.[1]

Password A special code word, or a string of characters, that a user must present before gaining access to a data system's resources. A sequence that an individual presents to a system for purposes of authentication.[1]

Password authentication protocol *See* **PAP**.

Password cracking A technique in which attackers try to guess or steal passwords to obtain access to computer systems.[1]

Paste To insert information from the clipboard. Information can be pasted multiple times. Many software programs allow for a shortcut from the keyboard by pressing and holding the control button or key and the 'V' button at the same time. *See also* **Cut**.[1]

Patch Vendors, in response to the discovery of security vulnerabilities, provide sets of files that have to be installed on computer systems. These files 'fix' or 'patch' the computer system or programs and remove the security vulnerability.[118]

Pathway *See* **Clinical pathway**.

Patient Person who is the target of healthcare activity.[4]

Patient administration system Information system or subsystem used for patient administration, billing, and reimbursement purposes.[4]

Patient centric A design goal or characteristic that establishes that all information in an application system shall be grouped and/or indexed according to the patient/person.[8]

Patient classification A classification of patients based on specific criteria or data elements.[4]

Patient demographic query *See* **PDQ**.

Patient identifier domain A single system or a set of interconnected systems that all share a common identification scheme for patients. Such a scheme includes (1) a single identifier-issuing authority; (2) an assignment process of an identifier to a patient; (3) a permanent record of issued patient identifiers with associated traits; and (4) a maintenance process over time. The goal of patient identification is to reduce errors.[56]

Patient experience Comprised of research reports and administrative information that reflect quality from the perspective of patients by capturing observations and opinions about what happened during the process of healthcare delivery. Patient experience encompasses various indicators of patient-centered care, including access (whether patients are obtaining appropriate care in a timely manner), communication skills, customer service, helpfulness of office staff, and information resources.[138]

Patient flow The movement of patients who seek care in an emergency department through the admission process. This is the process through which patients are granted entry for care at the hospital and seen by a physician.[138]

Patient information reconciliation *See* **PIR**.

Patient plan of care A roadmap to guide all services that are involved with a patient's care. The plan of care contains goals or outcomes related to treatment options. May also be based on the five-step nursing process: (1) assessment or problem list; (2) goals or outcomes; (3) specific planning with interventions described; (4) implementation; and (5) evaluation of care delivered.[26]

Patient privacy consent The act of a patient consenting to a specific privacy consent policy.[56]

Patient record Systematic record of the history of the health of a patient kept by a physician or other healthcare practitioner.[4]

Patient record system The set of components that form the mechanism by which patient records are created, used, stored, and retrieved; a patient record system is usually located within a healthcare provider setting. Includes people, dates, rules and procedures, processing and storage devices, and communication and support facilities.[30]

Patient registry A patient database maintained by a hospital, doctors' practice, or health plan that allows providers to identify their patients according to disease, demographic characteristics, and other factors. Patient registries can help providers better coordinate care for their patients, monitor treatment and progress, and improve overall quality of care.[138]

Patient safety Freedom from accidental or preventable injuries produced by medical care.[14]

Patient synchronized applications *See* **PSA**.

Patient-centered care Considers patients' cultural traditions, personal preferences and values, family situations, and lifestyles. Responsibility for important aspects of self-care and monitoring is put in patients' hands—along with the tools and support they need. Patient-centered care also ensures that transitions between different healthcare providers and care settings are coordinated and efficient. When care is patient-centered, unneeded and unwanted services can be reduced.[138]

Patient-specific data All data captured and stored in the system pertaining to a patient, such as clinical assessments, medications, insurance information, etc.[6]

Pay for performance *See* **P4P**.

Payer Indicates a third party entity who pays for or underwrites coverage for healthcare expenses. A payer may be an insurance company, a health maintenance organization (HMO), a preferred provider organization (PPO), a government agency, or an agency such as a third party administrator (TPA). *See also* **NPI**.[16]

PC Personal computer.[1] A computer designed for use by one person at a time. PC is also commonly used to describe an IBM-compatible personal computer in contrast to an Apple Macintosh computer.[1]

PC card slot The port in a computer in which a smart card is inserted via a 68-pin socket connector. They are available in type I, II, and III form factors. Type II form factor is the most prevalent.[1] *See also* **PCMCIA**.

PCI Peripheral component interconnect. Standard CPU to I/O device interface with 32-, 64-, and 128-bit data paths. PCI motherboards automatically configure interrupts. Introduced in 1993.[1]

PCMCIA Personal Computer Memory Card International Association. Association that has worked to standardize and promote PC card technology.[1]

PCP Primary care provider. 1. PCPs specialize in internal medicine, pediatrics, family practice, or obstetrics/gynecology. They provide primary care to members and make referrals to specialty care providers. **2.** A nurse practitioner, a state licensed registered nurse with specialized education, can also provide this basic level of healthcare.[15,102]

PDA Personal digital assistant. A handheld computing device capable of containing streamlined versions of healthcare software that is compatible with other major systems, and capable of communicating through a direct serial connection, modem, or wireless interface.[1]

PDC Primary domain controller. First operational computer in a Windows NT domain, and only PDC in a domain. Authenticates all users and maintains the master security accounts database.[1]

PDF Portable document format. A PDF file is an electronic facsimile of a printed document; the filename extension for a packed data file.[1]

PDF 417 A two-dimensional barcode symbology, enabling error-free transmission of larger blocks of data than is feasible with one-dimension barcode.[99]

PDI Portable data for imaging. Specifies actors and transactions that provide the distribution of diagnostic and therapeutic imaging information on interchange media. The goal of this profile is to provide reliable interchange of evidence objects and diagnostic reports for import, display, or print by a receiving actor. *See also* **Profile**.[56]

PDP Policy decision point. The system entity that evaluates applicable policy and renders an authorization decision.[125] *See also* **ACS**.

PDQ Patient demographic query. Provides ways for multiple distributed applications to query a central patient information server for a list of patients, based on user-defined search criteria. Patient demographics data can be entered directly into the application from which the user is querying by picking the appropriate record from a list of possible matches, called a patient pick list. *See also* **Profile**.[56]

Peer-to-peer network LAN with no central computer where 10 or fewer user computers are connected together. This network setup allows every computer to both offer and access network resources, such as shared files. Also called a *workgroup*.[1]

Penetration A successful and repeatable extraction and identification of recognizable privileged (i.e., clinical) data from a protected resource of a data system.[1]

PEP Policy enforcement point. The system entity that performs access control by making decision requests and enforcing authorization decisions.[125] *See also* **ACS.**

Performance assessment Involves the analysis and interpretation of performance measurement data to transform it into useful information for purposes of continuous performance improvement.[102]

Performance indicator Measure that allows observing the progress of a particular change, and evaluating its impact.[94]

Performance measure Sets of established standards against which health care performance is measured. Performance Measures are now widely accepted as a method for guiding informed decision making as a strong impetus for improvement.[138]

Perioperative nursing data set *See* **PNDS.**

Peripheral A piece of hardware that is outside the main computer. It usually refers to external hardware, such as disk drives, printers, and scanners.[1]

Perl Practical extraction and report language. An interpreted procedural programming language designed by Larry Wall. Perl has a unique set of features, some borrowed from imperative computer programming language (C), and some from others. *See also* **CGI.**[1]

Permanent virtual circuit *See* **PVC.**

Persistent data Data which are stored on a permanent basis.[116]

Person identification service *See* **PIDS.**

Personal computer *See* **PC.**

Personal computer memory card international *See* **PCMCIA.**

Personal digital assistant *See* **PDA.**

Personal health information *See* **PHI.**

Personal health record *See* **PHR** and **ePHR.**

Personal identification number *See* **PIN.**

Personal identity verification *See* **PIV.**

Personal representative Person(s) who has the authority, under applicable state law, to act on behalf of an individual who is an adult or an emancipated minor in making decisions related to the program, service, or activity that an entity provides to the individual. If, under applicable state law, a parent, guardian, or other person acting in loco parentis has authority to act on behalf of an individual who is an unemancipated minor in making decisions related to the program, service, or activity, this person should be treated as the personal representative of the individual.[48]

Personal system 2 *See* **PS/2.**

Personally identifiable health information Health information that contains an individual's identifiers (e.g., name, Social Security number, birth date) or contains a sufficient number of variables to allow identification of an individual.[1]

Personnel white pages *See* **PWP.**

Pervasive computing Promoters of this idea hope that embedding computation into the environment would enable people to move around and interact with computers more naturally than they currently do. One of the goals of ubiquitous computing is to enable devices to sense changes in their environment, and to automatically adapt and act based on these changes, based on user needs and preferences. Some simple examples of this type of behavior include GPS-equipped automobiles that give interactive driving directions, and RFID store checkout systems. *See* **Ubiquitous computing.**[7]

PET scan Positron emission tomography. A digital imaging modality capable of detecting subtle differences in temperature.[36]

PGP Presentation of grouped procedures. Addresses what is sometimes referred to as the linked studies problem: viewing image subsets resulting from a single acquisition with each image subset related to a different requested procedure (e.g., CT chest, abdomen, and pelvis). It provides a mechanism for facilitating workflow when viewing images and reporting on individual requested procedures that an operator has grouped (often for the sake of acquisition efficiency and patient comfort). A single acquired image set is produced, but the combined use of the scheduled workflow transactions and the consistent presentation of images allow separate viewing and interpretation of the image subsets related to each of the requested procedures. *See also* **Profile**.[56]

PGP Pretty good privacy. A public key encryption program used to encrypt and decrypt e-mail over the Internet. Also, PGP may be used for digital signatures to let the receiver know the sender's identity and that the transmission was not changed en route.[1]

Pharmacy informatics Pharmacy informatics is the scientific field that focuses on medication-related data and knowledge within the continuum of healthcare systems, including its acquisition, storage, analysis, use, and dissemination in the delivery of optimal medication-related patient care and health outcomes.[45]

Pharmacy information systems Health information system that deals with the pharmacy. Such systems can be linked to prescribing systems for electronic processing of requests for medications and can provide inventory control.[4]

Pharmacy management system An application used by a pharmacy to manage fulfillment of prescriptions, claims processing, and other administrative functions.[8]

PHI Protected/personal health information. Any individually identifiable health information, whether oral or recorded in any form or medium, that is created or received by a healthcare provider, health plan, public health authority, employer, life insurer, school or university, or healthcare clearinghouse; it relates to the past, present, or future physical or mental health or condition of an individual; the provision of healthcare to an individual; or the past, present, or future payment for the provision of healthcare to an individual. Any data transmitted or maintained in any other form or medium by covered entities, including paper records, fax documents and all oral communications, or any other form (i.e., screen prints of eligibility information, printed e-mails that have identified individual's health information, claim or billing information, hard copy birth or death certificate). Protected health information excludes school records that are subject to the Family Educational Rights and Privacy Act, and employment records held in DHS' role as an employer.[118]

PHIN Public health information network. CDC's vision for advancing fully capable and interoperable information systems in the many organizations that participate in public health. PHIN is a national initiative to implement a multi-organizational business and technical architecture for public health information systems. *See also* **CDC**.[46]

PHIN-MS Public health information network-messaging system. A protocol for secure transmission of data, based on the ebXML model. Developed and supported by Centers for Disease Control and Prevention (CDC). The protocol allows for rapid and secure messages to send sensitive health information over the Internet to other local, state, and federal organizations, as well as the CDC.[46]

PHO Physician health organization. Physician group that unifies for the purpose of negotiating healthcare contracts as a group.[15]

PHR Personal health record. 1. An electronic personal health record (ePHR) is a universally accessible, layperson comprehensible, lifelong tool for managing relevant health information, promoting health maintenance, and assisting with chronic disease management via an interactive, common data set of electronic health information and e-health tools. The ePHR is owned, managed, and shared by the individual or his or her legal proxy(s) and must be secure to protect the privacy and confidentiality of the health information it contains. It is not a legal record unless so defined and is subject to various legal limitations. **2.** Usually used when referring to the version of the health/medical record owned by the consumer/patient.[45,15] *See also* **Appendix A**.

Physical access The ability and the means to approach and use any hardware component of a clinical data system.[1]

Physical access control Refers to an automated system that controls an individual's ability to access to a physical location, such as a building, parking lot, office, or other designated physical space. A physical access control system requires validation of an individual's identity through some mechanism, such as a personal identification number (PIN), card, biometric, or other token prior to providing access. It has the capability to assign different access privileges to different persons, depending on their roles and responsibilities in an organization.[114]

Physical layer   First layer in the OSI model. Defines the physical characteristics of a link between communicating devices.[1]

Physical safeguards   The physical measures, policies, and procedures to protect a covered entity's electronic information systems and related buildings and equipment from natural and environmental hazards and unauthorized intrusion.[118]

Physical security   The measures taken against all physical threats to a clinical data system, including its remote facilities and operational area; including control of access and exit, protection against fire, explosion, natural disaster, sabotage, social protests, and power problems, and protection of all the stored clinical data from malicious destruction or theft.[1]

Physician dashboard   An application that allows physicians to designate the type of data they want to see and where they want to see it on the graphical user interface they use for accessing their patients' information. It allows physicians to design the display and interaction of the data they use to diagnose and treat patients. It is extremely flexible and can be modified by each individual doctor to suit his or her needs.[2]

Physician health organization   *See* **PHO**.

Physician online directory   A type of physician referral service that can be accessed from a computer, through a variety of online services.[1]

Picosecond   One trillionth of a second.[1]

Picture archiving and communication system   *See* **PACS** and **Radiology PACS**.

PIDS   **Person identification service.** Defines a set of interfaces to an interchangeable set of services that provides a best match or ordered list of best matches to possibly incomplete or conflicting data about a person.[124]

Piggyback   Interception of messages between a user and the computer system and then releasing them, modifying them, or returning error messages.[1]

PIM   **Platform independent model.** A model of a software or business system that is independent of the specific technological platform used to implement it. For example, HTML defines a model for hypertext that includes concepts such as title, headings, paragraphs, etc. This model is not linked to a specific operating system or Web browser and is, therefore, being successfully implemented on a variety of different computing systems. The term *platform-independent model* is most frequently used in the context of model-driven architectures.[144]

PIN   **Personal identification number.** Used to authenticate or identify a user.[1]

PING   **Packet Internet groper.** Utility used to test destination reachability. Sends an Internet control message protocol (ICMP) echo request to the destination and waits for a reply.[1]

PIP   **Policy information point.** Point that can provide external information to a policy decision point.[125] *See also* **ACS**.

PIR   **Patient information reconciliation.** Extends the scheduled workflow integration profile by offering the means to match images, diagnostic reports, and other evidence objects acquired for a misidentified or unidentified patient (e.g., during a trauma case) with the patient's record. *See also* **Profile**.[56]

PIV   **Personal identification verification.** A physical artifact (e.g., identity card, smart card) issued to an individual that contains stored identity credentials (e.g., photograph, cryptographic keys, digitized fingerprint representation) that the claimed identity of the cardholder can be verified against the stored credentials by another person (human readable) or an automated process (computer readable).[114]

PIX   **Patient identifier cross-referencing.** Provides cross-referencing of patient identifiers from multiple patient identifier domains. These patient identifiers can then be used by identity consumer systems to correlate information about a single patient from sources that know the patient by different identifiers. *See also* **Profile**.[56]

Pixel   The smallest unit of data for defining an image in the computer. The computer reduces a picture to a grid of pixels.[1]

Pixel skipping   A means of reducing image resolution by simply deleting pixels throughout the image.[1]

PKC   **Public key certificate.** X.509 public key certificates (PKCs) which bind an identity and a public key; the identity may be used to support identity-based access control decisions after the client proves that it has access to the private key that corresponds to the public key contained in the PKC.[121]

PKI Public key infrastructure. 1. Technology, facilities, people, operational procedures, and policy to support public key-based security mechanisms. It is an enabler for these encryption and digital signatures. **2.** Infrastructure used in the relation between a key holder and a relying party that allows a relying party to use a certificate relating to the key holder for at least one application using a public key dependent security service, and that includes a certification authority, a certificate data structure, means for the relying party to obtain current information on the revocation status of the certificate, a certification policy, and methods to validate the certification practice.[1,121]

PKZip Disk compression program.[1]

Plain text The original communication form, also called clear text, or readable text.[1]

Plan of care The plan of care (also interdisciplinary plan of care) is a plan based on data gathered during patient assessment that identifies the participant's care needs, describes the strategy for providing services to meet those needs, documents treatment goals and objectives, outlines the criteria for terminating specified interventions, and documents the participant's progress in meeting goals and objectives. Patient-specific policies and procedures, protocols, clinical practice guidelines, clinical paths, care maps, or a combination thereof may guide the format of the plan in some organizations. The care plan may include care, treatment, habilitation, and rehabilitation.[31]

Platform independent model *See* **PIM**.

Plenum cable Fire-resistant cable that is installed in false ceilings. Uses a coating that will not emit toxic fumes in the event of a fire.[1]

Plotter Output device that produces graphs and diagrams.[1]

Plug-and-play Software that can be plugged into the operating system, or other software, and used immediately, without any adaptation or reconfiguration on the part of the user.[1]

Plug-in A software tool that extends the capabilities of a Web browser, allowing the browser to run multimedia files.[1]

PNDS Perioperative nursing data set. A standardized nursing vocabulary of nursing diagnoses, nursing interventions, and nurse-sensitive patient outcomes that addresses the perioperative patient experience from pre-admission to discharge.[52]

PNG Portable network graphics. A lossless bitmap image format. PNG was created to both improve upon and replace the GIF format with an image file format that does not require a patent license to use. PNG is officially pronounced as 'ping' (/pɪŋ/ in IPA), but it is often just spelled out — possibly to avoid confusion with the Internet tool ping. PNG is supported by the PNG reference library, a platform independent library that contains C functions for handling PNG images.[7]

Point-of-care system Hospital information system that includes bedside workstations or other devices for capturing and entering data at the locations where patients receive care.[4]

Point-to-multipoint connection A communications architecture in which multiple devices are connected to a link that branches from a single point called an intelligent controller, which manages the flow of information.[1]

Point-to-point connection A communications link between two specific end devices, such as two computers or two modems.[1]

Point-to-point protocol *See* **PPP**.

Point-to-point tunneling protocol *See* **PPTP**.

Policy Overall intention and direction as formally expressed by management.[124]

Policy decision point *See* **PDP**.

Policy enforcement point *See* **PEP**.

Policy information point *See* **PIP**.

POP Post office protocol. A server using this protocol to hold users' incoming e-mail until they read or download it.[1]

Pop To remove data from the top of a stack.[1]

POP server Point of presence. A description for a server supporting POP, serving as a dial-up modem for an Internet service provider (ISP) or e-mail service provider. *See also* **ISP**.[1]

Pop-down list box   In a graphical user interface (GUI) environment, the list box that appears when the user selects an icon that represents a box with various choices.[1]

PORT   Patient outcomes research teams.

Portability   The capability of a program to be executed on various types of data processing systems with little or no modification, and without converting the program to a different language.[8]

Portability   The ability of a program to run on systems with different architectures.[4]

Portable data for imaging   *See* **PDI**.

Portable document format   *See* **PDF**.

Portable network graphics   *See* **PNG**.

Portable open systems interface   *See* **POSIX**.

Portal   *See* **Web portal**.[7]

Porting   Moving software and data files to other computer systems.[4]

POS   Point of service.

POS   Physician office system.[8]

Positron emission tomography   *See* **PET** scan.

POSIX   Portable open systems interface. IEEE standard for UNIX-like program implementation. Capable of case-sensitive file naming, last-access time stamping, and hard links. A standard, not an operating system. Windows NT supports POSIX.[1]

Post office protocol   *See* **POP**.

Post-processing workflow   *See* **PWF**.

Post-coordination   Describes representation of a concept using a combination of two or more codes.[19]

Post-coordination   Using more than one concept from one or many formal systems, combined using mechanisms within or outside the formal systems.[59]

Post-production   Part of the life-cycle of the product after the design has been completed and

the medical device has been manufactured and released.[68]

POTS   Plain old telephone system. *See also* **PSTN**.[1]

Power PC   RISC microprocessor developed by IBM with built-in features that allow it to emulate other microprocessors.[1]

PP   Prospective payment.

PPO   Preferred provider organization. A list of preferred providers that members utilize at a discounted fee.[1]

PPP   Point-to-point protocol. Protocol that links two networks for serial data transfer. Supports multiple network protocols (TCP/IP, IPX/SPX, and NetBEUI) compression and encryption.[1]

PPS   Prospective payment system. A system for paying for services which is not based on costs or charges, but on clinical characteristics of a case. DRGs are an example.[15]

PPTP   Point-to-point tunneling protocol. Protocol for data transfer over the Internet supporting secure communication through encryption.[1]

Practical extraction and report language   *See* **Perl**.

Practice management system   Generic term used to reference a management system. *See also* **Pharmacy management system, Physician management system**.[8]

PRAM   Parameter RAM. A small portion of the RAM set aside to hold basic information, such as the date and time, speaker volume, desktop pattern, and keyboard and mouse settings.[1]

Pre-coordination   Describes representation of a potentially complex concept using a single code.[19]

Predicate migration   Steps taken to enable pre-existing data retrieval predicates (including queries, standard reports, and decision support protocols) to be converted or utilized in a system using a mappable vocabulary.[19]

Preferred provider organization   *See* **PPO**.

Preferred term   The term that is deemed to be the most clinically appropriate way of expressing a concept in a clinical record. Preferred term is one of the three types of terms that can be indicated by the description type field.[19]

Prescriber Healthcare person authorized to issue prescriptions.[117]

Prescribing system An information system used in healthcare for processing the prescription of medication by a physician; such a system links the physician with pharmacies and others engaged in prescription of medication.[4]

Prescription Direction created by an authorized healthcare person to instruct a dispensing agent regarding the preparation and use of a medicinal product, or medicinal appliance to be taken or used by a patient.[117]

Prescription set Collection of one or more prescription items prescribed and/or dispensed as a unit.[117]

Presentation layer Sixth layer of the OSI model. Provides services to interface applications to the communications system in the form of encryption, compression, translation, and conversion. The network redirector resides here.[1]

Presentation of grouped procedures *See* **PGP**.

Presentation services **1.** Service that provides user interface capabilities and deals with formatting and presenting data to the user. May use user profiles/preferences, personalization, style sheets, etc. **2.** Client application systems that allow authorized users to access and view patient EHR data in an easily customizable manner. Also known as *presentation systems* or *EHR portal*.[8]

Pretty good privacy *See* **PGP**.

Prevalence The number of existing cases of a disease or condition, in a given population, at a specific time.[102]

PRG Procedure-related group.[9]

Primary care physician *See* **PCP**.

Primary domain controller *See* **PDC**.

Primary key A data element or combination of data elements in a table, whose values uniquely identify a row or record. The primary key must have a unique value for each record or row in the table.[1]

Primary patient record Primary record of care. The primary legal record documenting the healthcare services provided to a person in any aspect of healthcare delivery. This term is synonymous with medical record, electronic health record, client record, and resident record.[1]

Primitive A concept is primitive if its defining characteristics are insufficient to define it relative to its immediate supertype(s). For example, if the concept 'red sports car' is defined as [is a=car] + [color=red], this is the primitive, but the same definition applied to the concept 'red car' is fully defined.[19]

Print server A computer that manages print requests from many different users by holding them in a queue until they can be printed. It sends print requests to the appropriate printer in a multi-printer environment.[1]

Privacy **1.** The right to have all records and information pertaining to healthcare treated as confidential. **2.** Freedom from intrusion into the private life or affairs of an individual, when that intrusion results from undue or illegal gathering and use of data about that individual.[6,3]

Privacy consent policy One of the acceptable-use privacy consent policies that are agreed to and understood in the affinity domain.[56]

Privacy consent policy identifier An affinity domain assigned identifier (OID) that uniquely identifies the affinity domain privacy consent policy. There is one unique identifier (OID) for each privacy consent policy within the affinity domain.[56]

Privacy impact assessment Tells the 'story' of a project or policy initiative from a privacy perspective and helps to manage privacy impacts.[115]

Privacy officer Appointed by a covered entity to be responsible for developing and implementing policies and procedures for complying with the health information privacy requirements of the Health Insurance Portability and Accountability Act (HIPAA).[48]

Privacy rights Specific actions that an individual can take, or request to be taken, with regard to the uses and disclosures of their information.[48]

Private key A key in an asymmetric algorithm; the possession of this key is restricted, usually to one entity. Used for signing one's signature to a block of data, which is an HTML document, an e-mail message, or a photograph. *See also* **Digital signature**.[1]

Private key cryptography Encryption methodology in which the encryptor and decryptor use the same key, which must be kept secret.[1]

Privilege An individual's right to hold private and confidential the information given to a healthcare provider in the context of a professional relationship. The individual may, by overt act of consent or by other means, waive the right to privilege.[1]

Privileged information A datum or data combination for which adequate technological and administrative safeguards for handling, disclosure, storage, and disposal are required by law or by administrative policy.[1]

PRO **Professional review organization, or Peer review organization.** A group which provides utilization review and quality oversight to provider organizations.[32]

Problem domain The field of healthcare under consideration in a modeling process.[4]

Problem-oriented medical record Healthcare record in which all data may be linked to a list of health problems of an individual patient.[4]

Procedure Act or conduct of diagnosis, treatment, or operation. Method or technique[32]

Procedure-related group *See* **PRG**.

Process Set of interrelated or interacting activities, which transform inputs into outputs.[68]

Process model A number of tasks that have to be carried out, and a set of conditions that determine the order of the tasks.[111]

Process standard Standard that specifies requirements to be fulfilled by a process, to establish fitness for purpose.[4]

Processor The logic circuitry that responds to and processes the basic instructions that drive a computer. The term *processor* has generally replaced the term *central processing unit (CPU)*.[1]

Product standard Standard that specifies requirements to be fulfilled by a product or groups of products, to establish fitness for purpose.[4]

Professional review organization, or Peer review organization *See* **PRO**.

Profile A set of selected parameters that describes a particular reimplementation of a standard.[4]

Program A set of instructions which can be recognized by a computer system and used to carry out a set of processes.[4]

Program manager The person ultimately responsible for the overall procurement, development, integration, modification, or operation and maintenance of an IT system.[97]

Program security controls Controls designed to prevent unauthorized changes to programs in systems that are already in production.[1]

Programmable read-only memory *See* **PROM**.

Programmers Highly trained technical specialists who write computer software instructions.[1]

Project management A set of principals, methods, tools, and techniques for effective planning of work, thereby establishing a sound basis for effective scheduling, controlling, and preplanning in the management of programs and products.[6]

Project Sentinel A project of the National Biosurveillance Testbed, Project Sentinel takes de-identified HIPAA compliance data from participating emergency departments, aggregates it for a specific area, and allows for regional and national comparison for identification of emerging diseases and bioterrorism threats.[1]

PROM **Programmable read-only memory.** Subclass of ROM, non-volatile memory chip used in control devices because it can be programmed once.[1]

Prompt A message displayed on the monitor screen, which asks the customer to perform some action, and shows that the computer is ready to accept a command or instruction.[4]

Properties   Information about an object or file, including settings or options for that object. For example, user looks at properties of a file for information, such as the date created, file size, file type, and file attributes.[1]

Proprietary   Privately owned and controlled, typically by a single party. In the computer industry, proprietary is the opposite of open. A proprietary design or technique is one that is owned by a company. It also implies that the company has not divulged specifications that would allow other companies to duplicate the product.[1]

Protected health information   *See* **PHI**.

Protocol   In information technology, a protocol is a special set of rules using end points in a telecommunication connection for communication. Protocols exist at several levels.[14]

Protocol stack   Set of combined protocols that accomplish the communications process.[1]

Provider   Any supplier of a healthcare service.[8]

Proximity   Refers to a technology used to provide physical access control. This technology uses a contact-less interface with a card reader.[114]

PS/2   Personal System 2. Second generation series of IBM computers that used Micro Channel architecture.[1]

PSA   Patient synchronized applications. A means for viewing data for a single patient using independent and unlinked applications on a user's workstation, reducing the repetitive tasks of selecting the same patient in multiple applications. Data can be viewed from different identifier domains when used with the Patient Identifier Cross-referencing Integration profile to resolve multiple identifications for the same patient. This profile leverages the HL7 CCOW standard specifically for patient subject context management. *See also* **Profile**.[56]

PSTN   Packet switched telephone network. Regular dial-up telephone lines. Also known as plain old telephone system (POTS). The international telephone system, based on copper wires carrying analog voice data, in contrast to newer telephone networks, based on digital technologies.[1]

Psychotherapy notes   Recorded in any medium by a healthcare provider who is a mental health professional, documenting or analyzing the contents of conversation during a private counseling session, or a group, joint, or family counseling session, when notes are separated from the rest of the individual's record.[48]

Public health agency   An agency that performs or conducts one or more of the following essential functions that characterize public health programs, services, or activities: (a) monitor health status to identify community health problems; (b) diagnose and investigate health problems and health hazards in the community; (c) inform, educate, and empower people about health issues; (d) mobilize community partnerships to identify and solve health problems; (e) develop policies and plans that support individual and community health efforts; (f) enforce laws and regulations that protect health and ensure safety; (g) link people to needed personal health services and ensure the provision of healthcare when otherwise unavailable; (h) ensure a competent public health and personal healthcare workforce; (i) evaluate effectiveness, accessibility, and quality of personal and population-based health services; and (j) research for new insights and innovative solutions to health problems.[118]

Public health information network   *See* **PHIN**.

Public information   Data which, by their nature, require nonspecific handling, limited disclosure, protected storage, and disposal.[1]

Public key   A key in an asymmetric algorithm that is publicly available. Used for verifying a signature after it has been signed. *See also* **Digital signature**.[1]

Public key algorithms   A method of cryptography in which one key is used to encrypt a message and another key is used to decrypt it.[1]

Public key certificate   *See* **PKC**.

Public key cryptography   Encryption system that uses a linked pair of keys; one key encrypts, the other key decrypts.[1]

Public key infrastructure   *See* **PKI**.

Push   Putting data on a stack.[1]

PVC   Permanent virtual circuit. A fixed circuit between two users in a packet-switched network. PVCs are more efficient for connections between hosts that communicate frequently. *See also* **SVC**.[1]

PWF   Post-processing workflow. Addresses the need to schedule, distribute, and track the status of typical post-processing workflow steps, such as computer-aided detection or image processing. Work lists for each of these tasks are generated and can be queried, work items can be selected, and the status returned from the system performing the work to the system managing the work. *See also* **Profile**.[56]

PWP   Personnel White Pages. Provides access to basic human workforce user directory information. This information has broad use among many clinical and nonclinical applications across the healthcare enterprise. The information can be used to enhance the clinical workflow (contact information), enhance the user interface (user friendly names and titles), and ensure identity (digital certificates). This Personnel White Pages directory will be related to the user identity provided by the Enterprise User Authentication (EUA) Integration Profile previously defined by IHE. *See also* **Profile**.[56]

Q

QMF   Query management facility. Ad hoc query tool to extract data from some mainframe systems.[15]

QMR   Quick medical reference. Search system for the National Library of Medicine.[141]

Qualified certificate   In public key infrastructure security information technology, a qualified certificate is used to describe a certificate with a certain qualified status within applicable governing law.[121]

Quality   The totality of features and other characteristics of a product or service that bear on its ability to satisfy stated or implied needs.[123]

Quality assessment   The act of detecting and measuring the differences between efficacy and effectiveness that can be attributed to care, including variations across regions and people.[4]

Quality assurance   The formal and systematic exercise of identifying problems in medical care delivery, designing activities to overcome the problems, and carrying out follow-up steps to ensure that no new problems have been introduced, and that corrective actions have been effective.[4]

Quality control   A process to control the quality of care and services.[4]

Quality design   Systematic approach to service design that identifies the key features needed or desired by both external and internal clients; creates design options for the desired features, and then selects the combination of options that will maximize satisfaction within available resources.[123]

Quality improvement   An approach to the study and improvement of the processes of providing healthcare services to meet needs of clients.[123]

Quality indicator   An agreed-upon process to outcome measurement that is used to determine the level of quality achieved. A measurable variable, or characteristic, that can be used to determine the degree of adherence to a standard or achievement of quality goals.[123]

Quality management   An ongoing effort to provide services that meet or exceed customer expectations through a structured, systematic process for creating organizational participation in planning and implementing quality improvements.[123]

Quality measures   Mechanisms used to assign a quantity to quality of care by comparison to a criterion.[138]

Quality monitoring   The collection and analysis of data for selected indicators which enable managers to determine whether key standards are being achieved as planned, and are having the expected effect on the target population.[123]

Quality of care   Degrees of excellence of care in relation to actual medical knowledge, identified by quality tracers based on outcomes of care, as well as on structure and process.[4]

Quantity   Attribute of a phenomenon, body, or substance that may be distinguished qualitatively and determined quantitatively (e.g., length).[4]

Query **1.** The process by which a Web client requests specific information from a Web server, based on a character string that is passed along. **2.** A request for information that results in the aggregation and retrieval of data.[1,6]

Query management facility *See* **QMF.**

Queue A storage concept in which data are ordered in such a manner that the next data item to be retrieved is the one stored first. This concept is characterized as 'first-in-first-out' (FIFO).[8]

Queuing services This service provides store and forward capabilities. It can use message queues, as well as other persistence mechanisms, to store information. This service can be used for asynchronous types of operations.[8]

Quick medical reference *See* **QMR.**

QWERTY Keyboard layout named after the first six letters on the top left row of keys.[1]

R

R&C **Reasonable & customary.** An amount charged by a provider for services or supplies that is not in excess of the charge made by most providers in the same locality.[15]

RA **Registration authority. 1.** Body responsible for assigning healthcare coding scheme designators and for maintaining the Register of Health Care Coding Schemes as described in a standard. **2.** Entity that is responsible for identification and authentication of certificate subjects, but that does not sign or issue certificates (i.e., an RA is delegated certain tasks on behalf of a CA).[4,121]

Radio frequency identification *See* **RFID.**

Radio frequency interference Disruption caused by radio and television. A subset of electromagnetic interference.[1]

Radiology information system *See* **RIS.**

Radiology PACS **Picture archiving communications system.** Rather than using film, computed radiography uses an imaging plate. This plate contains photostimulable storage phosphors, which retain the latent image. When the imaging plate is scanned with a laser beam in the digitizer, the latent image information is released as visible light. This light is captured and converted into a digital stream to compute the digital image.[2]

RAID **Redundant array of independent disks.** A method of storing data on multiple hard disks. When disks are arranged in a RAID configuration, the computer sees them all as one large disk. However, they operate much more efficiently than a single hard drive. Since the data is spread out over multiple disks, the reading and writing operations can take place on multiple disks at once, which can speed up hard drive access time significantly.[2]

RAM **Random access memory. 1.** Primary storage of data or program instructions that can directly access any randomly chosen location in the same amount of time. **2.** The data in RAM stays there only as long as the computer is running. When the computer is turned off, RAM loses its data.[1]

Random access memory *See* **RAM.**

RARP **Reverse address resolution protocol.** Discovers the IP address of a device by broadcasting a request on a network. Hardware address to IP address resolution.[1]

RAS **Remote access server.** Dial-in capability of Windows NT providing remote access to the server or the entire network from a remote location. Allows the use of modems, ISDN, and X.25 adapters for connectivity.[1]

Raster A synonym for grid. Sometimes used to refer to the grid of addressable positions in an output device.[1]

Raster graphics Digital images created or captured as a set of samples of a given space. A raster is a grid of x and y coordinates on a display space. Examples of raster image file types are BMP, TIFF, GIF, and JPEG files.[1]

Rate A special form of proportion that includes specification of time.[123]

Ratio The relationship between two numbers.[123]

RDBMS **Relational database management system.** A type of DBMS that stores data in the form of related tables. Relational databases are powerful because they require few assumptions about how data are related or how they will be extracted from the database. As a result, the same database can be viewed in many different ways. *See also* **DBMS**.[1]

RDF Resource description framework.

RDISK Windows NT command to initiate the creation or updating of an emergency repair disk (ERD).[1]

Read codes Clinical terminology system used in United Kingdom, now NHS Clinical Terms, Version 3.[73]

Reader/writer A smart card reader/writer device provides a means for passing information from the smart card to a larger computer, and for writing information from the larger computer onto the smart card.[1]

Reader/writer driver layer The layer in various reader and writer devices that pulls information from, writes to, or erases segments and/or zones of a smart card.[1]

Read-only memory *See* **ROM**.

Realm A sphere of authority, expertise, or preference that influences the range of concepts and descriptions required, or the frequency with which they are used. A realm may be a nation, an organization, a professional discipline, a specialty, or an individual user.[19]

Real-time system Online computer that generates a nearly simultaneous output from the inputs received.[1]

Reasonable & customary *See* **R&C**.

REC Recommendation.

Record **1.** Document stating results achieved or providing evidence of activities performed. **2.** A collection of fields that are related to, or associated with, a focal point.[68,6]

Reduced instruction set computer *See* **RISC**.

Redundant array of independent disks *See* **RAID**.

Reference architecture Generalized architecture of several end systems that share one or more common domains. The reference architecture defines the infrastructure common to the end systems and the interfaces of components that will be included in the end systems. The ref-

erence architecture is then instantiated to create a software architecture of a specific system.[8]

Reference information model *See* **RIM**.

Reference model A structure used to describe a logical process.[4]

Reference model for open distributed processing *See* **RM-ODP**.

Reference terminology Standardized terminology that comprises a set of terms to which the terminology in the interface terminologies is mapped, enabling comparisons to be made even when different terminologies are used.[11]

Reference terminology model *See* **RTM**.

Refreezing Integrating the changes with existing behavioral frameworks to recreate a natural, whole, and stable entity.[6]

Regional health information organization *See* **RHIO**.

Registration authority *See* **RA**.

Registry Directory-like system that focuses solely on managing data pertaining to one conceptual entity. In an EHR, registries store, maintain, and provide access to peripheral information not categorized as clinical in nature, but required to operationalize an EHR. The primary purpose of a registry is to respond to searches using one or more predefined parameters in order to find and retrieve a unique occurrence of an entity.[8]

Regression model A data mining statistical method that predicts a value based on the correlation between two or more independent predictor values.[1]

Regression testing A hypothesis testing event that attempts to determine whether a recent change in one part of the application affects another specific event.[6]

Relational data model A logical database model that treats data as if they were stored in two-dimensional tables. It can relate data stored in one table to data in another, as long as the two tables share a common data element.[1]

Relational database A flexible collection of data stored in various locations that are held together by common elements.[6]

Relational database management system *See* **RDBMS**.

Relational online analytical processing (OLAP) *See* **ROLAP**.

Relationship Link between two or more concepts.[4]

Relationships table A data table consisting of rows, each of which represents a relationship.[19]

Relative value unit *See* **RVU**.

Reliability A measure of consistency of data items based on their reproducibility and an estimation of their error of measurement.[1]

Relying party Recipient of a certificate who acts in reliance on that certificate and/or digital signature verified using that certificate.[121]

Remote access Access to a system or to information therein, typically by telephone or communication network, by a customer who is physically removed from the system.[4]

Remote access server *See* **RAS**.

Remote access software The software that enables remote or mobile users to dial into a network and access the network resources.[1]

Remote boot Windows NT network service that can boot MS-DOS and Windows 95 computers from across the network.[1]

Remote hosting A form of outsourcing where a client's personal computers are networked into a vendor's remote data processing center via high-speed phone lines. Rapid response times allow the client to access software at the vendor's site. Thus, a client avoids hardware costs and shares processing and software costs with the vendor's other remote processing clients. If this is done with a Web-based architecture, it is referred to as *application service provisioning (ASP)*.[2]

Remote method invocation *See* **RMI**.

Remote network monitor *See* **RMON**.

Remote procedure call *See* **RPC**.

Remote service A support service (e.g., testing, diagnostics, software upgrades) which is not physically or directly connected to the device (e.g., remote access via modem, network, Internet).[45]

Removable media *See* **Electronic media**.

Rendering Process of formatting a print job by the print processor in Windows NT before delivery to a print device.[1]

Repeater Device that extends a LAN by increasing the signal of a LAN segment and joining it with another. The repeater forwards every packet appearing on one network to another.[1]

Repetition separator The repetition separator is used in some data fields to separate multiple occurrences of a field. It is used only where specifically authorized in the descriptions of the relevant data fields.[16]

Replication Periodic push duplication of specific data over the network from one server (export) to another (import).[1]

Reporting workflow *See* **RWF**.

Repository 1. A repository is a central place where data is stored and maintained. A repository can be a place where multiple databases or files are located for distribution over a network, or a repository can be a location that is directly accessible to the user without having to travel across a network. 2. An implementation of a collection of information along with data access and control mechanisms, such as search, indexing, storage, retrieval, and security.[7,8]

Repudiation Denial by one of the entities involved in a communication of having participated in all, or part of, the communication.[1]

Request for information *See* **RFI**.

Request for proposal *See* **RFP**.

Request to send *See* **RTS**.

Requirements A set of needs, functions, and demands, which need to be satisfied by a particular software implementation or specification.[4]

Research Systematic investigation, including research development, testing, and evaluation, designed to develop or contribute to generalized knowledge.[48]

Resident virus A computer virus that installs itself as part of the operating system to infect all suitable hosts that are accessed.[1]

Residual risk   Risk remaining after risk control measures have been taken.[68]

Resolution   Measure of graphical image dot density sharpness on a monitor. The higher the density, the sharper the display.[1]

Resource description framework   *See* **RDF**.

Retention   The maintenance and preservation of information in some form (e.g., paper, microfilm, or electronic storage) for a given period of time. There are no federal laws outlining time frames for the retention of health information.[1]

Retrieve information for display   *See* **RID**.

Return on investment   *See* **ROI**.

Reusability   The ability to use code developed for one application in another application, traditionally achieved using program libraries.[8]

Reverse address resolution protocol   *See* **RARP**.

Revocation   The process of permanently ending the operational period of a certificate from a specified time forward. Generally, revocation is performed when a private key has been compromised.[114]

RFI   **Request for information.** A standard business process, the purpose of which is to collect written information about the capabilities of various suppliers. Normally it follows a format that can be used for comparative purposes.[7]

RFID   **Radio frequency identification.** The RFID tag is attached to the patient, medications, or supplies. The tag consists of a microchip with an antenna, and an interrogator or reader with an antenna. The reader sends out electromagnetic waves. The tag antenna is tuned to receive these waves. A passive RFID tag draws power from the field created by the reader and uses it to power the microchip's circuits. The chip then modulates the waves that the tag sends back to the reader, and the reader converts the new waves into digital data.[2]

RFP   **Request for proposal.** An RFP typically asks for more than a price, including basic corporate information and history, financial information, and product information, such as stock availability and estimated completion period. The bidder returns a quote or proposal by a set date and time, known as a tender closing. The proposals are used to evaluate the suitability as a supplier, vendor, or institutional partner.[7]

RHIN   **Regional health information network.** *See* **RHIO**.[1]

RHIO   **Regional health information organization. 1.** A legally defined, neutral organization that adheres to a defined governance structure, which is composed of and facilitates collaboration among stakeholders in a given medical trading area, community, or region; and is dedicated to the promotion and use of secure digital health information exchange, in order to advance the effective and efficient delivery of healthcare for individuals and communities. **2.** A RHIO can be described as a network of stakeholders within a defined region who are committed to improving the quality, safety, access, and efficiency of healthcare through use of HIT. No two RHIOs look alike, and each reflects the unique nature and interests of its region and resources. **3.** A group of organizations with a business stake in improving the quality, safety, and efficiency of healthcare delivery. The purpose of a RHIO is to electronically exchange health information in a secure format so that the receiver can use the information. The terms 'RHIO' and 'health information exchange' or 'HIE' are often used interchangeably.[45]

Rich text format   *See* **RTF**.

RID   **Retrieve information for display.** A simple and rapid read-only access to patient information necessary for provision of better care. It supports access to existing persistent documents in well-known presentation formats, such as CDA, PDF, JPEG, etc. It also supports access to specific key patient-centric information, such as allergies, current medications, summary of reports, etc., for presentation to a clinician. *See also* **Profile**.[56]

RIM   **Reference information model.** A static model of health and healthcare information as viewed within the scope of HL7 standards development activities. It is the combined consensus view of information from the perspective of the HL7 working group and the HL7 international affiliates. The RIM is the ultimate source from which all HL7 Version 3.0 protocol specification standards draw their information-related content.[16]

Ring network Network topology in which all computers are linked by a closed loop in a manner that passes data in one direction, from one computer to another.[1]

RIP Routing information protocol. Used to advertise and exchange information between routers within an autonomous system.[1]

RIS Radiology information system. The components of radiology software, hardware, and network infrastructure to support patient documentation, retrieval, and analysis. *See also* **PACS**.[1]

RISC Reduced instruction set computer. Non-microcode computer that uses a simplified set of instructions in internal firmware to speed operation. Digital Equipment Corporation (DEC, now a part of Compaq), Alpha, IBM, Power PC, and MIPS are RISC computers.[1]

Risk Combination of the probability of an event and its consequences.[124]

Risk analysis A method for assessing risk. This may be used to subsequently compare the cost of achieving something (such as hospital system security) against the risk of losing something.[4]

Risk assessment 1. Process of analyzing threats to, and vulnerabilities of, an IT system, and the potential impact that the loss of information or capabilities of a system would have on national security. The resulting analysis is used as a basis for identifying appropriate and effective measures. 2. Overall process of risk analysis and risk evalution.[97,124]

Risk control Process in which decisions are made and measures implemented, by which risks are reduced to, or maintained within, specified levels.[68]

Risk estimation Process used to assign values to the probability of occurrence of harm and the severity of that harm.[68]

Risk evaluation Process of comparing the estimated risk against given risk criteria to determine the significance of the risk.[124]

Risk management 1. Systematic application of management policies, procedures, and practices to the tasks of analyzing, evaluating, controlling, and monitoring risk. 2. Coordinated activities to direct and control an organization with regard to risk.[68,124]

Risk treatment Process of selection and implementation of measures to modify risk.[124]

RMI Remote method invocation. An adaptation of the remote procedure call paradigm for object-oriented environments.[32]

RM-ODP Reference Model for Open Distributed Processing. The RM-ODP efforts began in 1987 as part of the International Standards Organization (ISO) Object Management Group (OMG) to enable the inter-working of applications and sharing of data across computer networks spanning organizational and national boundaries. As it relates to the healthcare domain, the uppermost two of five layers deal with the information viewpoint (such as HL7, X12, DICOM, CPT) and the enterprise viewpoint (such as patient registration, order communications, results retrieval).[1]

RMON Remote network monitor. Device that collects network traffic information for use by remote monitoring stations.[1]

Roadmap Technology road mapping is a technology management tool that attempts to plan and forecast the necessary steps toward achieving one or more technology goals. Technology roadmaps are different from project plans, in that roadmaps attempt to emphasize the uncertainty in the forecast, rather than create a linked set of tasks. The value of a technology roadmap includes communicating vision, encouraging collaborative thinking, garnering necessary resources to solve technology challenges, creating contingency approaches, and consensus view for decision making. One of the most common extensions of the technology roadmap is to link it to product roadmaps and market roadmaps to provide the complete picture of 'what, why, and how' in relation to the achievement and delivery of a particular technology goal. *See also* **Transition plan**.[7]

ROI Return on investment. A calculation used to determine whether a proposed investment is wise, and how well it will repay the investor. It is calculated as the ratio of the amount gained (taken as positive) or lost (taken as negative), relative to the basis.[7]

ROLAP Relational online analytical processing (OLAP). A technical OLAP approach where data are presented dimensionally, but stored and accessed using traditional two-dimensional relational DBMS technology allowing for very high flexibility. *See also* **OLAP**.[1]

Role **1.** Roles are attributes. These terms are synonymous. **2.** Set of behaviors that are associated with a task.[19,121]

ROM **Read-only memory.** Non-volatile permanent memory written in firmware. Contents usually cannot be changed.[1]

Root cause analysis A process for identifying the basic or causal factors that underlie variation in performance, including the occurrence, or possible occurrence, of an adverse event.[31]

Root directory System base directory. All other directories and files are found under the root directory.[1]

RPC **Remote procedure call.** Essentially an M code that may use optional parameters to do some work, and then return either a single value or an array back to the client application.[12]

Router Device that attaches multiple networks, LANs, and WANs and routes packets between the networks through the use of software. *See* **Routing switch**.[1]

Routing information protocol *See* **RIP**.

Routing services This service will route messages to the various internal integration channels, based on a publish/subscribe model.[8]

Routing switch Device that attaches multiple networks, LANs, and WANs, and routes packets between the networks through the use of hardware. Ten times faster than a conventional router.[1]

Routing table Lists maintained by routers that include the most recent information on routes advertised by other routers for different destinations.[1]

RSA A public key crypto-system, invented and patented by Ronald Rivest, Ade Shamir, and Leonard Adelman, based on large prime numbers. RSA is the best-known asymmetric algorithm.[1]

RTF **Rich text format.** A minimum file format for text files that includes formatting instructions, the text itself, and very little additional information. Also called *interchange format*.[1]

RTM **Reference terminology model.** Integration of a reference terminology model for nursing is an essential first step in creating comparable nursing data across settings and countries. Without such data, it is impossible to identify and implement 'best nursing practices' (i.e., those most likely to result in positive health outcomes for patients, families, and communities, or to determine how scarce nursing resources should be spent).[3]

RTS **Request to send.** Modem control operation from DTE requesting clearance to transmit.[1]

Rule A formal way of specifying a recommendation, directive, or strategy, expressed as 'IF premise THEN conclusion' or 'IF condition THEN action.'[4]

Run chart A visual display of data that enables monitoring of a process to determine whether there is a systematic change in that process over time.[123]

RVU **Relative value unit.** A comparable service measure used by hospitals to permit comparison of the amounts of resources required to perform various services within a single department or between departments. It is determined by assigning weight to such factors as personnel time, level of skill, and sophistication of equipment required to render patient services. RVUs are a common method of physician bonus plans based partially on productivity.[139]

RWF **Reporting workflow.** Addresses the need to schedule, distribute, and track the status of the reporting workflow tasks, such as interpretation, transcription, and verification. Work lists for each of these tasks are generated and can be queried; work items can be selected, and the resulting status returned from the system performing the work to the system managing the work. *See also* **Profile**.[56]

S

S/MIME **Secure MIME.** Extends the Multipurpose Internet mail extensions (MIME) standard to allow for encrypted e-mail.[1]

Sabotage Damage to another's systems on purpose.[1]

Safeguard A protective measure to mitigate against the effect of system vulnerability.[1]

Safety Freedom from unacceptable risk of harm.[4]

Salami A technique by which criminals steal resources a little at a time. Programs may adjust payroll deductions by just a few cents in each transaction and then collect the funds. This type of transaction is very difficult to detect.[1]

SAML **Security assertion markup language.** An XML standard for exchanging authentication and authorization data between security domains; that is, between an identity provider and a service provider.[91]

Sample One or more parts taken, or to be taken from a system, and intended to provide information on that system or a subsystem, or to provide a basis for decision on either.[4]

SAN **Storage area network.** A high-speed special purpose network (or sub-network) that interconnects different kinds of data storage devices with associated data servers on behalf of a larger network of users. Typically, a storage area network is part of the overall network of computing resources for an enterprise.[2]

Sanitization Erasing all identifiers from certain files (i.e., clinical files).[1]

SATAN **Security administrator tool for analyzing networks.**[1]

Scalability The ability to support the required quality of service as load increases.[8]

Scanner A device used to digitize a picture of a document so that it can be stored in memory and on a disk. Fax machines use this process to transmit documents to other fax machines.[1]

Scatter diagram A graphic display of data plotted along two dimensions.[123]

Scenario Formal description of a class of business activities, including the semantics of business agreements, conventions, and information content.[4]

Scheduled workflow *See* **SWF.**

Scheduler Portion of the operating system that moves programs from input to ready.[1]

Schema In general, a schema is an abstract representation of an object's characteristics and relationship to other objects. An XML schema represents the interrelationship between the attributes and elements of an XML object (e.g., a document or a portion of a document). To create a schema for a document, one would analyze its structure, defining each structural element as it is encountered (e.g., within a schema for a document describing a Web site, one would define a Web site element, a Web page element, and other elements that describe possible content divisions within any page on that site). Just as in XML and HTML, elements are defined within a set of tags.[33,42]

Schmeist head Person who executes a system command without knowing what the command will do.[1]

Science of clinical informatics The transformation of clinical data into information, then knowledge, which supports clinical decision making. This transformation requires an understanding of how clinicians structure decision making and what data are required to support this process.[6]

SCOS **Smart card operating system.** Organizes data on the integrated circuit chip into files, and protects them from unauthorized access.[1]

Screen saver A moving picture or pattern that is displayed on the screen when no activity takes place for a specified period of time; also called a *time out*.[1]

Script A type of code or program that consists of a set of instructions for another application or utility to use.[1]

SCUI **Smart card user interface.** Provides a standard interface between applications and the data on the chip. Multiple applications can reside on the chip, and the SCUI allows an application to access its own data without affecting another application's data.[1]

SDLC **System design life cycle.** The process used by a systems analyst to develop an information system, including requirements, validation, training, and user ownership through investigation, analysis, design, implementation, and maintenance. SDLC is also known as information systems development or application development. An SDLC should result in a high quality system that meets or exceeds customer expectations, within time and cost estimates, works effectively and efficiently in the current and planned information technology infrastructure, is inexpensive to maintain, and cost-effective to enhance.[7]

SDO Standard development organization. Standardization in the field of information for health, and health information and communications technology, to achieve compatibility and interoperability between independent systems. Also, to ensure compatibility of data for comparative statistical purposes (e.g., classifications) and to reduce duplication of effort and redundancies.[3]

Search engine A type of software that creates indexes of databases or Internet sites based on the titles or files, keywords, or the full text of files. The result of a search on the engine is a list of documents in which the keywords were found.[1]

Search/resolution services This service is used to interface with resolution services present in registries, such as client, provider, and other registries. It is also used to resolve situations where clinical data about a client resides in different locations and systems across an interoperated network of EHRs.[8]

Searchable identifiers Characteristics that uniquely identify an information object, support persistent access to that object, and support access to information about the object (i.e., metadata).[44]

Seat license The fee is paid per user or 'per seat,' or per concurrent user, through negotiations with a vendor to allow a fixed number of copies of copyrighted software. *See also* **Site license**.[1]

SEC Security. Establishes basic security measures that can, as part of an institution's overall security policies and procedures in the enterprise, help protect the confidentiality of patient information. It also provides institutions with a mechanism to consolidate audit trail events on user activity across several systems interconnected in a secure manner. *See also* **Profile**.[56]

Secondary data use Use of data for additional purposes than the primary reason for their collection, adding value to this data.[94]

Secondary record A record that is derived from the primary record and contains selected data elements.[1]

Secrecy The intentional concealment or withholding of information.[1]

Secret key A key in a symmetric algorithm; the possession of this key is restricted, usually to two entities.[1]

Secure communications channel Ensure the authenticity, the integrity, and the confidentiality of transactions, and the mutual trust between communicating parties.[48]

Secure electronic transmission *See* **SET**.

Secure HTTP *See* **S-HTTP**.

Secure MIME *See* **S/MIME**.

Secure shell *See* **SSH**.

Secure socket layer *See* **SSL**.

Secure Web server A program that implements certain cryptographic protocols to prevent eavesdropping on information transferred between a Web server and a Web browser. A server resistant to a determined attack over the Internet or from corporate insiders.[1]

Security Measures and controls that ensure confidentiality, integrity, availability, and accountability of the information processed and stored by a computer.[97]

Security administration control Includes all management control measures and appropriate policies necessary to provide an acceptable level of protection of data stored in the data system.[1]

Security administrator A member of the data system management team trained in data security matters, authorized to enforce the data security measures, and to create a confidentiality-/privacy-conscious working environment.[1]

Security and control testing A testing event that examines the presence and appropriate functioning of the application's security and controls to ensure integrity and confidentiality of data.[6]

Security architecture A plan and set of principles for an administrative domain and its security domains that describe the security services a system is required to provide to meet the needs of its users, the system elements required to implement the services, and the performance levels required in the elements to deal with the threat environment.[8]

Security assertion markup language *See* SAML.

Security compromise A specific loss of a component of the security system, due to an unauthorized person obtaining classified information.[1]

Security incident The attempted or successful unauthorized access, use, disclosure, modification, or destruction of information or interference with system operations in an information system.[118]

Security level Categorization of a controlled resource or defined data user.[1]

Security manager The person assigned responsibility for management of the organization's security program.[1]

Security overhead The total cost, in dollars, of the added hardware features and software drafting/running to serve the safeguarding purposes.[1]

Security policy The framework within which an organization establishes needed levels of information security to achieve the desired confidentiality goals.[1]

Security process The series of activities that monitor, evaluate, test, certify, accredit, and maintain the system accreditation throughout the system life-cycle.[97]

Security requirements Types and levels of protection necessary for equipment, data, information, applications, and facilities to meet security policy.[97]

Security service A processing or communication service that is provided by a system to give a specific kind of protection to resources, where said resources may reside with said system or reside with other systems (e.g., an authentication service, or a PKI-based document attribution and authentication service).[8]

Security system of a data system The integrated combination of technological means, security administrator's activities, and the related statutory laws intended to prevent accidental or unauthorized disclosure of clinical data, modification, or destruction of stored clinical data, or damage to the clinical data system, or at least to reduce the risk to an acceptable level.[1]

Security tool A program run to evaluate or enhance the security of a site.[1]

Security, design-in The provision of hardware and software features for security from the inception of the system.[1]

Segment A logical grouping of data fields. Segments of a message may be required or optional. They may occur only once in a message or they may be allowed to repeat. Each segment is identified by a unique character code known as the segment identifier.[16]

Semantic A subfield of linguistics that is traditionally defined as the study of meaning of (parts of) words, phrases, sentences, and texts.[7]

Semantic correspondence Measure of similarity between concepts.[126]

Semantic interoperability **1.** Ability for data shared by systems to be understood at the level of fully defined domain concepts. **2.** The ability to preserve the meaning of exchanged information.[124]

Semantic link Formal representation of a directed associative relation or partitive relation between two concepts.[126]

Semantic network A formalism (often expressed graphically) for representing relational information, the arcs of the network representing the relationships, and the nodes of objects in the network.[4]

Semantic Web The Semantic Web is a project that intends to create a universal medium for information exchange by giving meaning (semantics), in a manner understandable by machines, to the content of documents on the Web. Currently under the direction of the Web's creator, Tim Berners-Lee of the World Wide Web Consortium, the Semantic Web extends the ability of the World Wide Web through the use of standards, markup languages, and related processing tools.[7]

Semantics Meaning of symbols and codes.[4]

Sensitivity label A security level associated with the content of the information. Society has historically considered as sensitive that information which has a heightened potential for causing harm to the patient or data subject, or to others, such as the subject's spouse, children, friends, or partners.[1]

Sentinel event Unexpected occurrences involving death, serious physical or psychological injury, or risk thereof. Serious injury specifically includes loss of limb or function. The phrase 'risk thereof' includes any process variation for which a recurrence would carry a significant chance of serious adverse outcomes. Sometimes called a "never" event.[31]

Sequence A task in a process is enabled after the completion of a preceding task in the same process.[112]

Serial line Internet protocol *See* **SLIP**.

Serial transmission Sequential transmission of the signal elements of a group representing a character or other entity of data. The characters are transmitted in a sequence over a single line, rather than simultaneously over two or more lines, as in parallel transmission.[57]

Server Centralized network computer that provides an array of resources and services to network users. Also, a program that responds to a request from a client.[1]

Service Discrete units of application logic that expose loosely coupled message-based interfaces suitable for being accessed across a network.[8]

Service event The act of providing a health-related service.[8]

Service-oriented architecture *See* **SOA**.

Session A period of interaction. **1.** In computer science, in particular, networking. A session is either a lasting connection using the session layer of a network protocol or a lasting connection between a user (or user agent) and a peer, typically a server. **2.** In healthcare, a period of treatment, a 'therapy session.' **3.** Government: legislative, judicial, or executive session.[8]

Session layer Fifth layer of the OSI model. Provides file management needed to support intersystem communication through the use of synchronization and data stream checkpoints.

Also responsible for the establishment, management, and termination of sessions.[1]

Session management service This service manages user sessions. A user session will contain information such as ticket number, function and role information, authorization information, and other information that the system may choose to store to provide efficient access to information.[8]

SET Secure electronic transmission. A cryptographic protocol designed for sending encrypted credit card numbers over the Internet.[1]

Severity Measure of the possible consequences of a hazard.[68]

Severity system Expected likelihood of disease progression independent of treatment. Systems attempting to measure severity may use diagnostic codes, such as ICD, and/or additional clinical information.[53]

sFTP Secure File Transport Protocol. Standard for secure transfer of packets of information from one computer system to another. Commonly used in the transport of files of information containing confidential information.[99]

SGML Standardized general markup language. A metalanguage in which one can define markup languages for documents. SGML is a descendant of IBM's Generalized Markup Language (GML), developed in the 1960s by Charles Goldfarb, Edward Mosher, and Raymond Lorie (whose surname initials also happen to be GML). SGML should not be confused with the Geography Markup Language (GML) developed by the Open GIS Consortium, cf, or the Game Maker scripting language, GML. SGML provides a variety of markup syntaxes that can be used for many applications.[3]

SGMP Simple gateway monitoring protocol. Allows commands to be issued to application protocol entities to set or retrieve values (integer or octet string types) for use in monitoring the gateways on which the application protocol entities reside. SGMP was replaced by SNMP (simple network management protocol).[7]

Shared environment A computing environment in which a midrange or mainframe computer at a remote location provides the main information systems processing for several clients. Terminals are linked to the shared host computer.[2]

Shared service An approach to computerization provided by service organizations that offer remote computer services with supporting software functions for the full range of hospital business and clinical applications.[2]

Shared space A mechanism that provides storage of, and access to, data for users with bounded network space. Enterprise-shared space refers to a store of data that is accessible within or across security domains on the global information grid. A shared space provides virtual access to any number of data assets (catalogs, Web sites, registries, document storage database). Any user, system or application that posts data, uses shared space.[18]

Shareware Software that can be tried before purchase. It is distributed through online services and user groups.[1]

Shielded twisted pair See **STP**.

Shockwave A set of programs that allows Macromedia Director animation files to be played over the Internet with a Web browser.[1]

S-HTTP Secure HTTP. A system for signing and encrypting information sent over the Web's HTTP protocol. See **HTTP**.[1]

SIG Special interest group. Subset of professional computer organizations that concentrates on a specific technical computing area.[1]

SIMM Single in-line memory module. A type of RAM chip.[1]

Simple gateway monitoring protocol See **SGMP**.

Simple image and numeric report See **SINR**.

Simple mail transfer protocol See **SMTP**.

Simple merge The convergence of two or more branches into a single subsequent branch, such that each enablement of an incoming branch results in the thread of control being passed to the subsequent branch.[112] See **Exclusive choice**.

Simple network monitoring protocol See **SNMP**.

Simple object access protocol See **SOAP**.

Simplex Communication channel/circuit that allows data transmission in one direction only.[1]

Simulation Resembles a real-life situation that the learner might encounter; learners can engage in safe decision making.[6]

Simultaneous peripheral operation online See **SPOOL**.

Single in-line memory module See **SIMM**.

Single sign-on A specialized form of software authentication that enables a user to authenticate once and gain access to the resources of multiple software systems.

SINR Simple image and numeric report. Facilitates the growing use of digital dictation, voice recognition, and specialized reporting packages, by separating the functions of reporting into discrete actors for creation, management, storage, and viewing. Separating these functions while defining transactions to exchange the reports between them enables a vendor to include one or more of these functions in an actual system. See also **Profile**.[56]

Site license A renewable fee that has been paid through negotiations with a vendor to allow a fixed number of copies of copyrighted software at one site. See **Seat license**.[1]

SLIP Serial line Internet protocol. Minimal overhead protocol for TCP/IP-only data transfer over serial links, such as telephone circuits or RS-232 cables. Does not support multiple protocols, encryption, or compression. The precursor to PPP.[1]

Slow-scan video A device that transmits and receives still video pictures over a narrow telecommunications channel.[106]

Smart card An integrated circuit card which incorporates a processor unit. The processor may be used for security algorithms, data access, or for other functions according to the nature and purpose of the card.[4]

Smart card operating system See **SCOS**.

Smart card user interface See **SCUI**.

SMAU Multiple station access unit. A token-ring network hub.[1]

SME Subject matter expert. An individual who has expertise on a particular topic.

SMP **Symmetrical multi-processing.** A computing platform technology in which a single server uses multiple CPUs in a parallel fashion, managed by a single operating system.[1]

SMTP **Simple mail transfer protocol.** Protocol used to transfer mail between systems and from one computer to another. SMTP specifies how two mail systems interact, and the format of control messages they exchange to transfer mail.[1]

SNA **System network architecture.** Network architecture developed by IBM for mainframe networking. Does not interoperate with TCP/IP.[1]

Sniffer Network tool that collects network traffic packets to provide analysis on network and protocol usage, and generates statistics to assist in monitoring and optimizing networks.[1]

Sniffers Programs used to intercept clear text data in packets transmitted through local area networks. A method of eavesdropping on communications.[1]

SNMP **Simple network monitoring protocol.** Used to monitor hosts, routers, and networks. Enables a monitoring management station to configure, monitor, and receive alarms from network devices.[1]

SNMP **System network management protocol.** Forms part of the Internet protocol suite as defined by the Internet Engineering Task Force. The protocol can support monitoring of network-attached devices for any conditions that warrant administrative attention.[7]

SNOMED CT **Systematic Nomenclature of Medicine.** A controlled healthcare terminology developed by the College of American Pathologists in collaboration with the United Kingdom's National Health Service. SNOMED CT includes comprehensive coverage of diseases, clinical findings, therapies, procedures, and outcomes. Nursing experts from SNOMED and the international nursing community have worked to specify nursing requirements within SNOMED that will ensure that the mappings between the NANDA diagnoses concepts, the NIC intervention concepts, and the NOC outcome concepts will be appropriate.[19]

SOA **Service-oriented architecture. 1.** An infrastructure where many N-tier applications are deployed, sharing common software services that are accessible from any user interface. In this environment, any application can access any service, provided the application has the proper security permissions. The greatest strength of a service-oriented architecture is the potential for repeatable rapid development of new applications. It depends on interoperable services for the provision of high-value business logic processing. **2.** A software architectural concept that defines the use of services to support the requirements of software users. In an SOA environment, nodes on a network make resources available to other participants in the network as independent services that the participants access in a standardized way.[7,8]

SOAP **Simple object access protocol.** A third-generation programmable Web service built on top of standards-based Internet protocols that can be implemented on any platform, in any language.[1]

Socket The logical address of a communications access point to a specific device or program on a host. A socket is defined as the endpoint in a connection. Also, the communication between a client program and a server program in a network. *See also* **API, SSL.**[1]

Soft copy File maintained on disk in electronic storage format.[1]

Software A computer program encoded in such a fashion that the program (the instruction set) contents can be changed with minimal effort. Computer software can have various functions, such as controlling hardware, performing computations, communication with other software, human interaction, etc., all of which are prescribed in the program.[7]

Software access The ability and the means to communicate with the operating system or any file/database controlled by the operating system of a clinical data sytem.[1]

Software architecture The software architecture of a program or computing system is the structure or structures of the system, which comprise software components, the externally visible properties of those components, and the relationships among them.[8]

Software asset management A management process for making software acquisition and disposal decisions. It includes strategies that identify and eliminate unused or infrequently used software, consolidating software licenses, or moving toward new licensing models.[1]

Software security system A computer operating system certified as incorporating those hardware and software functions and features that are necessary to prohibit accidental or malicious access.[1]

SONET Synchronous optical network. ANSI standard for high-speed, high-quality digital optical transmission on optical media. The international equivalent of SONET is synchronous digital hierarchy. *See also* **ATM, Frame relay.**[1]

SOP Standard operating procedure. Formalized way of uniformly carrying out a process.[15]

Source systems Application systems where service encounter data is collected (e.g., laboratory information systems, pharmaceutical information systems, immunization systems). This clinical data is extracted from the source system and transformed prior to it being used in the electronic health record. *See also* **Feeder systems.**[8]

SOW Statement of work. A document describing the specific tasks and methodologies that will be followed to satisfy the requirements of an associated contract or memorandum of understanding (MOU).[10]

SP Subportal. A subportal provides highly targeted aggregate content and interactive capabilities that focus on a specific vertical healthcare market segment, as opposed to overall portals, such as Yahoo or Microsoft Network.[1]

Spam Trash e-mail. The practice of blindly or intentionally posting commercial messages or advertisements to a large number of unrelated and uninterested newsgroups.[1]

SPD Summary plan description. Document that explains the product and services a subscriber purchased.[15]

Special interest group *See* **SIG.**

Specification An explicit statement of the required characteristics for an input used in the healthcare system. The requirements are usually related to supplies, equipment, and physi-

cal structures used in the delivery of health services.[123]

Spider *See* **Web crawler.**[7]

SPIN Standard Prescriber Identification Number. National Council for Prescription Drug Programs sponsored the Standard Prescriber Identification Number from the early- to mid-1990s in an effort to address the need for a unique prescriber identifier for the retail pharmacy industry. However, the Health Insurance Portability and Accountability Act of 1996 (HIPAA) contained a provision for a National Provider Identifier (NPI). Years passed with no National Provider Identifier (NPI). Unfortunately, the need that NCPDP and others had identified in the early to mid-1990s did not diminish, but steadily grew over these years. By early 2001, NCPDP launched the HCIdea™ project, which is now ready for general release. On January 23, 2004, HHS published the Final Rule for the HIPAA NPI in the *Federal Register.*[54]

SPOOL Simultaneous peripheral operation online. It refers to putting jobs in a buffer, a special area in memory, or on a disk where a device can access them when it is ready. This is similar to a sewing machine spool, which a person puts thread onto, and a machine pulls at its convenience. Spooling is useful because devices access data at different rates. The buffer provides a waiting station where data can reside while the slower device catches up. Material is only added and deleted at the ends of the area; there is no random access or editing. This also allows the CPU to work on other tasks, while waiting for the slower device to do its task.[7]

Spooler Service that buffers data for low-speed output devices.[1]

Spreadsheet A spreadsheet is a rectangular table (or grid) of information, often financial information. (It is, therefore, a kind of matrix.) Spreadsheet programs can be used to tabulate many kinds of information, not just financial records; so the term 'spreadsheet' has developed a more general meaning as information (= data = facts) presented in a rectangular table, usually generated by a computer.[7]

Sprite An element that can be manipulated in an animation. Each different object in an animation is called a sprite.[57]

SQL   Structured query language. A syntax used by many database programs to retrieve and modify information (pronounced either *see-kwell* or as separate letters). SQL is a standardized query language for requesting information from a database.[1]

SRAM   Static random access memory. A type of memory that is faster and more reliable than the more common dynamic RAM or DRAM. The term static is derived from the fact that it does not need to be refreshed like dynamic RAM.[1]

SSH   Secure shell. Encrypted remote terminal that provides confidentiality and authentication.[1]

SSL   Secure socket layer. Secure method and protocol for managing the secure transfer of data between a Web browser and a Web server. *See also* **Socket, API**.[1]

Stack   Last in first out (LIFO) data holding structure.[1]

Standard   1. A document established by consensus and approved by a recognized body that provides, for common and repeated use, rules, guidelines, or characteristics for activities or their results, aimed at the achievement of the optimum degree of order in a given context. **2.** A definition or format that has been approved by a recognized standards organization, or is accepted as a de facto standard by the industry. Standards exist for programming languages, operating systems, data formats, communications protocols, and electrical interfaces.[117,7]

Standard development organization   *See* **SDO**.

Standard of care   1. The Standard of Care is the expected level and type of care provided by the average caregiver under a certain given set of circumstances. These circumstances are supported through findings from expert consensus and based on specific research and/or documentation in scientific literature. **2.** In the law of negligence, the degree of care which a reasonable, prudent, or careful person should exercise under the same or similar circumstances. If the standard falls below that established by law for the protection of others against unreasonable risk of harm, the person may be liable for damages resulting from such conduct.[138]

Standard operating procedure   *See* **SOP**.

Standard prescriber identification number *See* **SPIN**.

Standardization   Activity of establishing, with regard to actual or potential problems, provisions for common and repeated use, aimed at the achievement of the optimum degree of order in a given content.[4]

Standardization of terminology   Official recognition of a terminology by an authoritative body.[4]

Standardized general markup language *See* **SGML**.

Standardized taxonomy   Use of common standardized definitions, criteria, terminology, and data elements for treatment processes, outcomes, data collection, and electronic transmission, with the goal of saving much time, effort, and misunderstanding in communicating these elements.[1]

Standards body   Body that is recognized at national, regional, or international level that has as a principle function, by virtue of statutes, for the preparation, approval, or adoption of standards that are made generally available.[4]

Standing orders   Physicians' orders preestablished and approved for use by nurses and other professionals under specific conditions, in the absence of a physician.[123]

Star network   Type of LAN topology in which networked nodes are connected to a hub at a central point.[1]

Star schema   A data modeling technique and relational DBMS extension that is optimized for ad hoc, unpredictable, and denormalized data queries. It facilitates simple and speedy access to information by decision support users. *See also* **OLTP**.[1]

Start of care   *See* **admission date**.

Statement of work   *See* **SOW**.

Static audit tool   System scanner that looks for and reports weaknesses.[1]

Static memory   Memory that does not need to be refreshed while power is maintained. Faster than dynamic memory.[1]

Static random access memory *See* **SRAM**.

Statistical healthcare classification Exhaustive set of mutually exclusive categories to support aggregation of data at a pre-prescribed level of specialization for specific healthcare purposes.[126]

Stealth virus A type of resident virus that attempts to evade detection by concealing its presence in infected files. To achieve this, the virus intercepts system calls, which examine the contents and attributes of infected files.[1]

Steganography Hiding information in innocuous files and documents (e.g., insertion of instructions that modify portions of a program's output to carry information).[1]

Stemming A process that determines the morphological root of a given inflected (or, sometimes, derived) word form. A stemmer for English, for example, should identify the string 'cats' (and possibly 'catlike,' 'catty,' etc.) as based on the root 'cat,' and 'stemmer,' 'stemming,' and 'stemmed,' as based on 'stem.' Used by search engines and for natural language processing.[7]

Storage The function of storing records for future retrieval and use.[95]

Storage area network *See* **SAN**.

Store-and-forward Transmission of static images or audio-video clips to a remote data storage device, from which they can be retrieved by a medical practitioner for review and consultation at any time, obviating the need for the simultaneous availability of the consulting parties and reducing transmission costs due to low bandwidth requirements.[106]

Storyboard Originally developed in the Disney Studios in the 1930s, storyboards allow action elements to be identified and organized into various sequences to form a story. Storyboards are used to brainstorm and capture all the ideas before taking action. The process of visual thinking and planning allows a group of people to brainstorm together, placing their ideas on storyboards, and then arranging the storyboards on the wall. This fosters more ideas and generates consensus inside the group.[7]

STP Shielded twisted pair. Type of cabling 1.5 inches in diameter, in which the wire pairs are twisted together in a shielded protective jacket to reduce the effects of EMI. Used to implement 10BaseT - 100BaseT networks.[1]

Stream algorithms Algorithms that encrypt data byte-by-byte.[1]

Streaming A technique for delivering data used with audio and video, in which the recipient is able to hear or see part of the file before the entire file is delivered. Involves a method for the recipient computer to be able to do a smooth delivery, despite the uneven arrival of data.[11]

Structural role Role of an individual within an organization.[122]

Structured data Coded, semantically interoperable data that is based on a reference information model. The consent directive may be captured as a scanned image, which is not semantically interoperable and would preclude the ability of the consent repository to analyze it for conflicts with previously persisted consent directives.[48]

Structured query language *See* **SQL**.

Subject field Domain; field of special knowledge.[98]

Subject matter expert *See* **SME**.

Subject of care Person or defined groups of persons receiving, or registered as eligible to receive, healthcare services, or having received healthcare services.[117]

Subject of care identifier A unique number or code issued for the purpose of identifying a subject of (health)care.[95]

Subnet mask 32-bit portion of an IP address that identifies a specific network or host within a subnetwork.[1]

Subportal *See* **SP**.

Subscription services Services that provide capabilities to subscribe to events and manage the alerts and notifications functions when enabled.[8]

Subset Subsets represent groups of components that share specified characteristics that affect the way they are displayed or otherwise accessible within a particular realm, specialty, application, or context.[19]

Substitution A method of cryptography based on the principle of replacing each letter in the message with another one.[1]

Substitution cipher A cipher that replaces the characters of the original plain text. The characters retain their original position, but are altered.[1]

Subtype A specialization of a concept, sharing all the definitional attributes of the parent concept, with additional granularity. For example, bacterial infectious disease is a subtype of infectious disease. Bacterial septicemia, bacteremia, bacterial peritonitis, etc., are subtypes of bacterial infectious disease (and infectious disease as well).[19]

Summary plan description *See* **SPD.**

Sundial A common type of electronic mail used over the Internet.[1]

Super user Individuals identified within the end user groups as advocates for the new system; individuals better able to interact with, teach, and provide peer support for the new system.[6]

Super video graphics array *See* **SVGA.**

Superzapping The unauthorized use of utility computer programs to modify, copy, disclose, destroy, insert, use, or deny use of data stored in a computer or computer media. Type of computer crime.[1]

Surge suppressor A device to protect systems against power spikes.[1]

Surveillance The word 'surveillance' is commonly used to describe observation from a distance by means of electronic equipment or other technological means. *See also* **Biosurveillance.**[7]

Surveillance data source Application system or services that provide clinical and demographic data to be used by health surveillance systems.[8]

SVC **Switched virtual circuit.** A temporary virtual circuit that is set up and used only as long as data are being transmitted. Once the communication between the two hosts is complete, the SVC disappears. In contrast, a perma-nent virtual circuit (PVC) remains available at all times.[1]

SVGA **Super video graphics array.** Color display system providing high-resolution graphics of multiple colors at various resolutions.[1]

SWF **Scheduled workflow.** Establishes the continuity and integrity of basic departmental imaging data acquired in an environment where examinations are generally being ordered. It specifies a number of transactions that maintain the consistency of patient and ordering information, as well as defining the scheduling and imaging acquisition procedure steps. This profile also makes it possible to determine whether images and other evidence objects associated with a particular performed procedure step have been stored (archived), and are available to enable subsequent workflow steps, such as reporting. It may also provide central coordination of the completion of processing and reporting steps. *See also* **Profile.**[56]

Switch Within the Open Systems Interconnection (OSI) standard, as defined by the International Standards Organization, a switch is a high throughput network communications device that functions within the second layer, or data-link layer, to direct packets of information to specific destinations or network nodes.[1]

Switched virtual circuit *See* **SVC.**

Symbol Designation of a concept by letters, numerals, pictograms, or any combination thereof.[4]

Symmetric digital subscriber line *See* **Symmetric DSL/SDSL.**

Symmetric DSL/SDSL **Symmetric digital subscriber line.** A new technology that allows more data to be sent over existing copper telephone lines. *See also* **DSL.**[1]

Symmetric key algorithms Encryption algorithm in which the same key is used to encrypt and decrypt the message.[1]

Symmetric multiprocessing Multiprocessing technique that utilizes all available processors in a computer to execute the operating system and applications.[1]

Symmetrical multi-processing *See* **SMP.**

Synchronization The convergence of two or more branches into a single subsequent branch, such that the thread of control is passed to the subsequent branch when all input branches have been enabled.[112]

Synchronous optical network *See* **SONET**.

Synchronous transmission High-speed simultaneous transmission of large blocks of data.[1]

Synonym A term which is an acceptable alternative to the preferred term as a way of expressing a concept.[19]

Synonymy Relation between designations representing only one concept in one language.[3]

Syntax The rules of grammar; an organized set of rules for use. The rules and conventions that one needs to know or follow in order to validly record information, or interpret previously recorded information, for a specific purpose. Thus, a syntax is a grammar. Such rules and conventions may be either explicit or implicit. In X12 transactions, the data-element separators, the sub-element separators, the segment terminators, the segment identifiers, the loops, the loop identifiers (when present), the repetition factors, etc., are all aspects of the X12 syntax. When explicit, such syntactical elements tend to be the structural, or format-related, data elements that are not required when a direct data entry architecture is used. Ultimately, though, there is not a perfectly clear division between the syntactical elements and the business data content.[10]

System The combination of hardware and software which processes information for the customer.[4]

System architecture Describes the systems, capabilities, and information exchanges to support the business requirements and processes.[20]

System audit A systematic investigation of the effectiveness of an information resource in meeting its original goals.[6]

System design A specification of human factors, and hardware and software requirements, for an information system.[6]

System design life cycle *See* **SDLC**.

System developmental life cycle A structured and systematic process for the development and installation of an information system comprised of the following phases: analysis, design, development, implementation, and evaluation.[6]

System integration The ability of computers, instrumentation, and equipment to share data or applications with other components in the same or other functional areas. *See also* **EAI**.

System network architecture *See* **SNA**.

System network management protocol *See* **SNMP**.

System security The result of all safeguards, including hardware, software, personnel policies, information practice policies, disaster preparedness, and oversight of these components.[1]

System security administrator The person who controls access to computer systems by entering commands to perform such functions, such as assigning user access codes and privileges, revoking user access privileges, and setting file protection parameters.[1]

System testing A multi-faceted testing event that evaluates the functionality, performance, and fit of the whole application. System testing encompasses usability, final requirements, volume and stress, security and controls, recovery, documentation and procedures, and multi-site testing.[6]

Systematic Nomenclature of Medicine *See* **SNOMED CT**.

Systems administrator The individual who maintains the system and has system administrator privileges. In order to avoid errors and mistakes done by this individual while not acting as an administrator, he/she should limit the time he/she acts as an administrator (as known to the system) to a minimum.[118]

System's analysis The process of analyzing a user's needs to drive functional requirements.[6]

Systems integration Generally refers to the outsourcing of certain information systems tasks to a consultant, which may include customer support for users, operations, the design and development of system interface requirements and software, product and vendor selection, system testing and evaluation, modeling, software and/or hardware configuration and installation, project management, and other services.[1]

Systems integrator A firm that delivers the various services of systems integration.[1]

T

Table Database object with a unique name, and structured in columns and rows.[1]

TAG Technical advisory group. A group of topic experts working in a particular area and building consensus among the group for specific positions. Used mainly in consensus standards work.[3,48]

Tag image file format *See* **TIFF.**

Tags Information within a Web page contained between angle brackets (<>) which indicate document elements, structure, formatting, and hyperlinks. HTML tags are generally used to surround the text that they affect.[1]

Tampering Unauthorized modification that alters the proper functioning of a smart card.[1]

Task A logical unit of work that is carried out as a whole. Tasks can be executed based on sequential, parallel, or conditional routing.[111]

Task manager Provides information on CPU usage, memory usage, and physical memory statistics.[1]

Taxonomy A method of classifying a vocabulary of terms for a specific topic according to specific laws and principles.[6]

TC Technical committee. A term, often used by consensus standards organizations, including HL7, CEN, and ISO.[3,48]

T-Carrier High-speed, point-to-point, full duplex communications line identified in different levels: T-1, T-2, T-3, and T-4.[1]

TCO Total cost ownership. A document that describes the cost of a project or initiative that usually includes hardware, software, development, and ongoing expenses.[15]

TCP Transmission control protocol. Connection-oriented data transmission mode portion of TCP/IP.[1]

TCP/IP Transmission control protocol/ Internet protocol. Routable protocol required for Internet accesses. TCP portion is associated with data. IP is associated with source to destination packet delivery.[1]

TDR Time-domain reflectometer. Testing device that sends sound waves along cabling to detect shorts or breaks in the cable.[1]

Technical advisory group *See* **TAG.**

Technical architecture Describes the minimal set of rules governing the arrangement, interaction, and interdependence of system parts or elements.[20]

Technical committee *See* **TC.**

Technical framework The document that defines integration profiles, the problems and use cases they address, and the actors and transactions involved. It provides detailed implementation instructions for each transaction.[56]

Technical report A collection of informative data on a particular topic. Examples are survey data, implementation guide, a literature review of a specific topic, or an overview of a technical product or service.[3]

Technical safeguards Policies and procedures to protect electronic health information and control access.[48]

Technical specification A technical description of the desired behavior of a system, as derived from its requirements. A specification is used to develop and test an implementation of a system.[1]

Technical specification A second level ISO deliverable. Contains both normative and informative knowledge.[3]

Telecommunications The use of wire, radio, optical, or other electromagnetic channels to transmit or receive signals for voice, data, and video communications.[106]

TELecommunications NETwork *See* **TELNET.**

Teleconsultation Geographic separation between two or more providers during a consultation.[106]

Telediagnosis The detection of a disease by evaluating data transmitted to a receiving station from instruments monitoring a distant patient.[106]

Telehealth Using communications networks to provide health services including, but not limited to, direct care, health prevention, consulting, and home visits to patients in a geographical location different than the provider of these services. Any delivery of health services to a client in a geographical location different than that of the provider.[11]

Telematics The use of computer-based information processing in telecommunications, and the use of telecommunications to allow computers to transfer programs and data to one another.[106]

Telemedicine Part of telehealth that is defined as a health professional in one location, using electronic technologies for the diagnosis and/or treatment of a patient in another location.[11]

Telementoring The use of audio, video, and other telecommunications and electronic information processing technologies to provide individual guidance or instruction (e.g., involving a consultant guiding a distant clinician in a new medical procedure).[106]

Telemonitoring The use of audio, video, and other telecommunications and electronic information processing technologies to monitor patient status at a distance.[106]

Telenursing Practice of nursing over distance using telecommunications technology.[11]

Telepresence The use of robotic and other devices that allow a person (e.g., a surgeon) to perform a task at a remote site by manipulating instruments (e.g., lasers or dental hand pieces) and receiving sensory information or feedback (e.g., pressure akin to that created by touching a patient) that creates a sense of being present at the remote site, and allows a satisfactory degree of technical performance (e.g., dexterity).[106]

TELNET **TEL**ecommunications **NET**work. Protocol for remote terminal service connectivity. Connectivity from one site to interact with a remote system. A method of logging one computer onto another. A program that allows users to remotely use computers across networks.[1]

Terabyte Approximately one trillion bytes; unit of computer storage capacity.[1]

Term **1.** Verbal designation of a concept in a specific subject field. **2.** The word or phase in a particular language used to represent a concept (e.g., the concept doctor is represented in English by the term 'doctor' or 'physician,' and in Italian by the term 'il medico.')[98,4]

Terminal Not a PC, but rather a video terminal connected to a mainframe. Also called a *dumb terminal*, since no processing is accomplished at the local level, and the terminal has a dependency upon the mainframe computer. *See also* **Workstation**.[1]

Terminal printing suppression Suppressing the printing of passwords or other access control information.[1]

Terminal server Network communications device that allows one or more serial devices to connect to an Ethernet LAN. Used extensively throughout CHCS with the LAT protocol.[1]

Terminology A system of words used to name things in a particular discipline.[32]

Terminology identifier Unique permanent identifier of a healthcare terminology for use in information interchange.[98]

Test log A thorough record of testing, results, and follow-up.[6]

Test objectives Descriptions of what a specific testing event seeks to validate. The objectives state each feature of function to be tested and describe, at a high level, the expected results.[6]

TFTP **Trivial file transfer protocol.** Minimal overhead file transfer used to upload or download bootstrap files to diskless workstations through the use of UDP.[1]

Thesaurus The vocabulary of a controlled indexing language, formally organized so that the a priori relationships between concepts (e.g., broader and narrower) are made explicit.[3]

Thin client/dumb terminal A thin client is a low-cost, centrally managed computer, devoid of CD-ROM players, diskette drives, and expansion slots. Since the idea is to limit the capabilities of these computers to only essential applications, they tend to be purchased and remain 'thin' in terms of the client applications they include. This device can be used to access data on a mainframe, but does not process data locally on the device.[2]

Third party Party, other than data originator or data recipient, required to perform a security function as part of a communication protocol.[121]

Third party administrator *See* **TPA**.

Third party vendor *See* **TPV**.

Threat **1.** Any circumstance or event with the potential to cause harm to an IT system in the form of destruction, disclosure, adverse modification of data, and/or denial of service. **2.** Exploitation or compromise of a security of systems or networks.[97,48]

Threshold A level of achievement that determines the difference between what is deemed to be acceptable quality or not.[123]

Thunking Translation that takes place from 32- to 16-bit code.[1]

TIFF **Tag image file format.** A common format for exchanging raster graphics (bitmap) images between application programs, including those used for scanner images.[57]

Tightly coupled Tightly coupled application roles assume that common information about the subject classes participating in a message are available to system components outside of the specific message.[8]

Time bomb A subclass of logic bombs that explode at a certain event, such as a certain date. Can be used to damage disk directories on a certain date.[1]

Time to live *See* **TTL**.

Time-domain reflectometer *See* **TDR**.

TLAlgia Term composed of 'TLA' for three-letter acronym and '-algia' meaning 'pain'; thus, pain induced by excessive use of three-letter acronyms.[99]

tn3270 The tn3270 program is a TELNET program used to connect to an IBM mainframe and emulate a 3270 terminal, which is dumb terminal. *See also* **TELNET**.[1]

Token 1. A physical authentication device that the user carries (e.g., smart card, SecureID™). Often combined with a PIN to provide a two-factor authentication method that is generally thought of as superior to simple password authentication. **2.** Packet used for LAN access in a token-based network. The node that possesses the token controls the transmission medium, and is allowed to transmit on the network.[45,1]

Token-bus network Type of LAN topology in which networked nodes are connected to the main cable of the network. Uses a token for transmission access.[1]

Token-ring network Type of LAN topology in which networked nodes are connected at points to form a ring in which data packets travel. Uses a token for transmission access.[1]

Top-level concept A concept that is directly related to the root concept by a single relationship of the relationship type 'IS-A.' All other concepts are descended from one top-level concept via at least one series of relationships of the relationship type 'ISA' (i.e., all other concepts are subtypes of one top-level concept).[19]

Topology Physical layout or architecture of a network. Bus, Star, Ring, and Hybrid are network topologies.[1]

Total cost ownership *See* **TCO**.

Total quality management *See* **TQM**.

Touch screen Input technology that permits the entering or selecting of commands and data by touching the surface of a sensitized video display monitor with a finger or pointer.[1]

TPA **Third-party administrator.** A company that provides claim processing and administrative services for hospital or physicians groups.[15]

TPV **Third party vendor.** A company designated to support specific services for healthcare.[15]

TQM **Total quality management.** An approach to quality assurance that emphasizes to all members of a production unit of the needs and desires of the ultimate service recipients in the chain of service, and acknowledges how to use specific data-related techniques to assess and improve the quality of their own and the team's outputs.[123]

Traceroute A command causing the utility to initiate the sending of a packet, including in the packet a time limit that is designed to be exceeded by the first router that receives it, which will return a 'time exceeded' message.[1]

Trading partner agreement Related to the exchange of information in electronic transactions, specifically the communications protocols and transaction standards to be used.[48]

Train the trainer A core group of individuals are trained and then used to train other individuals who will be using the system. This is a common strategy when there are hundreds of users to be trained in a matter of weeks.[6]

Transaction **1.** The exchange of information between two parties to carry out clinical, financial, and administrative activities related to healthcare. **2.** An exchange of information between actors. For each transaction, the TF describes how to use an established standard, such as HL7, DICOM, or W3C.[10,56]

Transaction standard A standard specifying the format of messages being sent from or received by a system, rather than for how the information is stored in the system.[10]

Transition plan A written plan for a transition from the current organizational structure to a design that will minimize disruption, adverse impacts, capitalization, and startup requirements. A high level strategy/map to guide the adoption of systems or technologies. *See also* **Roadmap**.[150]

Transitions of care *See* **Care Transitions**.

Transmission The exchange of data between person and program, or program and program, when the sender and receiver are remote from each other.[1]

Transmission confidentiality Process to ensure that information in transit is not disclosed to unauthorized individuals, entities, or processes.[48]

Transmission control protocol *See* **TCP**.

Transmission control protocol/Internet protocol *See* **TCP/IP**.

Transmission integrity Process to guard against improper information modification or destruction while in transit.[48]

Transparent background Transparent GIF images can have one color designed to be transparent. Since all graphic images are stored as either square or rectangular shapes, even the background color will show up on a Web page. *See also* **GIF**.[1]

Transport layer Fourth layer of the OSI model. Handles the interface between hardware levels and software levels. Provides for end-to-end flow control and ensures that messages are delivered error-free.[1]

Transposition A method of cryptography based on the principle of scrambling the characters that are in the message.[1]

Transposition cipher A cipher in cryptography that rearranges the characters of the original plain message. Thus, the characters are unchanged, but their position is altered, making the text unintelligible.[1]

Trap doors Hardware features, software limitations, or specially planted entry points that can provide an unauthorized source with access to the system. *See also* **Back door**.[1]

Treatment The total bundle of services rendered to a patient in order to cope with a specific problem.[4]

Treatment protocols Precise and detailed plans for the study of a medical or biomedical problem and/or plans for a regimen of therapy.[5]

Trial implementation supplement A specification candidate for addition to an IHE Domain Technical Framework (e.g., a new profile) that is issued for early implementation by any interested party. The authoring technical committee expects developers' feedback.[93]

Trigger event An event such as the reception of a message or completion of a process, which causes another action to occur.[56]

Trivial file transfer protocol *See* **TFTP**.

Trojan horse A program that appears to have one ubiquitous function, but actually has a hidden malicious function. A program that performs a desired task, but also includes unexpected and usually undesirable functions. Does not replicate.[1]

Trunk Single circuit between two switching center points. Handles many channels simultaneously.[1]

Trust Windows NT domain association with another Windows NT domain, where the domains trust each other with resources.[1]

Trust-based security Security management and access provision based on trusted domains or facilities.[8]

Trusted system A system delivered to enforce a given set of attributes to a stated degree of assurance or confidence.[1]

Trusted third party *See* **TTP**.

Trusted user access level A system user who needs access to sensitive information.[1]

TTL Time to live. Length of active Internet time technique used to avoid endless loop packets. Every packet is assigned a decrementing TTL. Packets with expired TTLs are discarded by routers.[1]

TTP Trusted third party. Third party which is considered trusted for purposes of a security protocol.[121] (ENV 13608-1). Note: This term is used in many ISO/IEC International Standards and other documents describing mainly the services of a certification authority (CA). The concept is, however, broader and includes services such as time-stamping and possibly escrowing.

Tunneling *See* **Virtual private network**.[8]

Turnkey portal Refers to a Web application that provides access to various applications or content within a healthcare organization or to its consumers that has been developed by a vendor to facilitate easier implementation and support of the environment. The turnkey portal can have applications to support physicians and clinicians, patients/consumers, employers, etc. It can be used by internal employees (clinicians, executives, business, and marketing professionals) or external customers (patients/consumers, employers, payers, etc.).[7]

Tutorial A type of computer assisted learning (CAI) providing information which the learner interacts with by answering questions.

Responses provided by the learner may generate additional tutoring, or allow the learner to advance in the program.[6]

Twisted-pair cable Cable consisting of copper core wires surrounded by an insulator. A pair, consisting of two wires twisted together, forms a circuit that can transmit data. The twisting helps to prevent interference.[1]

U

UART Universal asynchronous receiver transmitter. The microchip with programming that controls a computer's interface to its attached serial devices.[42]

Ubiquitous computing Ubiquitous computing (ubicomp, or sometimes ubiqcomp) integrates computation into the environment, rather than having computers which are distinct objects. Another term for ubiquitous computing is 'pervasive computing.' Promoters of this idea hope that embedding computation into the environment would enable people to move around and interact with computers more naturally than they currently do. One of the goals of ubiquitous computing is to enable devices to sense changes in their environment, and to automatically adapt and act based on these changes, based on user needs and preferences. Some simple examples of this type of behavior include GPS-equipped automobiles that give interactive driving directions and RFID store checkout systems.[7]

UCC Uniform Code Council. European Article Numbering-Uniform Code Council (EAN-UCC) is the international organization of product barcodes that are printed on almost everything that is sold in stores worldwide, and is used in healthcare for pharmaceutical products and medical and surgical supplies for inpatient and outpatient healthcare areas. The UCC is the numbering organization in the U.S. to administer and manage the EAN·UCC system standards in the U.S. and Canada. In 2005, the organization changed its name to GS1.[7]

UDDI Universal Description, Discover, and Integration. An XML-based registry for businesses worldwide to list themselves on the Internet. Its ultimate goal is to streamline online transactions by enabling companies to find one another on the Web and make their systems interoperable for eCommerce. UDDI is often compared to a telephone book's white, yellow, and green pages. The project allows businesses to list themselves by name, product, location, or the Web services they offer.[8]

UDI Unique device identifier. A method of knowing a specific object apart from other objects like itself.[109]

UDK User defined keys. Used to store frequently used commands through the F6 to F20 keys on a video terminal keyboard.[1]

UDP User datagram protocol. A connectionless protocol that resides at the same level on the OSI model as TCP. Since it is connectionless, there is no handshaking or authentication.[1]

UI User interface. 1. The part of the application that allows the user to access the application and manipulate its functionality. It can include menus, forms, command buttons, etc. **2.** The part of the information system through which the end user interacts with the system; type of hardware and the series of on-screen commands and responses required for a user to work with the system.[107,1]

UM Utilization management. The evaluation of the necessity, appropriateness, and efficiency of the use of healthcare services, procedures, and facilities.[15]

UMDNS Universal medical device nomenclature system. The purpose of UMDNS is to facilitate identifying, processing, filing, storing, retrieving, transferring, and communicating data about medical devices. The nomenclature is used in applications ranging from hospital inventory and work order controls to national agency medical device regulatory systems, and from eCommerce and procurement to medical device databases.[55]

UMLS The Unified Medical Language System. A large project sponsored by the United States National Library of Medicine (NLM) to produce a unified thesaurus and cross reference linking various medical nomenclatures, including the MeSH headings, ICD-9-CM, SNOMED, and the Terminology of DXPlain and QMR.[4]

UMS Unified messaging system. The handling of voice, fax, and regular text messages as objects in a single mailbox that a user can

access either with a regular e-mail client or by telephone.[1]

UNC Universal naming convention. Text-based method to identify the path to a remote device, server, directory, or file. Implemented as: \\computername\sharename\directoryname\filename.[1]

Underuse Refers to the failure to provide a healthcare service when it would have produced a favorable outcome for a patient. Standard examples include failures to provide appropriate preventive services to eligible patients (e.g., Pap smears, flu shots for elderly patients, screening for hypertension) and proven medications for chronic illnesses (e.g., steroid inhalers for asthmatics, aspirin, beta-blockers, and lipid-lowering agents for patients who have suffered a recent myocardial infarction).[14]

Undirected information Information that is broadcast without regard to who reads it. Usenet and mailing lists are undirected.[1]

Unfreezing Requires information which discontinues the current behaviors or attitudes. It also requires some sense that change can be safely made.[6]

Unicode A standard character set that represents most of the characters used in the world using a 16-bit encoding. Unicode can be encoded in using UTF-8 to more efficiently store the most common ASCII characters.[19]

Unified messaging system *See* **UMS.**

Uniform Code Council *See* **UCC.**

Uniform resource locator *See* **URL.**

Uninterruptible power supply *See* **UPS.**

Unique device identifier *See* **UDI.**

Unique identifier *See* **NPI.**

Unit testing A document that guides a tester through a testing event and ensures consistency among separate executions of the testing event.[6]

Universal asynchronous receiver transmitter *See* **UART.**

Universal identifier A means to provide positive recognition of a particular individual for all people in a population. A universal healthcare or patient identifier provides the identifier for use in healthcare transactions.[1]

Universal medical device nomenclature system *See* **UMDNS**.

Universal naming convention *See* **UNC**.

Universal product code *See* **UPC**.

Universal product number *See* **UPN**.

Universal resource locator *See* **URL**.

UNIX Operating system for microcomputers, minicomputers, and mainframes that is machine-independent and supports multi-user processing, multi-tasking, and networking. UNIX was developed at AT&T's Bell Laboratories in 1969.[1]

UPC **Universal product code.** A unique 12-digit number assigned to retail merchandise that identifies both the product and the vendor that sells the product. The UPC on a product typically appears adjacent to its bar code, the machine-readable representation of the UPC. The first six digits of the UPC are the vendor's unique identification number. All of the products that one vendor sells will have the same first six digits in their UPCs. The next five digits are the product's unique reference number that identifies the product within any one vendor's line of products. The last number is called the check digit that is used to verify that the UPC for that specific product is correct.[58]

UPI **Unique patient identifier.** The identity of an individual consists of a set of personal characters by which that individual can be recognized. Identification is the proof of one's identity. Identifier verifies the sameness of one's identity. Patient identifier is the value assigned to an individual to facilitate positive identification of that individual for healthcare purposes. Unique patient identifier is the value permanently assigned to an individual for identification purposes, and is unique across the entire national healthcare system. Unique patient identifier is not shared with any other individual.[1]

Upload To send a file to another machine.[1]

UPN **Universal product number.** *See also* **UPC**.

UPS **Uninterruptible power supply.** Device that keeps a computer running by protecting against power outages and power sags by maintaining constant power via battery. Provides the opportunity for a graceful shutdown in a commercial power-out condition.[1]

URI **Uniform resource identifiers.** Provides a simple and extensible means for identifying a resource. A URI can be further classified as a locator, a name, or both.[8]

URL **Uniform resource locator.** Provides the unique location information by using a naming convention of protocol type, followed by a specific service.[1]

URL **Universal resource locator.** A standardized address name layout for resources, such as documents or images, on the Internet or elsewhere.[7]

Usability Quality attributed to an application system that describes its effectiveness and ease of use as determined by its users.[8]

Usability testing A testing event that determines how well the user will be able to use and understand the application.[6]

Use Sharing, employment, application, utilization, examination, or analysis of information within the entity that maintains such information.[48]

Use case Describes a set of activities of a system from the point of view of its actors, which lead to a perceptible outcome for the actors. A use case is always initiated by an actor. In all other respects, a use case is a complete, indivisible description.[8]

USENET A network of newsgroups. Thousands of newsgroups are available through USENET. Each one covers a specific topic or subject area.[1]

User **1.** A person, device, program, or computer system that uses a computer system for the purpose of data processing and information exchange. **2.** In electronic mail, a person or a functional unit that participates in message handling as a potential source or destination.[8]

User access A person or a group/organization in need of data for legitimate service function, teaching, or research, authorized to have access.[1]

User authentication The provision of assurance of the claimed identity of an individual or entity.[1]

User datagram protocol *See* **UDP**.

User defined keys *See* **UDK**.

User ID The string of characters that identifies a computer/system user. The user name by which the user is known to the network. Also called *username*.[1]

User interface *See* **UI**.

User profile A description of a user, typically used for access control. A user profile may include data such as user ID, user name, password, access rights, and other attributes. It is a pattern of a user's activity that can be used to detect changes in the activity.[3]

User-friendly Characteristics of a computer-human interface which contribute to its acceptance by users.[7]

Utility program System software consisting of programs for routine, repetitive tasks, which can be shared by many users.[1]

Utilization management *See* **UM**.

Utilization review An organized procedure carried out through committees to review admissions, duration of stay, professional services furnished, and to evaluate the medical necessity of those services and promote their most efficient use.[5]

UTP Type of cabling in which the insulated wire conductors are twisted together in an unshielded voice-grade cable. Used to implement 10BaseT and 100BaseT networks.[1]

V

Validation Determination of the correct implementation in the completed IT system, with the security requirements and approach agreed-upon by the users and the acquisition authority.[97]

Validity The extent to which data correspond to the actual state of affairs, or an instrument that measures what it purports to measure.[1]

Value-added network *See* **VAN**.

VAN Value-added network. A vendor of electronic data interchange (EDI) data communications and translation services.[10]

Vanilla Software implemented 'as is,' with no (or minimal) customization.

Vaporware Software that does not currently exist, but may be introduced sometime in the future.[1]

Variance analysis Data collection and aggregation techniques that are used to determine difference in care, outcomes, performance, budgets, and systems.[6]

Variant virus A type of virus generated by modifying a known virus. These modifications may add functionality, or ways to evade detection.[1]

Variation Differences in the output of a process resulting from the influences of people, equipment, materials, and /or methods.[123]

VAX Virtual address extension. An established line of mid-range server computers from the Digital Equipment Corporation (DEC, now a part of Hewlett-Packard). *See also* **VMS**.[1]

Vendor A company/consortium that provides products and/or services.[8]

Verification Confirmation, through the provision of objective evidence, that specified requirements have been fulfilled.[68]

Veronica A title search and retrieval system for use with the Internet Gopher.[147]

Veterans Health Information Systems Technology Architecture *See* **VistA**.

VGA Video graphics array. Color display system providing high-resolution graphics displays of 16 colors at a 640x480 resolution, and 256 colors at a 320x200 resolution.[1]

Video graphics array *See* **VGA**.

Video RAM or video random access memory *See* **VRAM**.

Virtual address extension *See* **VAX**.

Virtual card The data elements contained in the data indices without regard for physical addresses.[1]

Virtual community   A virtual community is a community of people sharing common interests, ideas, and feelings over the Internet of collaborative networks.[7]

Virtual memory system   *See* **VMS**.

Virtual private network   *See* **VPN**.

Virtual reality   An emerging technology that attempts to fully immerse the user in an interactive computer-generated environment. The participant, in a virtual reality experience, interacts with the system via a series of sensors and sophisticated output devices.[1]

Virtual reality modeling language   *See* **VRML**.

Virus   **1.** A type of programmed threat—a code fragment (not an independent program) that reproduces by attaching to another program. It may damage data directly, or it may degrade system performance by taking over system resources, which are then not available to authorized users. **2.** Code embedded within a program that causes a copy of itself to be inserted in one or more other programs; in addition to propagation, the virus usually performs some unwanted function.[118]

Virus scanner   A computer program (antivirus software) that detects a 'virus' computer program, or other kind of malware (e.g., worms and Trojans), warns of its presence, and attempts to prevent it from affecting the protected computer. Malware often results in undesired side effects generally unanticipated by the user.[45]

Visit   **1.** An episode of care at a healthcare facility. **2.** A visit to an individual care provider ('encounter').[8]

VistA   **Veterans Health Information Systems Technology Architecture.** An enterprise-wide system built around an electronic health record (EHR) and used throughout the Veterans Health Administration's 163 hospitals, 800+ clinics, and 135 nursing homes. Commonly considered to be one of the largest and most effective health IT systems in use today. Developed as the decentralized hospital computer system (DHCP), the name change to VistA signified deeper clinical content and increased GUI-zation (graphic user interface).[99]

VISTA   Microsoft's name for the latest version (2007) of its Windows operating system.[12]

VMS   **Virtual memory system.** An operating system from Digital Equipment Corporation (DEC) that runs on its computers. VMS originated in 1979 as a new operating system for DEC's new VAX computer, the successor to DEC's PDP-11.[1]

Vocabulary   A set of terms used for a particular purpose.[4]

Voice over Internet protocol   *See* **VoIP**.

Voice recognition   A software program that converts the voice audio analog to a digital signal for dictation. For a computer to decipher the signal, it must have a digital database, or vocabulary, of words or syllables and a speedy means of comparing this data with signals.[1]

Voice response system   A unit that allows a customer to call in by telephone and give instructions to a computer by speaking or by pressing digits on the phone.[1]

Voice response unit   *See* **VRU**.

VoIP   **Voice over Internet protocol.** A technology that allows users to make telephone calls using a broadband Internet connection instead of a regular (or analog) phone line. Some services using VoIP may only allow individuals to call other people using the same service, but others may allow calls to anyone who has a telephone number—including local, long distance, mobile, and international numbers. Also, while some services work only over a computer or a special VoIP phone, other services allow use of a traditional phone through an adaptor.[1]

Volume and stress testing   A testing event that determines the ability of the application to function under maximum volumes of data and peak loads.[6]

VPN   **Virtual private network. 1.** Refers to a network in which some of the parts are connected using the public Internet, but the data sent across the Internet is encrypted, so the entire network is 'virtually' private. Secure and encrypted connection between two points across the Internet. **2.** VPNs transfer information by encrypting and encapsulating traffic in IP packets and sending the packets over the Internet. That practice is called 'tunneling.' Most VPNs are built and run by Internet service providers, and secure protocols like Point-to-Point Tunneling Protocol (PPTP) to ensure that data transmissions are not intercepted by unauthorized parties. *See also* **Tunneling**.[8]

VRAM **Video RAM** or **video random access memory.** Refers to all forms of random access memory used to store image data for a computer display. VRAM is a type of buffer between the computer and the display.[1]

VRML **Virtual reality modeling language.** A standard for describing interactive three-dimensional scenes delivered across the Internet.[1]

VRU **Voice response unit.** Same as IVR.

VT100 An intelligent terminal manufactured by Digital Equipment Corporation (DEC). The term often refers to the entire family of DEC intelligent terminals. Most PC terminal emulators offer VT100 emulation.[1]

Vulnerability A weakness in a system that can be exploited to violate the system's intended behavior. There may be security, integrity, availability, and other vulnerabilities.[1]

Vulnerability assessment Systematic examination of an information system or product to determine the adequacy of security measures, identify security deficiencies, provide data from which to predict the effectiveness of proposed security measures, and confirm the adequacy of such measures after implementation.[97]

Vulnerable user access level System users who need access to information only within their job responsibility.[1]

W

WAIS **Wide-area information server.** WAIS is best at searches for various sources of academic information that have been indexed based on content. Its indices consist of every word in a document, and each word carries the same weight in a search.[1]

Wallpaper A graphical pattern displayed on the desktop computer.[1]

WAN **Wide area network.** A collection of long-distance telecommunication links and networks used to connect local area networks and end stations across regional, national, or international distances. *See also* **LAN, MAN**.[2]

WAP **Wireless application protocol.** A specification for a set of communication protocols to standardize the way that wireless devices, such as cellular telephones and radio transceivers, can be used for Internet access, including e-mail, the World Wide Web, newsgroups, and Internet Relay Chat.[1]

WASP **Wireless application service provider.** A part of a growing industry sector resulting from the convergence of two trends: wireless communications and the outsourcing of services.[1]

WAV or WAVE **Waveform audio format (.wav).** A proprietary format sponsored by Microsoft and IBM, the Resource Interchange File Format Waveform Audio Format (.wav) was introduced in MS Windows Version 3.1 and is most commonly used on Windows-based PCs.[1]

Waveform audio format (.wav) *See* **WAV or WAVE.**

Wavelet A software compression algorithm, such as that used with radiological studies.[1]

Web address An IP number or uniform resource locator (URL); a string of characters that represents the location or address of a resource on the Internet, and how that resource should be accessed.[1]

Web crawler A program that browses the World Wide Web in a methodical, automated manner. Web crawlers are mainly used to create a copy of all the visited pages for later processing by a search engine that will index the downloaded pages to provide fast searches.[7]

Web master A person who maintains and administers a Web server; also a standard e-mail address at most Web hosts where comments and questions can be sent to reach the responsible Web engineer.[1]

Web page A document created with hypertext markup language (HTML) that is part of a group of hypertext documents or resources available on the World Wide Web. *See also* **HTML, WWW**.[1]

Web portal   A Web portal is a Web site that provides a starting point, a gateway, or portal to other resources on the Internet or an intranet.[7]

Web security   A set of procedures, practices, and technologies for protecting Web servers, Web users, and their surrounding organizations.[1]

Web server   1. More often refers to software than the physical hardware. A Web server is a program that uses the client/server model and the WWW HTTP to serve the files that form Web pages to Web users (whose computers contain hypertext transfer protocol [HTTP] clients that forward their requests). 2. Every computer on the Internet that contains a Web site must have a Web server program. References may be made to hardware, or the dedicated computers on which server software resides. *See also* **HTTP, S-HTTP**.[1]

Web services description language   *See* **WSDL**.

WEP   **Wired equivalent privacy.** A security protocol, specified in the IEEE wireless fidelity (Wi-Fi) standard, 802.11b, that is designed to provide a wireless local area network (WLAN) with a level of security and privacy comparable to what is usually expected of a wired LAN.[2]

Wet signature   Ink on paper signature.[56]

WG   **Workgroup.** A workgroup is a collection of individuals working together on a task. Workgroup computing occurs when all the individuals have computers connected to a network that allows them to send e-mail to one another, share data files, and schedule meetings. Sophisticated workgroup systems allow users to define workflows so that data is automatically forwarded to appropriate people at each stage of a process.[58]

What you see is what you get   *See* **WYSIWYG**.

White board   Display in which multiple computer users in different geographical locations can write or draw while others watch. They are often used in teleconferencing.[11]

Whois   Search provides domain name registration information by domain names, IP addresses, and/or NIC handle.[147]

Wide area network   *See* **WAN**.

Wide SCSI   **Wide small computer system interface.** 20-40 Mbps high-speed interface for connecting devices to the computer bus.[1]

Wide small computer system interface   *See* **Wide SCSI**.

Wide-area information server   *See* **WAIS**.

Wi-Fi   **Wireless fidelity.** Wireless network components that are based on one of the Wi-Fi Alliance's 802.11 standards. The Wi-Fi Alliance created the 802.11 standards so that manufacturers can make wireless products that work with other manufacturers' equipment.[2]

Wi-Fi protected access   *See* **WPA**.

Wiki   Piece of server software that allows users to freely create and edit Web page content using any Web browser.[32]

Wildcard   Used when searching for files, a wildcard is a character (usually * or ?) that can stand for one or more unknown characters during a search, and cause the search results to yield all files within a general description or type of software.[1]

Window   An object on the screen that presents information, such as a document or message.[12]

Wired equivalent privacy   *See* **WEP**.

Wireless application protocol   *See* **WAP**.

Wireless application service provider   *See* **WASP**.

Wireless e-mail device   A handheld wireless device providing e-mail, telephone, text messaging, Web browsing, and other wireless data access.[36]

Wireless fidelity   *See* **Wi-Fi**.

Wireless local area network   *See* **WLAN**.

Wireless technology   Recent radio frequency architecture that transmits signals from remote, lightweight workstations to the wireless local area network (LAN) in such a way that health-related work processes can be reengineered toward greater mobility with an improved focus on the patient, such as bedside patient registration. *See also* **LAN, MAN, WAN**.[1]

WLAN   **Wireless local area network.** A wireless local area network that uses radio waves as its carrier; the last link with the users is wireless, to give a network connection to all users in the surrounding area. Areas may range from a single room to an entire campus. The backbone network usually uses cables, with one or more wireless access points connecting the wireless users to the wired network.[7]

Workflow **1.** A process description of how tasks are done, by whom, in what order, and how quickly. Workflow can be used in the context of electronic systems or people (i.e., an electronic workflow system can help automate a physician's personal workflow). **2.** A graphic representation of the flow of work in a process and its related subprocesses, including specific activities, information dependencies, and the sequence of decisions and activities.[21]

Workflow services The workflow service is responsible for maintaining lists of active components and the workflow schedules/process. It assembles the components and uses an executable engine to execute the workflow.[8]

Workgroup *See* **WG**.

Workstation Node, terminal, or computer attached to a network that runs local applications, or connects to servers to access shared server resources. Usually a microcomputer. *See also* **Terminal**.[1]

World Wide Web *See* **WWW**.

World Wide Web Consortium An international organization that develops programming and interoperability standards for the Web. Among its many projects, W3C is involved in initiatives for digital signatures, XML, and Dynamic Hypertext Mark-up Language (DHTML).[7]

WORM **Write once, read many times.** Process used for applications where permanent data storage is required.[1]

Worm A self-replicating program that hides its existence and spreads copies of itself within a computer system or through networks. Worms do not integrate their code into host programs.[1]

WPA **Wi-Fi protected access.** The latest security standard for users of computers equipped with Wi-Fi wireless connection. It is an improvement on, and is expected to replace, the original Wi-Fi security standard, Wired Equivalent Privacy (WEP). WPA provides more

sophisticated data encryption than WEP and also provides user authentication.[2]

Write once, read many times *See* **WORM**.

WSDL **Web services description language.** Provides a model and an XML format for describing Web services. WSDL enables one to separate the description of the abstract functionality offered by a service from concrete details of a service description, such as 'how' and 'where' that functionality is offered.[8]

WWW **World Wide Web.** Global network of networks offering various services to users with browsing software (Web browsers). A project originated at CERN, aimed at providing hypertext-style access to information from a wide range of sources. **2.** The graphical interface with which millions of users access Internet files that conform to the hypertext protocol (HTTP). The Web is the most accessible and widely used branch of the Internet.[8]

WYSIWYG **What you see is what you get.** Some early systems yielded a screen image that was unlike a printed document or file. This term is used to confirm that the system presents a screen image that matches what prints on paper. Pronounced 'wizzy-wig.'[1]

X

X and Y coordinates X, Y coordinates are respectively the horizontal and vertical addresses of any pixel or addressable point on a computer display screen. The 'x' coordinate is a given number of pixels along the horizontal axis. The 'y' coordinate is a given number of pixels along the vertical axis.

X.25 Packet switching network protocol with extensive error checking and accounting capability. Employs the use of permanent virtual circuits (PVC), switched virtual circuits (SVC), and packet assemblers and dissemblers.[1]

X12 standard Used to describe any ASC X12 standard that has been balloted and approved.[1]

XDS **Cross enterprise clinical document sharing.** Focused on providing a standards-based specification for managing the sharing of documents that healthcare enterprises (anywhere from a private physician, to a clinic, to an acute care inpatient facility) have decided to explicitly share. This contributes to the foundation of a shared electronic health record. *See also* **Profile**.[56]

XML   Extensible markup language. 1. General-purpose markup language for creating special-purpose markup languages. It is a simplified subset of SGML, capable of describing many different kinds of data. Its primary purpose is to facilitate the sharing of data across different systems, particularly systems connected via the Internet. **2.** Describes a class of data objects, called XML documents, and partially describes the behavior of computer programs which process them. XML is an application profile or restricted form of SGML, the Standard Generalized Markup Language (ISO 8879). By construction, XML documents are conforming SGML documents.[7]

XOR   1. A digital logic gate that implements exclusive disjunction. **2.** A logic gate that simulates the function of the logical operator XOR.

XSL   Extensible Stylesheet Language (XSL). XSL is the eXtensible Stylesheet Language, a family of languages which allows one to describe how files encoded in the XML standard are to be formatted or transformed. XSL Transformation (XSLT) is used to transform the XML document, and XSL Formatting Objects (XSL-FO) is used to render the transformed document.[8]

Y

Y2K   The calendar year 2000. Y2K required analysis, detection, remedy, and testing of software applications that depended on a program in which the year was represented by a two-digit number, such as '98' for 1998.[1]

Yahoo   Popular Internet search engine.[32]

Z

.zip   The filename extension used by files compressed into the ZIP format common on PCs.[1]

Zip drive   A small, portable disk drive used primarily for backing up and archiving personal computer files. The trademarked 'Zip' drive was developed and sold by Iomega Corporation.[1]

Zip or zipping   To package or compress a set of files into an archive file that is called a zip file. The compressed file takes up less space in storage, or takes less time to send to someone. Several popular tools exist for zipping.[1]

Zombie   1. UNIX process that does not terminate. Must be removed by the kill command.[1] **2.** A compromised Web site that is used as an attack launch point to launch an overwhelming number of requests toward an attacked Web site, which will soon be unable to service legitimate requests from its users.[1]

# #

8-bit color   A monitor with 8-bit color can display 256 colors, which is fine for business and home use, but not good enough for producing high-quality graphics. For multimedia applications, 256 colors is the minimum needed.[7]

7-   7, 7dictionary, etc.; a Web application that allows users to add content, as on an Internet forum, but also allows anyone to edit the content. The term '7' also refers to the collaborative software used to create such a Web site. The name is based on the Hawaiian term '7 7,' meaning 'quick' or 'informal.' 7 (with an upper case W) and 77Web are both used to refer specifically to the Portland Pattern Repository, the first 7 ever created.[7]

Healthcare Organizations That Have a Focus on Healthcare IT

AAACN   American Association of Ambulatory Care Nurses
The association of professional nurses and associates who identify ambulatory care practice as essential to the continuum of high quality, cost-effective health care.

> *East Holly Avenue*
> *Box 56*
> *Pitman, NJ 08071-0056*
> *Tel: 800-262-6877*
> *www.aaacn.org*

AACN   American Association of Critical-Care Nurses
Patients and their families rely on nurses at the most vulnerable times of their lives. Acute and critical care nurses rely on AACN for expert knowledge and the influence to fulfill their promise to patients and their families. AACN drives excellence because nothing less is acceptable.

> *101 Columbia*
> *Aliso Viejo, CA 92656-4109*
> *Tel: 949-362-2000*
> *Toll free: 800-899-2226*
> *Fax: 949-362-2020*
> *www.aacn.org*

AACN   American Association of Colleges of Nursing
The national voice for America's baccalaureate- and higher-degree nursing education programs. AACN's educational, research, governmental advocacy, data collection, publications, and other programs work to establish quality standards for bachelor's- and graduate-degree nursing education, assist deans and directors to implement those standards, influence the nursing profession to improve health care, and promote public support of baccalaureate and graduate education, research, and practice in nursing—the nation's largest health care profession.

> *One Dupont Circle, NW*
> *Suite 530*
> *Washington, DC 20036*
> *Tel: 202-463-6930*
> *Fax: 202-785-8320*
> *www.aacn.nche.edu*

AADE   American Association of Diabetic Educators
A professional association dedicated to promoting the expertise of the diabetes educator, ensuring the delivery of quality diabetes self-management training to the patient and contributing to the future direction of the profession.

> *100 W. Monroe*
> *Suite 400*
> *Chicago, IL 60603*
> *Tel: 800-338-3633*
> *www.diabeteseducator.org*

AAFP   American Academy of Family Physicians
To improve the health of patients, families, and communities by serving the needs of members with professionalism and creativity.

> *11400 Tomahawk Creek Parkway*
> *Leawood, KS 66211-2672*
> *Tel: 913-906-6000*
> *www.aafp.org*

AAHAM American Association of Healthcare Administrative Management
To be the premier professional organization in healthcare administrative management. Through a national organization and local chapters, AAHAM provides quality member services and leadership in the areas of education, communication, representation, professional standards and certification.

11240 Waples Mill Road
Suite 200
Fairfax, VA 22030
Tel: 703-281-4043
Fax: 703-359-7562
www.aaham.org

AAHC American Association of Healthcare Consultants
To serve as the preeminent credentialing, professional, and practice development organization for the healthcare consulting profession; to advance the knowledge, quality, and standards of practice for consulting to management in the healthcare industry; and to enhance the understanding and image of the healthcare consulting profession and Member Firms among its various publics.

5938 N. Drake Avenue
Chicago, IL 60659
Tel: 888-350-2242
www.aahc.net

AAHC American Association for Homecare
Works to strengthen access to care for the millions of Americans who require medical care in their homes, representing healthcare providers, equipment manufacturers, and other organizations in the homecare community.

2011 Crystal Drive
Suite 725
Arlington, VA 22202
Tel: 703-836-6263
Fax: 703-836-6730
www.aahomecare.org

AAHN American Association for the History of Nursing
Provides current nurses with the same intellectual and political tools that determined nursing pioneers applied to shape nursing values and beliefs to the social context of their times. Nursing history is not an ornament to be displayed on anniversary days, nor does it consist of only happy stories to be recalled and retold on special occasions. Nursing history is a vivid testimony, meant to incite, instruct and inspire today's nurses as they bravely trod the winding path of a reinvented health care system.

P.O. Box 175
Lanoka Harbor, NJ 08734
Tel: 609-693-7250
Fax: 609-693-1037
www.aahn.org

AAHP American Association of Health Plans
See AHIP (AAHP is now AHIP).

AAIHDS American Association of Integrated Healthcare Delivery Systems
Founded in 1993 as a non-profit organization dedicated to the educational advancement of provider-based managed care professionals involved in integrated healthcare delivery.

4435 Waterfront Drive
Suite 101
Glen Allen, VA 23060
Tel: 804-747-5823
Fax: 804-747-5316
www.aaihds.org

AALNA American Assisted Living Nurses Association
Promoting successful nursing practice in assisted living benefiting nurses and residents.

P.O. Box 10469
Napa, CA 94581
Tel: 760-510-6624
Fax: 707-253-8228
www.alnursing.org

AALNC American Association Legal Nurse Consultants

A not-for-profit membership organization dedicated to the professional enhancement and growth of registered nurses practicing in the specialty area of legal nurse consulting and to advancing this nursing specialty.

401 N. Michigan Avenue
Chicago, IL 60611
Tel: 877-402-2562
Fax: 312-673-6655
www.aalnc.org

AAMA American Academy of Medical Administrators

To advance excellence in healthcare leadership through individual relationships, multi-disciplinary interaction, practical business tools and active engagement.

701 Lee Street
Suite 600
Des Plaines, IL 60016
Tel: 847-759-8601
Fax: 847-759-8602
www.aameda.org

AAMC Association of American Medical Colleges

To improve the health of the public by enhancing the effectiveness of academic medicine.

2450 N Street, NW
Washington, DC 20037-1126
Tel: 202-828-0400
Fax: 202-828-1125
www.aamc.org

AAMCN American Association of Managed Care Nurses

To be recognized as the expert and resource in managed care nursing, to establish standards for managed care nursing practice, to positively impact public policy regarding managed health care delivery, and to assist in educating the public on managed care.

4435 Waterfront Drive
Suite 101
Glen Allen, VA 23060
Tel: 804-747-9698
Fax: 804-747-5316
www.aamcn.org

AAMI Association for Advancement of Medical Instrumentation

A unique alliance of over 6,000 members united by the common goal of increasing the understanding and beneficial use of medical instrumentation.

1110 N. Glebe Road
Suite 220
Arlington, VA 22201
Tel: 703-525-4890
Fax: 703-276-0793
www.aami.org

AAN American Academy of Neurology

To advance the art and science of neurology, and thereby promote the best possible care for patients with neurological disorders by: ensuring appropriate access to neurological care; supporting and advocating for an environment which ensures ethical, high quality neurological care; providing excellence in professional education by offering a variety of programs in both the clinical aspects of neurology and the basic neurosciences to physicians and allied health professionals; and supporting clinical and basic research in the neurosciences and related fields.

1080 Montreal Avenue
St. Paul, MN 55116
Tel: 651-695-2717
Fax: 651-695-2791
www.aan.com

AANA American Association of Nurse Anesthetists

Advancing patient safety and excellence in anesthesia.

222 South Prospect Avenue
Park Ridge, IL 60068-4001
Tel: 847-692-7050
Fax: 847-692-6968
www.aana.com

AANA American Association of Nurse Attorneys

Provides resources, education and leadership to its members and the healthcare and legal communities: to promote and enhance AANA and the profession of the nurse attorney; to provide educational programs, products and services to members, chapters and the public; to facilitate communication, collaboration and leadership among members; and to serve as a resource for the healthcare and legal communities.

P.O. Box 515
Columbus, OH 43216-0515
Tel: 877-538-2262
Fax: 614-221-2335
www.taana.org

AANN American Association of Neuroscience Nurses

Committed to the advancement of neuroscience nursing as a specialty through the development and support of nurses to promote excellence in patient care.

4700 W. Lake Avenue
Glenview, IL 60025
Tel: 847-375-4733
Toll free: 888-557-2266 (U.S. only)
Fax: 877-734-8677
Int'l fax: 732-460-7313
www.aann.org

AANP American Academy of Nurse Practitioners

Promote excellence in NP practice, education and research; shape the future of healthcare through advancing health policy; serve as the source of information for NPs, the healthcare community and consumers; and build a positive image of the NP role as a leader in the national and global healthcare community.

National Administration Office
P.O. Box 12846
Austin, TX 78711
Tel: 512-442-4262, ext. 5211
Fax: 512-442-6469
www.aanp.org

AAOHN American Association of Occupational Health Nurses

Vision: Work and community environments will be healthy and safe.

2920 Brandywine Road
Suite 100
Atlanta, GA 30341
Tel: 770-455-7757
Fax: 770-455-7271
www.aaohn.org

AAOS American Academy of Orthaepedic Surgeons

Serve the profession, champion the interests of patients, and advance the highest quality musculoskeletal health. This mission defines AAOS's fundamental reason for being, and establishes the parameters for its major activities and the defensible criteria against which all goals are established.

6300 North River Road
Rosemont, IL 60018-4262
Tel: 847-823-7186
Fax: 847-823-8125
www.aaos.org

AAP American Academy of Pediatrics

Committed to the attainment of optimal physical, mental, and social health and well-being for all infants, children, adolescents, and young adults.

141 Northwest Point Boulevard
Elk Grove Village, IL 60007
Tel: 847-434-4000
www.aap.org

AAPA American Academy of Physician Assistants

To promote quality, cost-effective, accessible health care, and to promote the professional and personal development of physician assistants.

950 North Washington Street
Alexandria, VA 22314-2272
Tel: 703-836-2272
Fax: 703-684-1924
www.aapa.org

AAPM&R American Academy of Physical Medicine and Rehabilitation

Serves its member physicians by advancing the specialty of physical medicine and rehabilitation, promoting excellence in physiatric practice, and advocating on public policy issues related to persons with disabling conditions.

330 North Wabash Avenue
Suite 2500
Chicago, IL 60611-7617
Tel: 312-464-9700
Fax: 312-464-0227
www.aapmr.org

AAPPO American Association of Preferred Provider Organizations

To be the most valued and effective advocate for the PPO Industry by: educating and informing the federal and state legislative and regulatory bodies concerning the benefits and value the PPO delivery system provides in partnership with providers to consumers, employers and purchasers; promoting PPO Industry best practices by developing and advancing PPO practices and guidelines including the promotion of practices to purchase shared services in an effort to reduce administration cost; advancing the business needs of Preferred Provider Networks and Payers by providing the resources to support PPO advocacy, education and services that promote empowerment; and promoting Preferred Provider Networks and PPO benefit products to purchasers, consumers, employers and the healthcare industry at large as the preferred healthcare solution.

222 S. First Street
Suite 303
Louisville, KY 40202
Tel: 502-403-1122
Fax: 502-403-1129
www.aappo.org

AARC American Association for Respiratory Care

To be the leading national and international professional association for respiratory care. The AARC will encourage and promote professional excellence, advance the science and practice of respiratory care, and serve as an advocate for patients, their families, the public, the profession and the respiratory therapist.

9425 N. MacArthur Boulevard
Suite 100
Irving, TX 75063-4706
Tel: 972-243-2272
Fax: 972-484-2720, or
972-484-6010
www.aarc.org

AASCIN American Association of Spinal Cord Injury Nurses

Promotes quality care for individuals with spinal cord injuries (SCI) by advancing SCI nursing practice through education, research, advocacy, health care policy and collaboration with consumers and health care delivery systems.

801 18th Street NW
Washington, DC 20006
Tel: 202-416-7704
Fax: 202-416-7641
www.aascin.org

ABA American Board of Anesthesiology

Examines and certifies physicians who complete an accredited program of anesthesiology training in the United States and voluntarily apply to the Board for certification or maintenance of certification. Its mission is to maintain the highest standards of the practice of anesthesiology and to serve the public, medical profession and health care facilities and organizations.

4101 Lake Boone Trail
Suite 510
Raleigh, NC 27607-7506
Tel: 919-881-2570
Fax: 919-881-2575
www.theABA.org

ABAI American Board of Allergy and Immunology
To establish qualifications and examine physician candidates for certification and recertification as specialists in allergy/immunology; serve the public and the health care community by providing the names of physicians certified as allergists/immunologists; improve the quality of health care; establish and improve standards for the teaching and practice of allergy/immunology; and establish standards for training programs in allergy/immunology working with the Residency Review Committee for Allergy and Immunology of the Accreditation Council for Graduate Medical Education (ACGME).

111 S. Independence Mall East
Suite 701
Philadelphia, PA 19106
Tel: 215-592-9466
Toll free: 866-264-5568
Fax: 215-592-9411
www.abai.org

ABCGN American Board of Certification for Gastroenterology Nurses
A volunteer non-profit organization, its purpose is to maintain and improve the knowledge, understanding and skill of nurses in the fields of gastroenterology and gastroenterology endoscopy by developing and administering a certification program.

401 N. Michigan Avenue
Chicago, IL 60611-4267
Tel: 800-245-SGNA, Option 3
Fax: 312-673-6723
www.abcgn.org

ABCRS American Board of Colon and Rectal Surgery
To promote the health and welfare of the American people through the development and maintenance of high standards for certification in the specialty of colon and rectal surgery.

20600 Eureka Road
Suite 600
Taylor, MI 48180
Tel: 734-282-9400
Fax: 734-282-9402
www.abcrs.org/default.htm

ABD American Board of Dermatology
To serve the public interest by promoting excellence in the practice of dermatology through lifelong certification.

Henry Ford Health System
1 Ford Place
Detroit, MI 48202-3450
Tel: 313-874-1088
Fax: 313-872-3221
www.abderm.org

ABEM American Board of Emergency Medicine
To protect the public by promoting and sustaining the integrity, quality, and standards of training in and practice of Emergency Medicine.

3000 Coolidge Road
East Lansing, MI 48823-6319
Tel: 517-332-4800
Fax: 517-332-2234
www.abem.org

ABFM American Board of Family Medicine
The specialty of Family Practice, based on the heritage of General Practice, would have graduate programs (residencies) for physicians whose training would encompass 1) first-contact care; 2) continuous care; 3) comprehensive care; 4) personal care (caritas); 5) family care; and 6) competency in scientific general medicine.

2228 Young Drive
Lexington, KY 40505-4294
Tel: 859-269-5626
Toll free: 888-995-5700
Fax: 859-335-7501, or
859-335-7509
www.theabfm.org

ABIM   American Board of Internal Medicine
Through ABIM's Certification and Maintenance of Certification processes, successful candidates are awarded or maintain Board Certified status. These physicians—referred to as Diplomates—have demonstrated the ability and the commitment to lifelong learning necessary to provide the high quality medical care that every patient deserves.

510 Walnut Street
Suite 1700
Philadelphia, PA 19106-3699
Tel: 215-446-3500
Toll free: 800-441-2246
Fax: 215-446-3590
www.abim.org

ABMG   American Board of Medical Genetics
(a) To elevate the standards and advance the art and science of medical genetics by encouraging its study and improving its practice; (b) to conduct examinations to determine the qualifications of medical geneticists who voluntarily apply to the ABMG for certification as Diplomates; (c) to grant and issue Diplomate certificates in the field of medical genetics and its various specialty areas to those medical geneticists who have received adequate preparation in accordance with the ABMG's educational, training, and experience requirements, and who have passed the comprehensive Certification Examinations administered by the ABMG; (d) to maintain a registry of holders of such certificates; (e) to evaluate and accredit qualified training programs in the field of medical genetics; and (f) thereby, to improve the public health.

9650 Rockville Pike
Bethesda, MD 20814-3998
Tel: 301-634-7316
Fax: 301-634-7320
www.abmg.org

ABNM   American Board of Nuclear Medicine
The primary certifying organization for nuclear medicine in the United States. The Board serves the public health through assurance of high quality patient care by establishing standards of training, and certification of initial and continuing competence for physicians rendering nuclear medicine services.

4555 Forest Park Boulevard
Suite 119
St. Louis, MO 63108
Tel: 314-367-2225
http://abnm.snm.org

ABNS   American Board of Neurological Surgery
To encourage the study, improve the practice, elevate the standards, and advance the science of neurological surgery and thereby to serve the cause of public health.

6550 Fannin Street
Suite 2139
Houston, TX 77030
Tel: 713-441-6015
Fax: 713-794-0207
www.abns.org

ABOG   American Board Obstetrics and Gynecology
To arrange and conduct examinations and/or other procedures to test the qualifications of voluntary candidates for certification and recertification by this Corporation. The criteria for certification and recertification shall be applied equally to all candidates regardless of sex, race, color or national origin.

2915 Vine Street
Dallas, TX 75204
Tel: 214-871-1619
Fax: 214-871-1943
www.abog.org

ABOHN The American Board for Occupational Health Nurses

The Occupational Health Nurse brings a unique perspective to management and clinical roles, acting as an employee advocate while balancing the needs of the workplace. Employers and peers recognize certification in occupational health nursing as a prestigious achievement. Certified occupational health nurses have passed a challenging national examination designed to test for advanced knowledge in clinical care, management, employee education, case management and safety. Certification also demonstrates that the OHN is committed to competency, education, and growth—all necessary to keep pace with the changing healthcare industry.

201 East Ogden Avenue
Suite 114
Hinsdale, IL 60521-3652
Tel: 630-789-5799
Toll free: 888-842-2646
Fax: 630-789-8901
www.abohn.org

ABOP American Board of Ophthalmology

To serve the public by improving the quality of ophthalmic practice through a certification and maintenance of certification process that fosters excellence and encourages continual learning.

111 Presidential Boulevard
Suite 241
Bala Cynwyd, PA 19004-1075
Tel: 610-664-1175
Fax: 610-664-6503
www.abop.org

ABOS American Board of Orthopaedic Surgery

To serve the best interests of the public and of the medical profession by establishing educational standards for orthopaedic residents and by evaluating the initial and continuing qualifications and knowledge of orthopaedic surgeons.

400 Silver Cedar Court
Chapel Hill, NC 27514
Tel: 919-929-7103
Fax: 919-942-8988
www.abos.org

ABOto American Board of Otolaryngology

To assure that, at the time of certification and recertification, diplomates certified by the ABOto will have met the ABOto's professional standards of training and knowledge in otolaryngology—head and neck surgery.

5615 Kirby Drive
Suite 600
Houston, TX 77005
Tel: 713-850-0399
Fax: 713-850-1104
www.aboto.org

ABP American Board of Pathology

As a member of the American Board of Medical Specialties, the mission of ABP is to promote the health of the public by advancing the practice and science of pathology.

P.O. Box 25915
Tampa, FL 33622-5915
Tel: 813-286-2444
Fax: 813-289-5279
www.abpath.org

ABP American Board of Pediatrics

Certifies general pediatricians and pediatric subspecialists based on standards of excellence that lead to high quality health care for infants, children and adolescents. The ABP certification provides assurance to the public that a general pediatrician or pediatric subspecialist has successfully completed accredited training and fulfills the continuous evaluation requirements that encompass the six core competencies: patient care, medical knowledge, practice-based learning and improvement, interpersonal and communication skills, professionalism, and systems-based practice. The ABP's quest for excellence is evident in its rigorous evaluation process and in new initiatives undertaken that not only continually improve the standards of its certification but also advance the science, education, study, and practice of pediatrics.

111 Silver Cedar Court
Chapel Hill, NC 27514
Tel: 919-929-0461
Fax: 919-929-9255
www.abp.org

ABPM American Board of Preventive Medicine

Preventive medicine is the specialty of medical practice that focuses on the health of individuals, communities, and defined populations. Its goal is to protect, promote, and maintain health and well-being and to prevent disease, disability, and death. Preventive medicine specialists have core competencies in biostatistics, epidemiology, environmental and occupational medicine, planning and evaluation of health services, management of health care organizations, research into causes of disease and injury in population groups, and the practice of prevention in clinical medicine.

330 South Wells Street
Suite 1018
Chicago, IL 60606-7106
Tel: 312-939-2276
Fax: 312-939-2218
www.abprevmed.org

ABPMR American Board of Physical Medicine and Rehabilitation

Establishes the requirements for certification and maintaining certification, creates its examinations, strives to improve training, and contributes to setting the standards for physical medicine and rehabilitation.

3015 Allegro Park Lane, SW
Rochester, MN 55902-4139
Tel: 507-282-1776
Fax: 507-282-9242
www.abpmr.org

ABPN American Board of Psychiatry and Neurology

To serve the public interest and the professions of psychiatry and neurology by promoting excellence in practice through certification and maintenance of the certification process.

500 Lake Cook Road
Suite 335
Deerfield, IL 60015
Tel: 847-945-7900
Fax: 847-945-1146
www.abpn.com

ABPS American Board of Plastic Surgery

To promote safe, ethical, efficacious plastic surgery to the public by maintaining high standards for the education, examination, certification and recertification of plastic surgeons as specialists and subspecialists.

Seven Penn Center
Suite 400
1635 Market Street
Philadelphia, PA 19103-2204
Tel: 215-587-9322
www.abplsurg.org

ABR American Board of Radiology

To serve the public and the medical profession by certifying that its diplomates have acquired, demonstrated, and maintained a requisite standard of knowledge, skill and understanding essential to the practice of radiology, radiation oncology and radiologic physics.

5441 East Williams Boulevard
Suite 200
Tucson, AZ 85711
Tel: 520-790-2900
ABR MOC Services Division:
Tel: 520-519-2152
Fax: 520-790-3200
www.theabr.org

ABS American Board of Surgery

An independent, non-profit organization founded in 1937 for the purpose of certifying surgeons who have met a defined standard of education, training and knowledge. Surgeons certified by the ABS, known as diplomates, have completed a minimum of five years of surgical residency training following medical school and successfully completed a written and oral examination process administered by the ABS.

1617 John F. Kennedy Boulevard
Suite 860
Philadelphia, PA 19103
Tel: 215-568-4000
Fax: 215-563-5718
www.absurgery.org

ABTS American Board of Thoracic Surgery
The primary purpose and most essential function of the Board is to protect the public by establishing and maintaining high standards in thoracic surgery. To achieve these objectives, the Board has established qualifications for examination and procedures for certification and recertification. The requirements and procedures are reviewed regularly and modified as necessary.

633 North St. Clair Street
Suite 2320
Chicago, IL 60611
Tel: 312-202-5900
Fax: 312-202-5960
www.abts.org

ABU American Board of Urology
Belongs to the American Board of Medical Specialties.

2216 Ivy Road
Suite 210
Charlottesville, VA 22903
Tel: 434-979-0059
Fax: 434-979-0266
www.abu.org

ACAHO Association of Canadian Academic Healthcare Organizations
To provide national leadership, advocacy, and effective policy representation in the three separate, but related, areas of (1) the funding, organization, management and delivery of highly specialized tertiary and quaternary, as well as primary healthcare services; (2) the education and training of the next generation of Canada's healthcare professionals; and (3) providing the necessary infrastructure to support and conduct basic and applied health research, medical discovery and innovation.

780 Echo Drive
Ottawa, Ontario K1S 5R7
Canada
Tel: 613-730-5818
Fax: 613-730-4314
www.acaho.org

ACAP Alliance of Claims Assistance Professionals
A national, non-profit organization dedicated to the growth and development of the claims assistance industry. We act as a central resource for clients across the country seeking assistance with health insurance claims issues, we educate the media about medical claims issues and CAP services, and we support our membership with opportunities for development and information sharing.

25500 Hawthorne Boulevard
Suite 1158
Torrance, CA 90505
Tel: 888-394-5163
www.claims.org

ACC American College of Cardiology
To advocate for quality cardiovascular care through education, research promotion, development and application of standards and guidelines and to influence healthcare policy.

Heart House
2400 N Street, NW
Washington, DC 20037
Tel: 202-375-6000
Fax: 202-375-7000
www.acc.org

ACCE American College of Clinical Engineering
To establish a standard of competence and to promote excellence in clinical engineering practice; to promote safe and effective application of science and technology in patient care; to define the body of knowledge on which the profession is based; and to represent the professional interests of clinical engineers.

5200 Butler Pike
Plymouth Meeting, PA 19462
Tel: 610-825-6067
Fax: 480-247-5040
www.accenet.org

ACCP American College of Chest Physicians
To promote the prevention and treatment of diseases of the chest through leadership, education, research, and communication.

3300 Dundee Road
Northbrook, IL 60062-2348
Tel: 847-498-1400
Toll free: 800-343-2227
www.chestnet.org

ACEHSA Accrediting Commission on Education for Health Services Administration
See CAHME (ACEHSA is now CAHME).

ACGME Accreditation Council for Graduate Medical Education
To improve health care by assessing and advancing the quality of resident physicians' education through accreditation.

515 North State Street
Suite 2000
Chicago, IL 60610-4322
Tel: 312-755-5000
Fax: 312-755-7498
www.acgme.org

ACHA American College of Healthcare Architects
To improve the quality of medical care facilities by offering board certification in the specialized field of healthcare architecture.

P.O. Box 14548
Lenexa, KS 66285-4548
Street Address:
18000 W. 105th Street
Olathe, KS 66061-7543
Tel: 913-895-4604
Fax: 913-895-4652
www.healtharchitects.org

ACHCA American College of Health Care Administrators
To be the leading force in promoting excellence in leadership among long-term care administrators.

300 N. Lee Street
Suite 301
Alexandria, VA 22314
Tel: 703-739-7900
Fax: 703-739-7901
www.achca.org

ACHE American College of Healthcare Executives
To advance our members and healthcare management excellence through high ethical standards, pertinent knowledge, and a relevant credentialing program.

1 N. Franklin
Suite 1700
Chicago, IL 60606-3529
Tel: 312-424-2800
Fax: 312-424-0023
www.ache.org

ACHP Alliance of Community Health Plans
Improve the health of the communities we serve and actively lead the transformation of health care so that it is safe, effective, patient-centered, timely, efficient and equitable.

1729 H Street, NW
Suite 400
Washington, DC 20006
Tel: 202-785-2247
Fax: 202-785-4060
www.achp.org

ACMA American Case Management Association
To be THE Association that offers solutions to support the evolving collaborative practice of Hospital/Health System Case Management.

10310 W. Markham
Suite 209
Little Rock, AR 72205
Tel: 501-907-ACMA (2262)
Fax: 501-227-4247
www.acmaweb.org

ACNM American College of Nurse-Midwives
To promote the health and well-being of women and infants within their families and communities through the development and support of the profession of midwifery as practiced by certified nurse-midwives and certified midwives. The philosphy inherent in the profession states that nurse-midwives believe every individual has the right to safe, satisfying health care with respect for human dignity and cultural variations.

8403 Colesville Road
Suite 1550
Silver Spring, MD 20910
Tel: 240-485-1800
Fax: 240-485-1818
www.midwife.org

ACOG   American College of Obstetricians and Gynecologists

A professional membership organization dedicated to advancing women's health by building and sustaining the obstetric and gynecologic community and actively supporting its members. The College pursues this mission through education, practice, research and advocacy. ACOG will emphasize life-long learning, incorporate new knowledge and information technology, and evolve its governance structure. To achieve its strategic goals, ACOG will develop an operational plan that includes appropriate metrics.

409 12th Street, SW
P.O. Box 96920
Washington, DC 20090-6920
Tel: 202-638-5577
www.acog.org

ACP-ASIM   American College of Physicians - American Society of Internal Medicine

To enhance the quality and effectiveness of healthcare by fostering excellence and professionalism in the practice of medicine.

190 N. Independence Mall West
Philadelphia, PA 19106
Tel: 800-523-1546, ext. 2600
www.acponline.org

ACPE   American College of Physician Executives

To support physicians in acquiring the leadership skills and credentials necessary to effectively lead at all levels in organizations and in all sectors of the health care industry.

4890 W. Kennedy Boulevard
Suite 200
Tampa, FL 33609
Tel: 800-562-8088
Fax: 813-287-8993
www.acpe.org

ACR   American College of Radiology

To serve patients and society by maximizing the value of radiology, radiation oncology, interventional radiology, nuclear medicine and medical physics by advancing the science of radiology, improving the quality of patient care, positively influencing the socio-economics of the practice of radiology, providing continuing education for radiology and allied health professions and conducting research for the future of radiology.

1891 Preston White Drive
Reston, VA 20191
Tel: 703-648-8900
www.acr.org

ACS   American College of Surgeons

Dedicated to improving the care of the surgical patient and to safeguarding standards of care in an optimal and ethical practice environment.

633 North St. Clair Street
Chicago, IL 60611
Tel: 312-202-5000
Fax: 312-202-5001
www.facs.org

ADA   American Dental Association

The professional association of dentists committed to the public's oral health, ethics, science and professional advancement; leading a unified profession through initiatives in advocacy, education, research and the development of standards.

211 E. Chicago Avenue
Chicago, IL 60611
Tel: 312-440-2500
www.ada.org

ADA   American Diabetes Association

To prevent and cure diabetes and to improve the lives of all people affected by diabetes.

1701 N. Beauregard Street
Alexandria, VA 22311
Tel: 800-342-2383
www.diabetes.org

AeA   Advancing the Business of Technology
Founded in 1943, AeA (formerly the American Electronics Association) is a nationwide non-profit trade association that represents all segments of the technology industry and is dedicated solely to helping our members' top line and bottom line. We do this in partnership with our small, medium, and large member companies by lobbying governments at the state, federal, and international levels; providing access to capital and business opportunities; and offering select business services and networking programs.

601 Pennsylvania Avenue, NW
North Building, Suite 600
Washington, DC 20004
Tel: 202-682-9110
Fax: 202-682-9111
www.aeanet.org

AFEHCT   Association for Electronic Health Care Transactions
To lead change in the healthcare information and management systems field through knowledge sharing, advocacy, collaboration, innovation, and community affiliations. Merged with HIMSS in 2006.

230 E. Ohio Street
Suite 500
Chicago, IL 60611
Tel: 312-994-4467
www.himss.org

AfPP   Association for Perioperative Practice
Promotes perioperative practice through publishing literature reviews, research based articles, topical discussions, advice on clinical issues, current news items and product information.

Chicago Office:
33 West Monroe
Suite 1600
Chicago, IL 60603
Tel: 312-541-4999
Fax: 312-541-4998
www.afpp.org.uk

AHA   American Heart Association
To build healthier lives, free of cardiovascular diseases and stroke. That single purpose drives all we do. The need for our work is beyond question.

National Center
7272 Greenville Avenue
Dallas, TX 75231

AHA:
800-AHA-USA-1, or
800-242-8721

ASA:
888-4-STROKE, or
888-478-7653

AHA Professional Membership:
800-787-8984
Outside U.S.: 301-223-2307

AHA Instructor Network:
877-AHA-4CPR
www.americanheart.org

AHA   American Hospital Association
To advance the health of individuals and communities. The AHA leads, represents, and serves hospitals, health systems, and other related organizations that are accountable to the community and committed to health improvement.

1 N. Franklin
Chicago, IL 60606-3421
Tel: 312-422-3000
www.aha.org

AHCJ   Association of Health Care Journalists
An independent, nonprofit organization dedicated to advancing public understanding of health care issues. Its mission is to improve the quality, accuracy and visibility of health care reporting, writing and editing.

Missouri School of Journalism
10 Neff Hall
Columbia, MO 65211
Tel: 573-884-5606
Fax: 573-884-5609
www.healthjournalism.org

AHCPR Agency for Health Care Policy Research
See AHRQ (AHCPR is now AHRQ).

AHIC American Health Information Community
A federal advisory body, chartered in 2005 to make recommendations to the Secretary of the U.S. Department of Health and Human Services on how to accelerate the development and adoption of health information technology. AHIC was formed by the Secretary to help advance efforts to achieve President Bush's goal for most Americans to have access to secure electronic health records by 2014. Last meeting was November 2008. Succeeded by NeHC - National e-Health Collaborative.
www.hhs.gov/healthit/community/
background/

AHIMA American Health Information Management Association
To be the professional community that improves healthcare by advancing best practices and standards for health information management and the trusted source for education, research, and professional credentialing.
233 N. Michigan Avenue
21st Floor
Chicago, IL 60601-5800
Tel: 312-233-1100
Fax: 312-233-1090
www.ahima.org

AHIP America's Health Insurance Plans
To provide a unified voice for the healthcare financing industry, to expand access to high quality, cost effective healthcare to all Americans, and to ensure Americans' financial security through robust insurance markets, product flexibility and innovation, and an abundance of consumer choice.
601 Pennsylvania Avenue, NW
South Building
Suite 500
Washington, DC 20004
Tel: 202-778-3200
Fax: 202-331-7487
www.ahip.org

AHNA American Holistic Nurses Association
To unite nurses in healing.
323 N. San Francisco Street
Suite 201
Flagstaff, AZ 86001
Tel: 800-278-2462
www.ahna.org

AHQA American Health Quality Association
To improve health care quality and patient safety.
1155 21st Street, NW
Suite 202
Washington, DC 20036
Tel: 202-331-5790
Fax: 202-331-9334
www.ahqa.org

AHRMM Association for Healthcare Resource & Materials Management
To advance healthcare through supply chain excellence.
1 N. Franklin
Chicago, IL 60606
Tel: 312-422-3840
Fax: 312-422-4573
www.ahrmm.org

AHRQ Agency for Healthcare Research and Quality
To improve the quality, safety, efficiency, and effectiveness of healthcare for all Americans.
540 Gaither Road
Suite 2000
Rockville, MD 20850
Tel: 301-427-1364
www.ahrq.gov

AIM Association for Automatic Identification and Mobility
An international trade association representing automatic identification and mobility technology solution providers. Through the years, industry leaders continue to work within AIM to promote the adoption of emerging technologies.
125 Warrendale-Bayne Road
Suite 100
Warrendale, PA 15086
Tel: 724-934-4470
Fax: 724-934-4495
www.aimglobal.org

ALA American Lung Association
To prevent lung disease and promote lung health.

61 Broadway, 6th Floor
New York, NY 10006
Tel: 212-315-8700
Toll free: 800-548-8252
www.lungusa.org

Alliance HPSR Alliance for Health Policy and Systems Research
To promote the generation and use of health policy and systems research as a means to improve the health systems of developing countries.

20 Avenue Appia
1211 Geneva
Switzerland
Tel: +41 22 791 2973
Fax: +41 22 791 4169
www.who.int/alliance-hpsr

AMA American Medical Association
To promote the art and science of medicine and the betterment of public health.

515 N. State Street
Chicago, IL 60610
Tel: 800-621-8335
www.ama-assn.org

AMCP Academy of Managed Care Pharmacy
To empower its members to serve society by using sound medication management principles and strategies to improve health care for all.

100 N. Pitt Street
Suite 400
Alexandria, VA 22314
Tel: 703-683-8416
Toll free: 800-827-2627
www.amcp.org

AMDA American Medical Directors Association
The professional association of medical directors and physicians practicing in the long term care continuum, dedicated to excellence in patient care by providing education, advocacy, information, and professional development.

11000 Broken Land Parkway
Suite 400
Columbia, MD 21044
Tel: 410-740-9743
Toll free: 800-876-2632
Fax: 410-740-4572
www.amda.com

AMDIS Association of Medical Directors of Information Systems
To advance the field of applied medical informatics and direct physician use of information technology to improve the practice of medicine.

682 Peninsula Drive
Lake Almanor, CA 96137
Tel: 530-596-4477
Fax: 978-389-7729
www.amdis.org

AMGA American Medical Group Association
Advocates for multispecialty medical groups and other organized systems of care and for the patients served by these systems by continuously striving to improve patient care through innovation, information sharing, benchmarking, the creation of sound public policy, and leadership development.

1422 Duke Street
Alexandria, VA 22314-3403
Tel: 703-838-0033
Fax: 703-548-1890
www.amga.org

AMIA American Medical Informatics Association
Dedicated to promoting the effective organization, analysis, management and use of information in health care in support of patient care, public health, teaching, research administration, and related policy.

4915 St. Elmo Avenue
Suite 401
Bethesda, MD 20814
Tel: 301-657-1291
Fax: 301-657-1296
www.amia.org

Amerinet
To promote quality health care delivery, partner with all types of health care providers, help them better manage expenses through a suite of margin improvement tools. (Formerly known as ANC.)

500 Commonwealth Drive
Warrendale, PA 15086
Tel: 877-711-5600
www.amerinetcentral.org

AMP Applied Measurement Professionals
To provide certification organizations, governmental agencies, associations and private industry with psychometric consultation, testing and measurement, association management and publishing services that meet the highest professional and ethical standards; tailor these services to fulfill the unique requirements of each client; and personalize the delivery of these services by providing innovative and accessible professional and managerial staffs serving client organizations throughout all phases of the program.

18000 W. 105th Street
Olathe, KS 66061
Tel: 913-895-4600
Fax: 913-895-4650
www.goamp.com

AMPA American Medical Publishers Association
To advance health science publishing and scientific communication worldwide.

14 Fort Hill Road
Huntington, NY 11743
Tel: 631-423-0075
www.ampaonline.org

AMSN Academy of Medical-Surgical Nurses
To promote excellence in adult health.

East Holly Avenue
Box 56
Pitman, NJ 08071-0056
Tel: 866-877-2676
www.medsurgnurse.org

ANA American Nurses Association
Advances the nursing profession by fostering high standards of nursing practice, promoting the rights of nurses in the workplace, projecting a positive and realistic view of nursing, and by lobbying the Congress and regulatory agencies on healthcare issues affecting nurses and the public.

8515 Georgia Avenue
Suite 400
Silver Spring, MD 20910-3492
Tel: 301-628-5000
Fax: 301-628-5001
http://nursingworld.org

ANASA Association of Nursing Agencies for South Africa
An association representing member agencies that consistently maintain high ethical and professional standards, thereby ensuring that the acronym ANASA is synonymous with quality care rendered by all its members.

P.O. Box 12339
Clubview
0014
Pretoria, South Africa
Tel: +27-12-083-444-9227
Fax: +27-12-083-444-9667
Enquiries: Marie Jacobs
E-mail (enquiries): office@anasa.org.za
http://anasa.org.za

ANC Amerinet Central
See Amerinet (ANC is now Amerinet).

ANIA   American Nursing Informatics Association

To provide networking, education and information resources that enrich and strengthen the roles of nurses in the field of informatics. The field of nursing informatics includes domains of clinical information, education and administration decision support.

1908 S. El Camino Real
Suite H
San Clemente, CA 92672
www.ania.org

ANCC   American Nurses Credentialing Center

To promote excellence in nursing and health care globally through credentialing programs and related services.

P.O. Box 791333
Baltimore, MD 21279-1333
Tel: 301-628-5250
Toll free: 800-284-2378
www.nursecredentialing.org

ANI   Alliance for Nursing Informatics

A collaboration of organizations that represent a unified voice for nursing informatics. The Alliance represents more than 3,000 nurses and brings together over 25 distinct nursing informatics groups in the United States and provides a single contact point for informatics nurses and the healthcare community. ANI facilitates the involvement of informatics nurses in the development of resources, guidelines, research, public policy, certification, advocacy, and career development.

230 E. Ohio Street
Suite 500
Chicago, IL 60611
www.allianceni.org

ANNA   American Nephrology Nurses Association

The professional organization for registered nurses who specialize in the care of patients experiencing the real or threatened impact of renal dysfunction. ANNA sets forth and updates standards of patient care, educates its practitioners, stimulates and supports research, disseminates new ideas throughout the field, promotes interdisciplinary communication and cooperation, and monitors and addresses issues encompassing the practice of nephrology nursing.

East Holly Avenue
Box 56
Pitman, NJ 08071-0056
Tel: 856-256-2320
Toll free: 888-600-2662
Fax: 856-589-7463
www.annanurse.org

ANSI   American National Standards Institute

To enhance both the global competitiveness of U.S. business and the U.S. quality of life by promoting and facilitating voluntary consensus standards and conformity assessment systems, and safeguarding their integrity.

1819 L Street, NW
6th Floor
Washington, DC 20036
Tel: 202-293-8020
Fax: 202-293-9287
www.ansi.org

AONE   American Organization of Nurse Executives

To represent nurse leaders who improve healthcare. AONE members are leaders in collaboration and catalysts for innovation.

Liberty Place
325 Seventh Street, NW
Washington, DC 20004
Tel: 202-626-2240
Fax: 202-638-5499
www.aone.org

AORN Association of Peri-Operative Registered Nurses

To promote safety and optimal outcomes for patients undergoing operative and other invasive procedures by providing practice support and professional development opportunities to perioperative nurses. AORN will collaborate with professional and regulatory organizations, industry leaders, and other healthcare partners who support the mission.

2170 S. Parker Road
Suite 300
Denver, CO 80231
Tel: 303-755-6304
Toll free: 800-755-2676
www.aorn.org

APhA American Pharmacists Association

To serve society as the profession responsible for the appropriate use of medications, devices, and services to achieve optimal therapeutic outcomes.

1100 15th Street, NW
Suite 400
Washington, DC 20005
Tel: 202-628-4410
Fax: 202-783-2351
www.pharmacist.com

APHA American Public Health Association

To improve the health of the public and achieve equity in health status.

800 I Street, NW
Washington, DC 20001
Tel: 202-777-2742
Fax: 202-777-2533
www.apha.org

API Association for Pathology Informatics

To promote the field of pathology informatics as an academic and a clinical subspecialty of pathology.

9650 Rockville Pike
Bethesda, MD 20814-3993
Tel: 301-634-7820
Fax: 301-634-7990
www.pathologyinformatics.org

APNA American Psychiatric Nurses Association

To promote and improve mental health.

1555 Wilson Boulevard
Suite 602
Arlington, VA 22209
Tel: 866-243-2443
Fax: 703-243-3390
www.apna.org

APTA American Physical Therapy Association

To further the profession's role in the prevention, diagnosis, and treatment of movement dysfunctions and the enhancement of the physical health and functional abilities of members of the public.

1111 North Fairfax Street
Alexandria, VA 22314-1488
Tel: 703-684-2782
Toll free: 800-999-2782
TDD: 703-683-6748
Fax: 703-684-7343
www.apta.org

ARN Association of Rehabilitation Nurses

To promote and advance professional rehabilitation nursing practice through education, advocacy, collaboration, and research to enhance the quality of life for those affected by disability and chronic illness.

4700 W. Lake Avenue
Glenview, IL 60025-1485
Tel: 847-375-4710
Toll free: 800-229-7530
Fax: 877-734-9384
www.rehabnurse.org

ASAE American Society of Association Executives

To help associations transform society through the power of collaborative action; and to make sure associations continue to play a vital role in society by equipping association professionals with the tools they need to lead and manage.

1575 I Street, NW
Washington, DC 20005
Tel: 202-371-0940
Toll free: 888-950-2723
Fax: 202-371-8315
www.asaecenter.org

ASC X12 The Accredited Standards Committee
To be an innovative leader in the development of cross industry e-commerce standards that improve global business interoperability and facilitate business information exchange.

7600 Leesburg Pike
Suite 430
Falls Church, VA 22043
Tel: 703-970-4480
Fax: 703-970-4480
www.x12.org

ASCP American Society for Clinical Pathology
To provide excellence in education, certification, and advocacy on behalf of patients, pathologists, and laboratory professionals.

33 West Monroe
Suite 1600
Chicago, IL 60603
Tel: 312-541-4999
Fax: 312-541-4998
www.ascp.org

ASHE American Society for Healthcare Engineering
Dedicated to optimizing the healthcare physical environment.

1 N. Franklin
28th Floor
Chicago, IL 60606
Tel: 312-422-3800
Fax: 312-422-4571
www.ashe.org

ASHP American Society of Health-System Pharmacists
To advance and support the professional practice of pharmacists in hospitals and health systems and serve as their collective voice on issues related to medication use and public health.

7272 Wisconsin Avenue
Bethesda, MD 20814
Tel: 301-657-3000
www.ashp.org

ASHRM American Society for Healthcare Risk Management
To advance safe and trusted patient-centered healthcare delivery, ASHRM promotes proactive and innovative management of organization-wide risk.

1 N. Franklin Street
28th Floor
Chicago, IL 60606
Tel: 312-422-3980
Fax: 312-422-4580
www.ashrm.org

ASNC American Society of Nuclear Cardiology
To be the preeminent voice and resource of Nuclear Cardiology and Cardiovascular Computed Tomography.

4550 Montgomery Avenue
Suite 780 North
Bethesda, MD 20814-3304
Tel: 301-215-7575
Fax: 301-215-7113
www.asnc.org

ASPAN American Society of PeriAnesthesia Nurses
To advance the unique specialty of perianesthesia nursing.

10 Melrose Avenue
Suite 110
Cherry Hill, NJ 08003-3696
Tel: 856-616-9600
Toll free: 877-737-9696
Fax: 856-616-9601
www.aspan.org

ASQ American Society for Quality
By making quality a global priority, an organizational imperative and personal ethic, ASQ becomes the community for everyone who seeks quality concepts, technology and tools to improve themselves and their world.

P.O. Box 3005
Milwaukee, WI 53201-3005
or
600 North Plankinton Avenue
Milwaukee, WI 53203
Tel: 800-984-4323
Fax: 414-272-1734
www.asq.org

ASSE American Society of Safety Engineers, Healthcare Practice Specialty
Membership evokes a duty to serve and protect people, property and the environment. This duty is to be exercised with integrity, honor and dignity. Members are accountable for following the Code of Professional Conduct.

1800 E. Oakton Street
Des Plaines, IL 60018
Tel: 847-699-2929
Fax: 847-768-3434
www.asse.org

ASTM ASTM International
To be recognized globally as the premier developer and provider of voluntary consensus standards, related technical information, and services that promote public health and safety, support the protection and sustainability of the environment, and the overall quality of life; contribute to the reliability of materials, products, systems and services; and facilitate international, regional, and national commerce.

100 Barr Harbor Drive
P.O. Box C700
West Conshohocken, PA 19428
Tel: 610-832-9585
www.astm.org

ATA American Telemedicine Association
To bring together diverse groups from traditional medicine, academic medical centers, technology and telecommunications companies, e-health, medical societies, government and others to overcome barriers to the advancement of telemedicine through the professional, ethical and equitable improvement in healthcare delivery.

1100 Connecticut Avenue, NW
Suite 540
Washington, DC 20036
Tel: 202-223-3333
Fax: 202-223-2787
www.atmeda.org

ATSP Association of Telehealth Service Providers
To promote the appropriate use of telecommunications technologies in the provision of health care services and health education. We strive to advance the field of telehealth through advocacy, removal of barriers, health care delivery, health education and telemedicine business development. The Association will provide telehealth organizations with the information and resources needed to optimize the delivery of telehealth services.

4702 SW Scholls Ferry Road
#400
Portland, OR 97225
Tel: 503-922-0988
Fax: 315-222-2402
www.atsp.org

AUPHA Association of University Programs in Health Administration
To foster excellence and innovation in healthcare management education, research and practice by providing opportunities for member programs to learn from each other, by influencing practice, and by promoting the value of healthcare management education.

2000 N. 14th Street
Suite 780
Arlington, VA 22201
Tel: 703-894-0940
Fax: 703-894-0941
www.aupha.org

AWHONN Association of Women's Health, Obstetric and Neonatal Nurses
Promoting the health of women and newborns, our mission is to improve and promote the health of women and newborns and to strengthen the nursing profession through the delivery of superior advocacy, research, education and other professional and clinical resources to nurses and other health care professionals.

2000 L Street, NW
Suite 740
Washington, DC 20036
Tel: 202-261-2400
Toll free U.S.: 800-673-8499
Toll free Canada: 800-245-0231
Fax: 202-728-0575
www.awhonn.org

BACCN British Association of Critical-Care Nurses

To provide opportunities and services to our members which support personal and professional development and promote the art and science of critical care nursing.

Wessex House
Eastleigh Business Centre
Upper Market Street
Eastleigh, Hants SO50 9FD
United Kingdom
www.baccn.org

CAC Citizen Advocacy Center

To increase the accountability and effectiveness of health care regulatory, credentialing, oversight and governing boards by: Advocating for the inclusion of public members; improving the training and effectiveness of public members; developing and advancing positions on relevant administrative and policy issues; providing training and discussion forums for public members; and performing needed clearinghouse functions for public members and other interested parties.

1400 16th Street, NW
Suite 101
Washington, DC 20036
Tel: 202-462-1174
Fax: 202-354-5372
www.cacenter.org

CACCN Canadian Association of Critical-Care Nurses

A non-profit, specialty organization dedicated to maintaining and enhancing the quality of care provided to critically ill clients and their families. CACCN serves its membership, the public and the critical care nursing community by meeting the professional and educational needs of critical care nurses.

P.O. Box 25322
London, Ontario N6B 6B1
Canada
Tel: 519-649-5284
Toll free: 866-477-9077
Fax: 519-649-1458
www.caccn.ca

CADTH Canadian Agency for Drugs and Technologies

An independent, not-for-profit agency funded by Canadian federal, provincial, and territorial governments to provide credible, impartial advice and evidence-based information about the effectiveness of drugs and other health technologies to Canadian health care decision makers.

600-865 Carling Avenue
Ottawa, Ontario K1S 5S8
Canada
Tel: 613-226-2553
Fax: 613-226-5392
www.cadth.ca

CAHME Commission on Accreditation of Healthcare Management Education

To serve the public good through promoting, evaluating, and continuously improving the quality of academic healthcare management education in the United States and Canada and elsewhere as deemed appropriate by the Corporate Members and the Board of Directors. Through its partnership between academe and the field of practice, CAHME serves universities and programs in a voluntary peer review process as a means to continuously improve academic education. In so doing, CAHME's designation of "Accredited" becomes the benchmark by which students and employers determine the integrity of healthcare management education and the standard of measurement for the world community. (Formerly ACEHSA.)

2000 14th Street, North
Suite 780
Arlington, VA 22201
Tel: 703-894-0960
Fax: 703-894-0941
www.cahme.org

CAHTA   Catalan Agency for Health Technology Assessment and Research
Non-profit public agency founded in 1994 to promote production and use of scientific knowledge to prevent disease and promote better health in the autonomous region of Catalonia, Spain. Its specific objectives are to encourage the introduction, adoption, diffusion and utilization of health technologies according to proven scientific criteria of efficacy, safety, effectiveness and efficiency; to promote needs assessment and equity analysis in health service delivery and financing; and to promote research oriented to health need. Member of the International Network of Agencies of Health Technology Assessment.

> *Carrer de Roc Boronat*
> *81-95 (2a planta)*
> *08005 Barcelona*
> *Spain*
> *Tel: +34 935 513 888*
> *Fax: +34 935 517 510*
> *(WHO Regional Office for Europe)*
> *http://www.euro.who.int/HEN/*
> *Resources/CAHTA/20050428_1*

CAP   College of American Pathologists
To serve patients, pathologists, and the public by fostering and advocating excellence in the practice of pathology and laboratory medicine.

> *325 Waukegan Road*
> *Northfield, IL 60093-2750*
> *Tel: 847-832-7000*
> *Toll free: 800-323-4040*
> *Fax: 847-832-8000*
> *www.cap.org*

CAQH   Council for Affordable Quality Healthcare
To be the catalyst for industry collaboration on initiatives that simplify healthcare administration for health plans and providers, resulting in a better care experience for patients and caregivers.

> *601Pennsylvania Avenue, NW*
> *South Building*
> *Suite 500*
> *Washington, DC 20004*
> *Tel: 202-861-1492*
> *Fax: 202-861-1454*
> *www.caqh.org*

CARING   Capital Area Roundtable on Informatics in Nursing
A nursing informatics organization advancing the delivery of quality healthcare through the integration of informatics in practice, education, administration, and research. (Merged with ANIA)

> *Tel: 866-552-6404*
> *www.caringonline.org*

CCBH   Community Care Behavioral Health Organization
To improve the health and well-being of the community through the delivery of effective and accessible behavioral health services. Community Care believes that the highest quality services are best provided through a not-for-profit partnership with public agencies, experienced local providers, and involved members and families. Community Care also affirms that the success of these partnerships, as well as the achievement of the organization's goals, relies on the strong commitment of all parties involved to conduct business lawfully and ethically.

> *One Chatham Center*
> *Suite 700*
> *112 Washington Place*
> *Pittsburgh, PA 15219*
> *Tel: 412-454-2120*
> *www.ccbh.com*

CCHIT   Certification Commission for Healthcare Information Technology
To accelerate the adoption of health information technology by creating an efficient, credible and sustainable certification program.

> *233 N. Michigan Avenue*
> *21st Floor*
> *Chicago, IL 60601*
> *Tel: 312-233-1582*
> *Fax: 312-896-1466*
> *www.cchit.org*

CDC   Centers for Disease Control and Prevention
To promote health and quality of life by preventing and controlling disease, injury, and disability.

1600 Clifton Road
Atlanta, GA 30333
Tel: 404-498-1515
Toll free: 800-311-3435
www.cdc.gov

CDISC   Clinical Data Interchange Standards Consortium
To develop and support global, platform-independent data standards that enable information system interoperability to improve medical research and related areas of healthcare.

For information about joining CDISC, Member Benefits, User Networks, and Fundraising, please contact:

Tanyss Mason, Member Relations
Tel: 919-419-7100
Cell: 919 -744-5973
Fax: 919-489-4850
E-mail: tmason@cdisc.org
www.cdisc.org

CEN   European Committee for Standardization
Contributing to the objectives of the European Union and European Economic Area with voluntary technical standards which promote free trade, the safety of workers and consumers, interoperability of networks, environmental protection, exploitation of research and development programmes, and public procurement.

36 rue de Stassart
B -1050
Brussels
Tel: +32-2-550-08-11
Fax: +32-2-550-08-19
www.cen.eu

CHCA   Child Health Corporation of America
To reduce hospital costs, increase revenue, strengthen the competitive position of children's hospitals, and improve the quality of care for children. CHCA owner hospitals are widely known for their excellence in caring for America's children.

6803 W. 64th Street
Suite 208
Shawnee Mission, KS 66202
Tel: 913-262-1436
Fax: 913-262-1575
www.chca.com

CHI   Consolidated Health Informatics
This initiative adopts a portfolio of existing health information interoperability standards (health vocabulary and messaging) enabling all agencies in the federal health enterprise to "speak the same language" based on common enterprise-wide business and information technology architectures.

e-government initiative
Washington, DC
www.egov.usda.gov/Presidential_Initiatives/
Other_eGovernment_Initiatives/Consolidated_Health_Informatics/

CHIK   CHIK Services Pty Ltd.
To create global communications mechanisms of choice for the health ICT industry by publishing regular health ICT industry newsletters; networking existing stakeholders and new market entrants; conducting primary and applied research; and enhancing the industry's commercial and export potential.

Suite 3.11, Platinum Building
4 Ilya Avenue
P.O. Box 3307
Erina NSW 2250
Australia
Tel: +612-4365-7500
Fax: +612-4365-7566
www.chik.com.au

CHIM Center for Healthcare Information Management
To positively impact the industry through the promotion of health care information technology. By disseminating information, convening educational programming, and fostering a collaborative environment, CHIM members seek to bring a greater awareness and understanding among professionals on how information technology can be harnessed to improve the quality and cost effectiveness of health care. Merged with HIMSS in 2001.

230 E. Ohio Street
Suite 500
Chicago, IL 60611-3270
Tel: 312-664-4467
Fax: 312-664-6143
www.himss.org

CHIME College of Healthcare Information Management Executives
To serve the professional needs of healthcare Chief Information Officers; and to advance the strategic application of information technology in innovative ways aimed at improving the effectiveness of healthcare delivery.

3300 Washtenaw Avenue
Suite 225
Ann Arbor, MI 48104
Tel: 734-665-0000
Fax: 734-665-4922
www.cio-chime.org

CHITTA Canadian Healthcare Information Technology Trade Association
To strengthen the competitiveness of Canada's Healthcare Information and Communications Technology (ICT) industry through cooperative efforts among and between members and through direct contact with all levels of government and associated agencies.

5782-172 Street
Edmonton, Alberta T6M1B4
Canada
Tel: 780-489-4574
Fax: 780-489-3290
www.chitta.ca

CHT Center for Health and Technology
To discover and share knowledge to advance health.

UC Davis
Center for Health and Technology
2315 Stockton Boulevard
Sacramento, CA 95817
Tel: 916-734-5675
Fax: 916-734-1366
www.ucdmc.ucdavis.edu/cht/

CHT Center for Health Transformation
To grow a movement that will accelerate the adoption of transformational health solutions and policies that create better health and more choices at lower cost.

1425 K Street, NW
Suite 450
Washington, DC 20005
Tel: 202-375-2001
www.healthtransformation.net

CIHI Canadian Institute for Health Information
An independent, not-for-profit organization that provides essential data and analysis on Canada's health system and the health of Canadians. CIHI tracks data in many areas, thanks to information supplied by hospitals, regional health authorities, medical practitioners and governments. Other sources provide further data to help inform CIHI's in-depth analytic reports.

495 Richmond Road
Suite 600
Ottawa, Ontario K2A 4H6
Canada
Tel: 613-241-7860
Fax: 613-241-8121
www.cihi.ca

CINA Canadian Intravenous Nurses Association
See CVAA (CINA changed its name to CVAA, effective March 2007.)

CITL Center for Information Technology Leadership
The ultimate goal is to improve quality of care. Focus is on the impact that IT can have, and our main objective is to help healthcare providers make intelligent IT investments.

One Constitution Center
2nd Floor West
Charlestown, MA 02129
Tel: 617-643-4162
Fax: 617-643-4180
www.citl.org

CLMA Clinical Laboratory Management Association
Empowers laboratory professionals through forward-thinking educational, networking, and advocacy opportunities in leadership and healthcare management.

989 Old Eagle School Road
Suite 815
Wayne, PA 19087
Tel: 610-995-2640
Fax: 610-995-9568
www.clma.org

CLSI Clinical and Laboratory Standards Institute
To develop best practices in clinical and laboratory testing and promote their use throughout the world, using a consensus-driven process that balances the viewpoints of industry, government, and the healthcare professions. (Name changed from NCCLS in January 2005.)

940 W. Valley Road
Suite 1400
Wayne, PA 19087-1898
Tel: 610-688-0100
Fax: 610-688-0700
www.clsi.org

CMS Centers for Medicare & Medicaid Services
To ensure effective, up-to-date health care coverage and to promote quality care for beneficiaries.

7500 Security Boulevard
Baltimore, MD 21244
Tel: 410-786-3000
Toll free: 877-267-2323
www.cms.hhs.gov

CMSA Case Management Society of America
We envision case managers as pioneers of healthcare change...key initiators of and participants in the healthcare team who open up new areas of thought...research and development... leading the way toward the day when every American will know what a case/care manager does and will know how to access case and care management services.

6301 Ranch Drive
Little Rock, AR 72223
Tel: 501-225-2229
Fax: 501-221-9068
www.cmsa.org

CNA Canadian Nurses Association
The national professional voice of Registered Nurses, supporting them in their practice and advocating for healthy public policy and a quality, publicly funded, not-for-profit health system.

50 Driveway
Ottawa, Ontario K2P 1E2
Canada
Tel: 613-237-2133
Toll free: 800-361-8404
Fax: 613-237-3520
www.cna-nurses.ca

CNC Center for Nursing Classification and Clinical Effectiveness
To prepare the next generation of nursing leaders and to be a leader in the discovery, dissemination and application of nursing knowledge. As the only state-supported higher degree program in nursing, the College has a mandate to supply the next generation of nurses for the state of Iowa. As one of eleven colleges in a Research Extensive university, the College of Nursing has a responsibility to support its research mission through national leadership in both innovative educational programs and generation of new knowledge.

University of Iowa College of Nursing
101 Nursing Building
50 Newton Road
Iowa City, IA 52242-1121
Tel: 319-335-7018
Fax: 319-335-9990
www.nursing.uiowa.edu/cnc/

COACH   Canada's Health Informatics Association

To promote understanding and adoption of Health Informatics within the Canadian health system through leadership, professional development, advocacy, and a strong and diverse membership.

250 Consumers Road
Suite 301
Toronto, Ontario M2J 4V6
Canada
Tel: 416-494-9324
Fax: 416-495-8723
www.coachorg.com

COC   AHIMA's Council on Certification

To ensure that its members meet professional standards of excellence, AHIMA issues credentials in health information management, coding, and healthcare privacy and security. Members earn credentials through a combination of education and experience, and finally performance on national certification exams. Following their initial certification, AHIMA members must maintain their credentials and thereby the highest level of competency for their employers and consumers through rigorous continuing education requirements.

233 N. Michigan Avenue
21st Floor
Chicago, IL 60601-5800
Tel: 312-233-1100
Fax: 312-233-1090
www.ahima.org/certification

CPRI   Computer-based Patient Record Institute

The Computer-based Patient Record Institute Work Group on Confidentiality, Privacy, and Security was established to encourage creation of policies and the implementation of mechanisms that protect patient and caregiver privacy as well as preserve the confidentiality, protect the integrity, and ensure the availability of information in computer-based patient record systems. Merged with HIMSS in 2002.

230 E. Ohio Street
Suite 500
Chicago, IL 60611-3270
Tel: 312-664-4467
Fax: 312-664-6143
www.himss.org

CVAA   Canadian Vascular Access Association

Advocates for safe quality care across the health care continuum by providing leadership and promoting education, partnerships, knowledge and research in vascular access with a vision for optimal client outcomes.

685 McCowan Road
P.O. Box 66572
Toronto, Ontario M1J 3N8
Canada
Tel: 416-696-7761
Fax: 416-696-8437
www.cvaa.info

DAHTA   German Agency for Health Technology Assessment (part of the German Medical Documentation and Information Agency)

The term Health Technology Assessment (HTA) specifies a process of systematically evaluating medical procedures and technologies with relation to the health care of the population. Since the middle of the 1990s HTA has played an important role in German health policy. The German Agency for HTA at DIMDI - DAHTA@ DIMDI - was established in 2000. It runs the HTA information system and a programme for the production of HTA reports.

DIMDI's central mailbox is for general feedback or inquiries. Special questions will be forwarded.

E-mail: Central Mailbox
Tel: +49 221 4724-1
Fax: +49 221 4724-444
www.dimdi.de

DARPA   Defense Advanced Research Projects Agency

To maintain the technological superiority of the U.S. military and prevent technological surprise from harming our national security by sponsoring revolutionary, high-payoff research that bridges the gap between fundamental discoveries and their military use.

3701 N. Fairfax Drive
Arlington, VA 22203-1714
www.darpa.mil

DHHS   Department of Health and Human Services

The U.S. government's principal agency for protecting the health of all Americans and providing essential human services, especially for those who are least able to help themselves.

200 Independence Avenue, SW
Washington, DC 20201
Tel: 202-619-0257
Toll free: 877-696-6775
www.dhhs.gov

DICOM   Digital Imaging and Communications in Medicine

The DICOM Standards Committee exists to create and maintain international standards for the communication of biomedical, diagnostic and therapeutic information in disciplines that use digital images and associated data.

NEMA
1300 N. 17th Street
Suite 1752
Rosslyn, VA 22209
Tel: 703-841-3285
http://medical.nema.org

DIHTA   Danish Institute for Health Technology Assessment

As the central authority on health care in Denmark, the National Board of Health contributes, through monitoring, supervision, administration and development, to ensuring a high quality and efficiency within prevention and treatment so as to improve the possibilities for a healthy lifestyle for citizens in Denmark.

National Board of Health
Islands Brygge 67
DK - 2300 Copenhagen S
P.O. Box 1881
Denmark
Tel: +45-72-22-74-00
Fax: +45-72-22-74-11
www.sst.dk

DIMDI   German Institute of Medical Documentation and Information

Founded in 1969, DIMDI is an institute within the scope of the German Federal Ministry of Health (BMG). DIMDI's main task is to provide information in all fields of the life sciences to the interested public.

DIMDI's central mailbox is for general
feedback or inquiries. Special questions will
be forwarded.
E-mail: Central Mailbox
Tel: +49-221-4724-1
Fax: +49-221-4724-444
www.dimdi.de

DISA   Data Interchange Standards Association

Established as a not-for-profit, the Data Interchange Standards Association (DISA) is home for the development of cross-industry electronic business interchange standards.

7600 Leesburg Pike
Suite 430
Falls Church, VA 22043
Tel: 703-970-4480
Fax: 703-970-4488
www.disa.org

DMAA Disease Management Association of America

Standardizing definitions and outcome measures; promoting high quality standards for disease management and care coordination programs as well as support services and materials; identifying and sharing best practices of program components; fostering research and exploration of innovative approaches and best practices for care models and disease management services delivery; educating consumers, payors, providers, physicians, health care professionals, and accreditation bodies on the value propositions of disease management in the enhancement of individual and population-based health; advocating the principles and benefits of disease and care management before state and federal government entities; convening and aligning stakeholders in health care delivery, including international organizations and government entities; and promoting the six health care aims identified by the Institute of Medicine: safety, timeliness, effectiveness, efficiency, equity, and patient-centeredness.

701 Pennsylvania Avenue, NW
Suite 700
Washington, DC 20004-2694
Tel: 202-737-5980
Fax: 202-478-5113
www.dmaa.org

DNA Dermatology Nurses Association

A professional nursing organization comprised of a diverse group of individuals committed to quality care through sharing knowledge and expertise. The core purpose of the DNA is to promote excellence in dermatologic care.

East Holly Avenue
Box 56
Pitman, NJ 08071-0056
Tel: 800-454-4362
www.dnanurse.org

DoD Department of Defense - Health Affairs

To enhance the Department of Defense and our nation's security by providing health support for the full range of military operations and sustaining the health of all those entrusted to our care.

Skyline 5
5111 Leesburg Pike
Suite 810
Falls Church, VA 22041-3206
Tel: 888-647-6676
www.ha.osd.mil

ECRI Emergency Care Research Institute

To bringing the discipline of applied scientific research to discover which medical procedures, devices, drugs, and processes are best, all to enable you to improve patient care. As pioneers in this science, we pride ourselves in having the unique ability to marry practical experience and uncompromising independence with the thoroughness and objectivity of evidence-based research.

5200 Butler Pike
Plymouth Meeting, PA 19462
Tel: 610-825-6000
Fax: 610-834-1275
www.ecri.org

EDIA See DISA.

eHI eHealth Initiative

The missions of both the eHealth Initiative and its Foundation for eHealth are the same: to drive improvement in the quality, safety, and efficiency of healthcare through information and information technology.

818 Connecticut Avenue, NW
Suite 500
Washington, DC 20006
Tel: 202-624-3270
Fax: 202-429-5553
www.ehealthinitiative.org

eHealth Institute

Seeks to explore ways to use emerging technologies to improve the health and well being of all people, including the underserved. We develop initiatives to enhance the capacity of people to access and utilize eHealth resources, improve the state of knowledge and public understanding of eHealth-related issues, and improve the quality and effectiveness of eHealth resources.

www.ehealthinstitute.org

EMEA   European Medicines Agency

To foster scientific excellence in the evaluation and supervision of medicines, for the benefit of public and animal health.

7 Westferry Circus
Canary Wharf
London E14 4HB
United Kingdom
Tel: +44-20-74-18-84-00
www.emea.europa.eu

ENA   Emergency Nurse Association

A professional membership organization recognized internationally for promoting excellence in emergency nursing through leadership, research, education and advocacy.

915 Lee Street
Des Plaines, IL 60016-6569
Tel: 800-900-9659, or
800-243-8362
www.ena.org

ESQH   European Society for Quality in Healthcare

A not-for-profit organisation dedicated to the improvement of quality in European healthcare.

St. Camillus Hospital
Shelbourne Road
Limerick
Ireland
Tel: +353-61-483315
www.esqh.net

EUnetHTA   European Network for Health Technology Assessment

To establish the organisational and structural framework for the Network with a supporting secretariat; to develop and implement generic tools for adapting assessments made for one country to new contexts; to develop and implement effective tools to transfer HTA results into applicable health policy advice in the Member States and EU—including systems for identification and prioritisation of topics for HTAs and assessment of impact of HTA advice; to effectively disseminate and handle HTA results, information sharing and coordination of HTA activities through the development and implementation of elaborate communication strategies and clearinghouse activities; effective monitoring of emerging health technologies to identify those that will have greatest impact on health systems and patients; and to establish a support system to countries without institutionalised HTA activity.

Hosted by
Danish Centre for Evaluation and HTA
(DACEHTA)
National Board of Health
Islands Brygge 67
2300 Copenhagen
Denmark
Tel: +45-7222-7548
Fax: +45-7222-7411
www.eunethta.net

Project Leader (Project content issues):
Finn Børlum Kristensen
Director, Professor
DACEHTA
fbk@sst.dk

Project Coordinator (Project management issues):
Julia Chamova, MBA
juch@sst.dk
Tel: +45-7222-7861
Mob: +45-40-629-357
www.eunethta.net/HTA/

FAH   Federation of American Hospitals
To foster the public good through the creation and delivery of quality healthcare for all people.

801 Pennsylvania Avenue, NW
Suite 245
Washington, DC 20004-2604
Tel: 202-624-1500
Fax: 202-737-6462
www.fah.org

FCC   Federal Communications Commission
An independent United States government agency, directly responsible to Congress. The FCC was established by the Communications Act of 1934 and is charged with regulating interstate and international communications by radio, television, wire, satellite and cable. The FCC's jurisdiction covers the 50 states, the District of Columbia, and U.S. possessions.

7435 Oakland Mills Road
Columbia, MD 21046
Tel: 301-362-3000
Fax: 301-362-3290
www.fcc.gov

FDA   U.S. Food and Drug Administration
Responsible for protecting the public health by assuring the safety, efficacy, and security of human and veterinary drugs, biological products, medical devices, our nation's food supply, cosmetics, and products that emit radiation. The FDA is also responsible for advancing the public health by helping to speed innovations that make medicines and foods more effective, safer, and more affordable; and helping the public get the accurate, science-based information they need to use medicines and foods to improve their health.

5600 Fishers Lane
Rockville, MD 20857-0001
Tel: 888-463-6332
www.fda.gov

The George Institute for International Health
To improve global health through undertaking high quality research, and applying this research to health policy and practice.

MLC Centre
Level 56, 19 Martin Place
Sydney NSW 2000
Australia
Postal Address:
P.O. Box M201
Missenden Road
Sydney NSW 2050
Australia
Tel: +61-2-9657-0300
www.thegeorgeinstitute.org

GS1 US   Global Standards-1
To provide integrated solutions that improve our customers' supply chains across industries. We achieve this by taking a leadership role in establishing and promoting global standards and tools for collaborative commerce. (Formerly known as UCC.)

Princeton Pike Corporate Center 1009
Lenox Drive
Suite 202
Lawrenceville, NJ 08648
Tel: 609-620-0200
Fax: 609-620-1200
www.gs1us.org

HCCA   Health Care Compliance Association
Exists to champion ethical practice and compliance standards and to provide the necessary resources for ethics and compliance professionals and others who share these principles.

6500 Barrie Road
Suite 250
Minneapolis, MN 55435
Tel: 952-988-0141
Fax: 952-988-0146
www.hcca-info.org

HCCA Health Care Conference Administrators, LLC

Develops, organizes and administers conferences, audioconferences, trade shows, courses, customized learning and education, and Internet-based programming, alone, or in joint venture with or on behalf of sponsoring organizations. HCCA seeks to illuminate complex issues of healthcare practice and policy by bringing together leading-edge doers and thinkers—from operations to academia, from clinical practice to corporate management, from Main Street to Wall Street and from patient to politician.

1201 Third Avenue
Suite 2200
Seattle, WA 98101
Tel: 206-757-8053
Fax: 206-757-7053
www.ehcca.com

HCEA Healthcare Convention and Exhibitors Association

To improve the effectiveness and promote the value of all conventions, meetings and exhibitions for the healthcare industry.

1100 Johnson Ferry Road
Suite 300
Atlanta, GA 30342
Tel: 404-252-3663
Fax: 404-252-0774
www.hcea.org

HCEC Health Care eBusiness Collaborative

To enable healthcare organizations to understand and leverage the efficiencies of eBusiness strategies and technologies and reduce implementation and operations costs by providing: affordable education on eBusiness applications for healthcare; a central source for information on standards, specifications, technology and issues; updates on eBusiness initiatives and developments in healthcare; access to cost-effective eBusiness tools and resources; guidelines for eBusiness implementation; and support for collaborative eBusiness initiatives.

1405 North Pierce
Suite 100
Little Rock, AR 72207-3578
Tel: 800-905-4583
Fax: 501-661-0507
www.hcec.org

HCMA Healthcare Communication & Marketing Association

To enhance and optimize the careers of its members. The HCMA recognizes excellence in marketing, communications and education that impacts and improves health. (MMA merged with HCMA.)

19 Mantua Road
Mt. Royal, NJ 08061
Tel: 800-551-2173
Fax: 856-423-3420
www.mmanet.org

HDWA Healthcare Data Warehousing Association

To facilitate greater use of analytical information systems that help lower healthcare costs and improve quality of care; to advance the state of healthcare data warehousing and analytics by applying lessons and experience from other industries; a lack of emphasis by other professional organizations on the operational issues affecting data warehousing in healthcare; to assist other healthcare organizations that were just beginning or struggling to be successful with data warehousing and analytics; to influence vendors—the fairness of their pricing, the quality of their products and services, their willingness to share our risk, and their understanding of issues unique to healthcare; and to facilitate the development of standards and best practices that could lower the costs of development and operation for enterprise data warehouses in healthcare.

Intermountain Healthcare (IHC) hosts
the Web site.
Salt Lake City, UT
www.hdwa.org

Health Tech Health Technology Center

To create a trusted source of objective, expert and useful information about the future of healthcare technologies.

524 Second Street
2nd Floor
San Francisco, CA 94107
Tel: 415-537-6978
Fax: 415-537-6949
www.healthtechcenter.org

HFMA Healthcare Financial Management
Association
To define, realize and advance the financial
management of healthcare by helping members
and others improve the business performance of
organizations operating in or serving the healthcare field.

2 Westbrook Corporate Center
Suite 700
Westchester, IL 60154
Tel: 708-531-9600
Toll free: 800-252-4362
Fax: 708-531-0032
www.hfma.org

HIAA Health Insurance Association of America
See AHIP (HIAA is now AHIP.)

HIBCC Health Industry Business
Communications Council
An industry-sponsored and supported non-
profit organization. As an ANSI-accredited
organization, our primary function is to facilitate electronic communications by developing
appropriate standards for information exchange
among all healthcare trading partners. Our
broad mission has consistently expanded to
meet industry requirements and has involved
HIBCC in a number of critical areas, including
electronic data interchange message formats,
bar code labeling data standards, universal
numbering systems, and the provision of databases which assure common identifiers. HIBCC
plays a major advocacy and educational role in
the healthcare industry and serves as the forum
through which consensus can be reached as it
electronically transforms itself for 21st century
commerce.

2525 E. Arizona Biltmore Circle
Suite 127
Teloenix, AZ 85016
Tel: 602-381-1091
Fax: 602-381-1093
www.hibcc.org

HIMA Health Industry Manufacturers
Association
Organized in 1974 as a national trade association representing manufacturers of medical
devices, diagnostics, and health information
systems. It represents the industry before Congress and regulatory agencies including the
Food and Drug Administration and the Health
Care Financing Administration on issues of
interest to members.

1200 G Street, NW
Suite 400
Washington, DC 20005
Tel: 202-783-8700
Fax: 202-783-8750
www.health.gov/nhic/NHIC

HIMSS Healthcare Information and
Management Systems Society
To lead healthcare transformation through the
effective use of health information technology.

230 E. Ohio Street
Suite 500
Chicago, IL 60611-3270
Tel: 312-664-4467
Fax: 312-664-6143
www.himss.org

HITSP Health Informatics Technology
Standards Panel
To serve as a cooperative partnership between
the public and private sectors for the purpose
of achieving a widely accepted and useful set
of standards specifically to enable and support
widespread interoperability among healthcare
software applications, as they will interact in a
local, regional and national health information
network for the United States.

1819 L Street, NW
6th Floor
Washington, DC 20036
Tel: 202-293-8020
Fax: 202-293-9287
www.hitsp.org

HL7 Health Level Seven

Provides standards for interoperability that improve care delivery, optimize workflow, reduce ambiguity and enhance knowledge transfer among all of our stakeholders, including healthcare providers, government agencies, the vendor community, fellow SDOs and patients. In all of our processes we exhibit timeliness, scientific rigor and technical expertise without compromising transparency, accountability, practicality, or our willingness to put the needs of our stakeholders first.

3300 Washtenaw Avenue
Suite 227
Ann Arbor, MI 48104
Tel: 734-677-7777
Fax: 734-677-6622
www.hl7.org

HLC Healthcare Leadership Council

A coalition of chief executives from all disciplines within the health care system, HLC is the exclusive forum for the leaders of our nation's health care system to jointly develop policies, plans and programs to achieve their vision of a 21st century health care system.

1001 Pennsylvania Avenue, NW
Suite 550 South
Washington, DC 20004
Tel: 202-452-8700
Fax: 202-296-9561
www.hlc.org

HPNA Hospice and Palliative Nurses Association

Dedicated to quality end-of-life care through the promotion of excellence in hospice and palliative nursing. HPNA strives to promote excellence in hospice and palliative nursing through its mission, purpose, and strategic plan.

One Penn Center West
Suite 229
Pittsburgh, PA 15276-0100
Tel: 412-787-9301
Fax: 412-787-9305
www.hpna.org

HSC Center for Studying Health System Change

To inform policy makers and private decision makers about how local and national changes in the financing and delivery of health care affect people. HSC strives to provide high-quality, timely and objective research and analysis that leads to sound policy decisions, with the ultimate goal of improving the health of the American public.

600 Maryland Avenue, SW
#550
Washington, DC 20024
Tel: 202-484-5261
Fax: 202-484-9258
www.hschange.com

HTAi Health Technology Assessment International

To support the development, communication, understanding and use of HTA around the world as a means of promoting the introduction of effective innovations and effective use of resources in health care.

HTAi Secretariat
c/o Institute of Health Economics
1200, 10405 Jasper Avenue
Edmonton, Alberta T5J 3N4
Canada
Tel: 780-448-4881
Fax: 780-448-0018
www.htai.org

IAPP International Association of Privacy Professionals

To define, promote, and improve the privacy profession globally.

170 Cider Hill Road
York, ME 03909
Tel: 207-351-1500
Toll free: 800-266-6501
Fax: 207-351-1501
www.privacyassociation.org

ICCBBA International Council for Commonality in Blood Bank Automation
Enhances safety for patients by managing the ISBT 128 international information standard for use in transfusion and transplantation.

California, USA Office
P.O. Box 11309
San Bernardino, CA 92423-1309
Tel: 909-793-6516
Fax: 909-793-6214
http://iccbba.org/index.html

ICN International Council of Nurses
To represent nursing worldwide, advancing the profession and influencing health policy.

3, Place Jean Marteau
1201 - Geneva
Switzerland
Tel: +41-22-908-01-00
Fax: +41-22-908-01-01
www.icn.ch

IEC International Electrotechnical Commission
The leading global organization that prepares and publishes international standards for all electrical, electronic and related technologies. These serve as a basis for national standardization and as references when drafting international tenders and contracts.

3, rue de Varembé
P.O. Box 131
CH - 1211 Geneva 20
Switzerland
Tel: +41-22-919-02-11
Fax: +41-22-919-03-00
www.iec.ch

IEEE Institute of Electrical and Electronics Engineers
To foster technological innovation and excellence for the benefit of humanity.

1730 Massachusetts Avenue, NW
Washington, DC 20036-1992
Tel: 202-371-0101
Fax: 202-728-9614
www.ieee.org

IHE Integrating the Healthcare Enterprise
An initiative by healthcare professionals and industry to improve the way computer systems in healthcare share information. IHE promotes the coordinated use of established standards such as DICOM and HL7 to address specific clinical needs in support of optimal patient care. Systems developed in accordance with IHE communicate with one another better, are easier to implement, and enable care providers to use information more effectively. Physicians, medical specialists, nurses, administrators and other care providers envision a day when vital information can be passed seamlessly from system to system within and across departments and made readily available at the point of care. IHE is designed to make their vision a reality by improving the state of systems integration and removing barriers to optimal patient care.

HIMSS
230 E. Ohio Street
Suite 500
Chicago, IL 60611-3270
Tel: 312-664-4467
Fax: 312-664-6143

RSNA
820 Jorie Boulevard
Oak Brook, IL 60523-2251
Tel: 630-571-2670
Fax: 630-571-7837
www.ihe.net

IHF International Hospital Federation
To become a world leader in facilitating the exchange of knowledge and experience in health sector management. Through the dissemination of evidence-based information, IHF will help improve patient care quality around the globe.

Immeuble JB SAY
13 Chemin du Levant
F-01210 Ferney Voltaire
France
Tel: +33 (0) 450 42 6000
Fax: +33 (0) 450 42 6001
www.ihf-fih.org

IHTSDO   International Health Terminology Standards Development Organization

To acquire, own and administer the rights to SNOMED CT, other health terminologies and/or related standards, and other relevant assets (collectively, the "Terminology Products"); to develop, maintain, promote and enable the uptake and correct use of its Terminology Products in health systems, services and products around the world; and to undertake any or all activities incidental and conducive to achieving the purpose of the Association for the benefit of the Members.

Rued Langgaards Vej 7, 5A56
2300 Copenhagen S
Denmark
Tel: +45-36-44-87-36
Fax: +45-44-44-87-36
www.ihtsdo.org

IIE   International Institute of Education

Promoting closer educational relations between the people of the United States and those of other countries; strengthening and linking institutions of higher learning globally; rescuing threatened scholars and advancing academic freedom; and building leadership skills and enhancing the capacity of individuals and organizations to address local and global challenges.

Midwest Office:
25 E. Washington Street
Suite 1735
Chicago, IL 60602
Tel: 312-346-0026
Fax: 312-346-2574
E-mail: midwest@iie.org
www.iie.org

IIR   Institute for International Research

To facilitate the growth and advancement of our core client-partners by supplying the optimum business solutions—at the right time and in the right format—so that their goals can be surpassed and unique marketplace challenges overcome. We pride ourselves on our abilities to respond quickly to market needs and work in conjunction with each of our partners to provide you, our stakeholder, with quality learning experiences that are leading edge, dynamic, and fully customizable. Our Mission and Vision are fueled by a set of core values, to which all IIR associates are dedicated: Know our customers and strive to exceed their expectations; keep customer satisfaction as the one true measure of success; be the innovators of our industry, bringing new ideas in topic and format to our customers; and maintain a work environment that fosters the entrepreneurial spirit, work ethic, and teamwork for IIR and its associates.

708 3rd Avenue
4th Floor
New York, NY 10017
Tel: 212-599-2192
Fax: 212-661-3500
www.iirusa.com

IMIA   International Medical Informatics Association

To promote informatics in health care and research in health, bio and medical informatics; to advance and nurture international cooperation; to stimulate research, development and routine application; to move informatics from theory into practice in a full range of health delivery settings, from physician's office to acute and long term care; to further the dissemination and exchange of knowledge, information and technology; to promote education and responsible behaviour; and to represent the medical and health informatics field with the World Health Organization and other international professional and governmental organizations.

5782 - 172 Street
Edmonton, Alberta T6M 1B4
Canada
Tel: 780-489-4531
Fax: 780-489-3290
www.imia.org

INAHTA International Network of Agencies for Health Technology Assessment
To provide a forum for the identification and pursuit of interests common to health technology assessment agencies.

INAHTA Secretariat
c/o SBU P.O. Box 5650
Visiting address: Tyrgatan 7
SE-114 86 Stockholm
Sweden
Tel: +46-8-412-32-00
Fax: +46-8-411-32-60
www.inahta.org

INS International Neuropsychological Society
To promote the international and interdisciplinary study of brain-behavioral relationships throughout the lifespan. The Society's emphasis is on science, education, and the applications of scientific knowledge.

700 Ackerman Road
Suite 625
Columbus, OH 43202
Tel: 614-263-4200
Fax: 614-263-4366
www.the-ins.org

INS Intravenous Nursing Society
Sets the standard for excellence in infusion nursing by developing and disseminating standards of practice; providing professional development opportunities and quality education; advancing best practice through evidence-based research; supporting professional certification; and advocating for the public.

315 Norwood Park South
Norwood, MA 02062
Tel: 800-694-0298, ext. 330/331/334
After 5:00 pm:
800-694-0298, ext. 331
Fax: 781-440-9409
www.ins1.org

INCITS InterNational Committee for Information Technology Standards
To promote the effective use of information and communication technology through standardization in a way that balances the interests of all stakeholders and increases the global competitiveness of the member organizations.

c/o Information Technology Industry
Council
1101 K Street NW
Suite 610
Washington, DC 20005
Tel: 202-737-8888
Fax: 202-638-4922
www.incits.org

IOM Institute of Medicine of the National Academies
Serves as adviser to the nation to improve health.

500 Fifth Street, NW
Washington, DC 20001
Tel: 202-334-2352
Fax: 202-334-1412
www.iom.edu

IOMSN International Organization for Multiple Sclerosis Nurses
The establishment and perpetuation of a specialized branch of nursing in multiple sclerosis, to establish standards of nursing care in multiple sclerosis; to support multiple sclerosis nursing research; to educate the health care community about multiple sclerosis; and to disseminate this knowledge throughout the world.

P.O. Box 450
Teaneck, NJ 07666
or
359 Main Street
Suite A
Hackensack, NJ 07601
Tel: 201-487-1050, ext. 106
Fax: 201-678-2291
www.iomsn.org

ISNCC International Society of Nurses in Cancer Care

The protection and preservation of health and the relief of cancer-related sickness, and the promotion and coordination of the activities of cancer nursing through the advancement and improvement of: the delivery of nursing care to people affected by cancer; education in cancer nursing; and nursing research, including the publication of the useful results of such research.

375 West 5th Avenue
Suite 201
Vancouver, British Columbia V5Y 1J6
Canada
Tel: +1-604-630-5516
Fax: +1-604-874-4378
www.isncc.org

ISO International Organization for Standardization

To enable a consensus to be reached on solutions that meet both the requirements of business and the broader needs of society.

1, ch. De la Voie Creuse
Case Postale 56
CH-1211
Geneva 20
Switzerland
Tel:+41-22-749-01-11
Fax: +41-22-733-34-30
www.iso.org

ISPN International Society of Psychiatric-Mental Health Nurses

To unite and strengthen the presence and the voice of specialty psychiatric-mental health nursing while influencing health care policy to promote equitable, evidence-based and effective treatment and care for individuals, families and communities.

2810 Crossroads Drive
Suite 3800
Madison, WI 53718
Tel: 608-443-2463
Toll free: 866-330-7227
Fax: 608-443-2474 or 2478
www.ispn-psych.org

ISQUA International Society for Quality in Health Care

Driving continual improvement in the quality and safety of healthcare worldwide through education, research, collaboration and the dissemination of evidence-based knowledge.

Clarendon Terrace
212 Clarendon Street
East Melbourne, Victoria 3002
Australia
Tel: +61-3-9417-6971
Fax: +61-3-9417-6851
www.isqua.org.au

ISSA Information Systems Security Association

To promote management practices that will ensure the confidentiality, integrity and availability of information resources. The ISSA facilitates interaction and education to create a more successful environment for global information systems security and for the professionals involved.

9220 SW Barbur Boulevard
#119-333
Portland, OR 97219
Tel: 866-349-5818
Fax: 206-299-3366
www.issa.org

ITAC Information Technology Association of Canada

To identify and lead on issues that affect our industry and to advocate initiatives, which will enable its continued growth and development.

5090 Explorer Drive
Suite 801
Mississauga, Ontario L4W 4T9
Canada
Tel: 905-602-8345
Fax: 905-602-8346
www.itac.ca

ITU International Telecommunication Union
To enable the growth and sustained development of telecommunications and information networks, and to facilitate universal access so that people everywhere can participate in, and benefit from, the emerging information society and global economy. The ability to communicate freely is a prerequisite for a more equitable, prosperous and peaceful world. And ITU assists in mobilizing the technical, financial and human resources needed to make this vision a reality.

Place des Nations
1211 Geneva 20
Switzerland
Tel: +41-22-730-5111
Fax: +41-22-733-72-56
www.itu.int

JCAHO The Joint Commission on Accreditation of Healthcare Organizations
See The Joint Commission (JCAHO is now The Joint Commission).

The Joint Commission
To continuously improve health care for the public, in collaboration with other stakeholders, by evaluating health care organizations and inspiring them to excel in providing safe and effective care of the highest quality and value.

One Renaissance Boulevard
Oakbrook Terrace, IL 60181
Tel: 630-792-5000
Fax: 630-792-5005
www.jointcommission.org

JCR Joint Commission Resources
To continuously improve the safety and quality of health care in the United States and in the international community through the provision of education, publications, consultation, and evaluation services.

1515 W. 22nd Street
Oak Brook, IL 60523
Tel: 630-268-7400
www.jcrinc.com

The Leapfrog Group
To trigger giant leaps forward in the safety, quality and affordability of healthcare by supporting informed healthcare decisions by those who use and pay for healthcare; and promoting high-value healthcare through incentives and rewards.

c/o Academy Health
Suite 600
1150 17th Street, NW
Washington, DC 20036
Tel: 202-292-6713
Fax: 202-292-6813
www.leapfroggroup.org

LOINC Logical Observation Identifiers Names and Codes
To facilitate the exchange and pooling of clinical results for clinical care, outcomes management, and research by providing a set of universal codes and names to identify laboratory and other clinical observations.

Regenstrief Institute, Inc.
410 W. 10th Street
Suite 2000
Indianapolis, IN 46202
Tel: 317-630-7604
Fax: 317-423-5695
www.loinc.org

MEC Medical Education Collaborative
To deliver independent accreditation services and continuing education expertise that improve healthcare education and professional performance.

651 Corporate Circle
Suite 104
Golden, CO 80401
Tel: 866-420-3252
Fax: 303-420-3259
www.meccme.org

MGMA   Medical Group Management Association

To continually improve the performance of medical group practice professionals and the organizations they represent.

104 Inverness Terrace East
Englewood, CO 80112-5306
Tel: 303-799-1111
Fax: 303-643-4439
www.mgma.com

mHealth Initiative

To connect and coordinate the roles of all health participants, including patients, the wide range of healthcare providers, payers, pharma, wellness providers, and more.

398 Columbus Avene
Suite 295
Boston, MA 02116
Tel: 617-816-7513
Fax: 617-670-0708
www.mobih.org

MLA   Medical Library Association

Committed to educating health information professionals, supporting health information research, promoting access to the world's health sciences information, and working to ensure that the best health information is available to all.

Boston VA Healthcare System
150 S. Huntington Avenue
Boston, MA 02130
Tel: 857-364-5939
Fax: 857-364-6587
www.mlanet.org

MMA   Medical Marketing Association

See HCMA (MMA merged with HCMA).

MS-HUG   Microsoft Healthcare Users Group

To better serve MS-HUG members and the industry through a shared strategic vision to provide leadership and healthcare information technology solutions that improve the delivery of patient care.

230 E. Ohio Street
Suite 500
Chicago, IL 60611
Tel: 312-664-4467
www.mshug.org

MTPPI   Medical Technologies Practice Patterns Institute

A nonprofit organization dedicated to research, education, and the dissemination of information regarding current and emerging medical technologies.

4733 Bethesda Avenue
Suite 510
Bethesda, MD 20814
Tel: 301-652-4005
Fax: 301-652-8335
www.mtppi.org

NAFAC   National Association for Ambulatory Care

A national association of urgent and ambulatory care providers joined together for mutual benefit of education, networking and representing our concerns and needs to insurers and state and federal governments.

18870 Rutledge Road
Minneapolis, MN 55391
Tel: 952-476-0015
www.urgentcare.org - or - www.nafac.com

NAHC   National Association for Home Care

From professional development to fighting for better regulation, from knowing all angles of federal and state regulations to providing the latest information affecting home care and hospice, NAHC stands ready to serve your needs, enabling you to better serve your patients.

228 Seventh Street, SE
Washington, DC 20003
Tel: 202-547-7424
Fax: 202-547-3540
www.nahc.org

NAHDO National Association for Health Data Organizations
A national, not-for-profit membership organization dedicated to improving healthcare through the collection, analysis, dissemination, public availability, and use of health data. NAHDO provides leadership in healthcare information management and analysis, promotes the availability of and access to health data, and encourages the use of these data to make informed decisions and guide the development of health policy. NAHDO provides information on current issues and strategies to develop a nationwide, comprehensive, integrated health information system, sponsors educational programs, provides assistance, and serves as a forum to foster collaboration and the exchange of ideas and experiences among collectors and users of health data. By doing so, NAHDO works to increase the state of knowledge.

448 East 400 South
Suite 301
Salt Lake City, UT 84111
Tel: 801-532-2299
Fax: 801-532-2228
www.nahdo.org

NAHIT National Alliance for Health Information Technology
Operations stopped September 2009. Please *see* Appendix D for the consensus definitions from 2008.

NAHQ National Association for Healthcare Quality
Empowers healthcare quality professionals from every specialty by providing vital research, education, networking, certification and professional practice resources, and a strong voice for healthcare quality.

4700 W. Lake Avenue
Glenview, IL 60025-1485
Tel: 847-375-4720
Fax: 888-412-7576
www.nahq.org

NANDA North American Nursing Diagnosis Association
To increase the visibility of nursing's contribution to patient care by continuing to develop, refine and classify phenomena of concern to nurses.

100 N. 20th Street
4th Floor
Philadelphia, PA 19103
Tel: 215-545-8105
Fax: 215-564-2175
www.nanda.org

NAPCI National Alliance for Primary Care Informatics
I. To promote the creation of a national health information infrastructure (NHII) that identifies and supports the unique needs of primary care practitioners and provides incentives to primary care practitioners to participate in the NHII; II. To document and report on the use of informatics and information technology in primary care, and to promote primary care clinical research through the NHII in the most high-quality and cost-efficient manner possible; III. To educate primary care providers in the use of informatics and information technology in the practice of primary care; IV. To facilitate work within NAPCI and between NAPCI and other organizations to present a unified coalition representing the interests of primary care in the NHII and promoting the NHII; V. To take part in and sponsor meetings, publications, and other forums for the purpose of advancing the mission of NAPCI and its member organizations.

4915 St. Elmo Avenue
Suite 401
Bethesda, MD 20814
Tel: 301-657-1291
Fax: 301-657-1296
www.napci.org

NASN   National Association of School Nurses
Improves the health and educational success of children and youth by developing and providing leadership to advance school nursing practice.

8484 Georgia Avenue
Suite 420
Silver Spring, MD 20910
Tel: 240-821-1130
Toll free: 866-627-6767
Fax: 301-585-1791
www.nasn.org

NBDHMT   National Board of Diving and Hyperbaric Medical Technology
To provide board certification and ongoing support to hyperbaric technologists, hyperbaric nurses and diving medical technicians to ensure that the fields of hyperbaric medicine, hyperbaric chamber operation, and diving medicine are supported with the most highly qualified personnel possible.

1816 Industrial Boulevard
Harvey, LA 70058
Tel: 504-328-8871
www.nbdhmt.org

NCCA   National Commission for Certifying Agencies
Promotes excellence in competency assessment for practitioners in all occupations and professions by providing expertise and guidance; developing and implementing standards for accreditation of certification programs through NCCA (NOCA's accrediting body); providing educational and networking resources; and serving as an advocate on certification issues.

2025 M Street, NW
Suite 800
Washington, DC 20036
Tel: 202-367-1165
Fax: 202-367-2165
www.noca.org

NCCLS   National Committee for Clinical Laboratory Standards
See CLSI (NCCLS is now CLSI).

NCEMI   National Center for Emergency Medicine Informatics
To the advancement of Emergency Medicine through the application of information technology. At NCEMI, we believe that the greatest advances in medicine over the next two decades will result from the application of the tools and principles of information science to the problems of clinical medicine. New developments in informatics will drive advances in clinical care, medical administration, medical research, and medical education.

www.ncemi.org

NCHS   National Center for Health Statistics
To provide statistical information that will guide actions and policies to improve the health of the American people. As the nation's principal health statistics agency, NCHS leads the way with accurate, relevant, and timely data.

3311 Toledo Road
Hyattsville, MD 20782
Tel: 301-458-4000
www.cdc.gov/nchs

NCO/NITRD   National Coordination Office for Networking and Information Technology Research and Development
To formulate and promote federal information technology research and development to meet national goals.

Suite II-405
4201 Wilson Boulevard
Arlington, VA 22230
Tel: 703-292-4873
Fax: 703-292-9097
www.nitrd.gov

NCPDP National Council for Prescription Drug Program
Creates and promotes standards for the transfer of data to and from the pharmacy services sector of the healthcare industry. The organization provides a forum and support wherein our diverse membership can efficiently and effectively develop and maintain these standards through a consensus building process. NCPDP also offers its members resources, including educational opportunities and database services, to better manage their businesses.

9240 E. Raintree Drive
Scottsdale, AZ 85260-7518
Tel: 480-477-1000
Fax: 480-767-1042
www.ncpdp.org

NCQA National Committee for Quality Assurance
To improve the quality of healthcare.

1100 13th Street, NW
Suite 1000
Washington, DC 20005
Tel: 202-955-3500
Fax: 202-955-3599
www.ncqa.org

NCSBN National Council of State Boards of Nursing
Provides leadership to advance regulatory excellence for public protection.

111 East Wacker Drive
Suite 2900
Chicago, IL 60601
Tel: 312-525-3600
Fax: 312-279-1032
www.ncsbn.org

NCVHS National Committee on Vital and Health Statistics
To advise on shaping a national information strategy for improving the population's health.

200 Independence Avenue, SW
Washington, DC 20201
Tel: 202-619-0257
Toll free: 877-696-6775
www.ncvhs.dhhs.gov

NeHC National eHealth Collaborative
Integrity, Authenticity, Accuracy: Pillars for effective health information capture, exchange and use.

National eHealth Collaborative
P.O. Box 27225
Washington, DC 20038-7225
Tel: 877-835-6506
Fax: 202-719-5303
www.nationalehealth.org

NHCAA National Health Care Anti-Fraud Association
To protect and serve the public interest by increasing awareness and improving the detection, investigation, civil and criminal prosecution and prevention of healthcare fraud.

1201 New York Avenue, NW
Suite 1120
Washington, DC 20005
Tel: 202-659-5955
Fax: 202-785-6764
www.nhcaa.org

NHIC National Health Information Center
A health information referral service sponsored by the Office of Disease Prevention and Health Promotion. NHIC puts health professionals and consumers who have health questions in touch with those organizations that are best able to provide answers. Using a database that contains descriptions of health-related organizations, NHIC staff refer people to the most appropriate resource.

Referral Specialist
P.O. Box 1133
Washington, DC 20013-1133
Toll-free: 800-336-4797
Tel: 301-565-4167
Fax: 301-984-4256
http://www.health.gov/nhic

NHII   National Health Information
Infrastructure
An initiative set forth to improve the effectiveness, efficiency and overall quality of health and
healthcare in the U.S.

> *U.S. Dept. of Health & Human Services*
> *200 Independence Avenue, SW*
> *Washington, DC 20201*
> *Tel: 202-619-0257*
> *http://aspe.hhs.gov/sp/NHII/*

NHLBI   National Heart, Lung and Blood
Institute
Provides leadership for a national program in
diseases of the heart, blood vessels, lung, and
blood; blood resources; and sleep disorders.
Since October 1997, the NHLBI has also had
administrative responsibility for the NIH Wom-
an's Health Initiative.

> *Building 31, Room 5A48*
> *31 Center Drive MSC 2486*
> *Bethesda, MD 20892*
> *Tel: 301-592-8573*
> *TTY: 240-629-3255*
> *Fax: 240-629-3246*
> *www.nhlbi.nih.gov*

NIDSEC   Nursing Information and Data Set
Evaluation Center
Develops and disseminates standards pertaining to information systems that support the
documentation of nursing practice, and evaluates voluntarily submitted information systems
against these standards.

> *8515 Georgia Avenue*
> *Suite 400*
> *Silver Spring, MD 20910-3492*
> *Tel: 301-628-5000*
> *Fax: 301-628-5001*
> *www.nursingworld.org/nidsec*

NIH   National Institutes of Health
NIH is the steward of medical and behavioral
research for the nation. Its mission is science
in pursuit of fundamental knowledge about
the nature and behavior of living systems and
the application of that knowledge to extend
healthy life and reduce the burdens of illness
and disability.

> *9000 Rockville Pike*
> *Bethesda, MD 20892*
> *Tel: 301-496-4000*
> *www.nih.gov*

NIHR   National Institute of Health Research
Health Technology Assessment Program
The HTA programme produces independent
research about the effectiveness of different
healthcare treatments and tests for those who
use, manage and provide care in the NHS. It
identifies the most important questions that
the NHS needs the answers to by consulting
widely with these groups, and commissions the
research it thinks is most important through different funding routes. The HTA programme is a
programme of the National Institute for Health
Research (NIHR).

> *NCCHTA*
> *Mailpoint 728*
> *Boldrewood*
> *University of Southampton*
> *Bassett Crescent East*
> *Southampton SO16 7PX*
> *Tel: +44 (0)23-8059-5586*
> *Fax: +44 (0)23-8059-5639*
> *www.hta.nhsweb.nhs.uk/*

NINR   National Institute of Nursing Research

To promote and improve the health of individuals, families, communities and populations. NINR supports and conducts clinical and basic research and research training on health and illness across the lifespan. The research focus encompasses health promotion and disease prevention, quality of life, health disparities, and end of life. NINR seeks to extend nursing science by integrating the biological and behavioral sciences, employing new technologies to research questions, improving research methods, and developing the scientists of the future.

31 Center Drive
Room 5B10
Bethesda, MD 20892-2178
Tel: 301-496-0207
Toll free: 866-910-3804
TTY: 301-594-5605
Fax: 301-480-8845
www.ninr.nih.gov

NIST   National Institute of Standards and Technology

To promote U.S. innovation and industrial competitiveness by advancing measurement science, standards, and technology in ways that enhance economic security and improve our quality of life.

100 Bureau Drive
Stop 1070
Gaithersburg, MD 20899-1070
Tel: 301-975-6478
www.nist.gov

NKCHS   Norwegian Knowledge Centre for Health Services

Gathers and disseminates evidence about the effect and quality of methods and interventions within all parts of the health services. The uptake of this evidence by the health services is also an important goal for the Centre's activities.

P.O. Box 7004
St. Olavs plass
N-0130 Oslo, Norway
Tel: +47 23 25 50 00
Fax: +47 23 25 50 10
www.kunnskapssenteret.no

NKF   National Kidney Foundation

A major voluntary health organization, NKF seeks to prevent kidney and urinary tract diseases, improve the health and well-being of individuals and families affected by these diseases, and increase the availability of all organs for transplantation.

30 E. 33rd Street
New York, NY 10016
Tel: 800-622-9010
www.kidney.org

NLM   National Library of Medicine

On the campus of the National Institutes of Health in Bethesda, Maryland, the NLM is the world's largest medical library. The Library collects materials in all areas of biomedicine and health care, as well as works on biomedical aspects of technology, the humanities, and the physical, life, and social sciences. The collections stand at more than 9 million items—books, journals, technical reports, manuscripts, microfilms, photographs and images. Housed within the Library is one of the world's finest medical history collections of old and rare medical works. The Library's collection may be consulted in the reading room or requested on interlibrary loan. NLM is a national resource for all U.S. health science libraries through a National Network of Libraries of Medicine®.

8600 Rockville Pike
Bethesda, MD 20894
Tel: 301-594-5983
Fax: 301-402-1384
www.nlm.nih.gov

NLN   National League of Nursing

Promotes excellence in nursing education to build a strong and diverse nursing workforce.

61 Broadway
33rd Floor
New York, NY 10006
Tel: 212-363-5555
Fax: 212-812-0391
www.nln.org

NOA Nursing Organizations Alliance

Formed when two long-standing coalitions of nursing organizations united to create an enduring collaborative. The historic vote to create The Alliance occurred on November 17, 2001 at a special meeting with National Federation for Specialty Nursing Organizations (NFSNO) and the Nursing Organizations Liaison Forum (NOLF) member organizations in Salt Lake City, Utah. The purpose of the Alliance is to provide a forum for identification, education and collaboration building on issues of common interest to advance the nursing profession.

201 East Main Street
Suite 140
Lexington, KY 40507
Tel: 859-514-9157
Fax: 859-514-9166
www.nursing-alliance.org

NOCA National Organization for Competency Assurance

Promotes excellence in competency assessment for practitioners in all occupations and professions by providing expertise and guidance; developing and implementing standards for accreditation of certification programs through NCCA (NOCA's accrediting body); providing educational and networking resources; and serving as an advocate on certification issues.

2025 M Street, NW
Suite 800
Washington, DC 20036
Tel: 202-367-1165
Fax: 202-367-2165
www.noca.org

NSF National Science Foundation

An independent federal agency created by Congress in 1950 to promote the progress of science; to advance the national health, prosperity, and welfare; and to secure the national defense. With an annual budget of about $5.92 billion, we are the funding source for approximately 20 percent of all federally supported basic research conducted by America's colleges and universities. In many fields such as mathematics, computer science and the social sciences, NSF is the major source of federal backing.

4201 Wilson Boulevard
Arlington, VA 22230
Tel: 703-292-5111
FIRS: 800-877-8339
TDD: 800-281-8749
www.nsf.gov

NUBC National Uniform Billing Committee

Brought together by the American Hospital Association (AHA) in 1975, NUBC includes the participation of all the major national provider and payer organizations. The NUBC was formed to develop a single billing form and standard data set that could be used nationwide by institutional providers and payers for handling health care claims.

American Hospital Association
National Uniform Billing Committee
One N. Franklin
Chicago, IL 60606-3421
www.nubc.org

NUCC National Uniform Claim Committee
A voluntary organization that replaced the Uniform Claim Form Task Force in 1995. The committee was created to develop a standardized data set for use by the non-institutional healthcare community to transmit claim and encounter information to and from all third-party payers. It is chaired by the American Medical Association (AMA), with the Centers for Medicare & Medicaid Services (CMS) as a critical partner. The committee includes representation from key provider and payer organizations, as well as standards maintenance organizations, public health organizations, and a vendor.

American Medical Association
515 N. State Street
Chicago, IL 60610
Tel: 800-621-8335
www.nucc.org

NZHTA New Zealand Health Technology Assessment
A clearing house for health outcomes and health technology assessment. The mission of NZHTA is to assist New Zealand health and disability services through the production and dissemination of evidence-based information for decisions on health policy and purchasing, service management, and clinical practice.

Department of Public Health and
General Practice
School of Medicine and Health Sciences
University of Otago, Christchurch
St. Elmo Courts Building
Level 4, 47 Hereford Street
P.O. Box 4345
Christchurch
New Zealand
Tel: +64-3-364-3696
Fax: +64-3-364-3697
http://nzhta.chmeds.ac.nz/

OASIS Advancing Open Standards for the Information Society
An organization that engenders participation from industry, bringing together competitors and industry standards groups. Through open discussion and debate, the OASIS process reconciles conflicting perspectives to create XML implementations that are representative of the industry as a whole.

630 Boston Road
Suite M-102
Billerica, MA 01821
Tel: 978-667-5115
Fax: 978-667-5114
www.oasis-open.org

OMG Object Management Group
An international, open membership, not-for-profit computer industry consortium since 1989. Any organization may join OMG and participate in our standards-setting process. Our one-organization-one-vote policy ensures that every organization, large and small, has an effective voice in our process. Our membership includes hundreds of organizations, with half being software end-users in over two dozen vertical markets, and the other half representing virtually every large organization in the computer industry and many smaller ones. Most of the organizations that shape enterprise and Internet computing today are represented on our Board of Directors.

140 Kendrick Street
Building A
Suite 300
Needham, MA 02494
Tel: 781-444 0404
Fax: 781-444-0320
www.omg.org

ONC Office of the National Coordinator for Health Information Technology
Provides leadership for the development and nationwide implementation of an interoperable health information technology infrastructure to improve the quality and efficiency of healthcare and the ability of consumers to manage their care and safety.

200 Independence Avenue, SW
Washington, DC 20201
Tel: 202-619-0257
Toll free: 877-696-6775
www.hhs.gov/healthit/mission.html

ONS   Oncology Nursing Society

A professional organization of over 35,000 registered nurses and other healthcare providers dedicated to excellence in patient care, education, research, and administration in oncology nursing. It is also the largest professional oncology association in the world.

125 Enterprise Drive
RIDC Park West
Pittsburgh, PA 15275-1214
Tel: 412-859-6100
Toll free: 866-257-4ONS
Fax: 877-369-5497
www.ons.org

OSHA   Occupational Safety and Health Administration

To assure the safety and health of America's workers by setting and enforcing standards; providing training, outreach, and education; establishing partnerships; and encouraging continual improvement in workplace safety and health.

200 Constitution Avenue, NW
Washington, DC 20210
Tel: 800-321-6742
www.osha.gov

Perio   American Academy of Peridontology

Known for advancing oral health and well-being through expertise in periodontics, implants, periodontal medicine, periodontal plastic surgery, and oral reconstructive surgery.

737 N. Michigan Avenue
Suite 800
Chicago, IL 60611-6660
Tel: 312-787-5518
Fax: 312-787-3670
www.perio.org

PHII   Public Health Informatics Institute

To improve the performance of the public health system by advancing public health practitioners' ability to strategically manage and apply health information systems.

750 Commerce Drive
Suite 400
Decatur, GA 30030
Tel: 866-815-9704
Fax: 800-765-7520
www.phii.org

PITAC   President's Information Technology Advisory Committee

Provides the President, Congress, and the federal agencies involved in networking and information technology research and development with expert, independent advice on maintaining America's preeminence in advanced information technologies, including such critical elements of the national information technology infrastructure as high performance computing, large-scale networking, cyber security, and high assurance software and systems design. As part of this assessment, the PITAC reviews the Federal Networking and Information Technology Research and Development (NITRD) Program. Comprised of leading IT experts from industry and academia, the Committee helps guide the Administration's efforts to accelerate the development and adoption of information technologies vital for American prosperity in the 21st century.

4201 Wilson Boulevard
Suite ll-405
Arlington, VA 22230
Tel: 703-292-4873
Fax: 703-292-9097
www.nitrd.gov/pitac/

PMI   Project Management Institute

Actively engaged in advocacy for the profession, setting professional standards, conducting research and providing access to a wealth of information and resources.

Four Campus Boulevard
Newtown Square, PA 19073-3299
Tel: 610-356-4600
Fax: 610-356-4647
www.pmi.org

RCN Royal College of Nursing

To deliver our mission we aim to: *Represent* the interests of nurses and nursing and be their voice locally, nationally and internationally; *Influence* and lobby governments and others to develop and implement policy that improves the quality of patient care, and builds on the importance of nurses, health care assistants and nursing students to health outcomes; *Support and protect* the value of nurses and nursing staff in all their diversity, their terms and conditions of employment in all employment sectors, the interests of nurses professionally; *Develop* and educate nurses professionally and academically, building our resource of professional expertise and leadership, the science and art of nursing and its professional practice; and *Build* a sustainable, member-led organisation with the capacity to deliver our mission effectively, efficiently and in accordance with our values, the systems, attitudes and resources to offer the best possible support and development to our staff.

20 Cavendish Square
London W1G 0RN
United Kingdom
Tel: +020-7409-3333
www.rcn.org.uk

Regenstrief Institute

An internationally recognized informatics and healthcare research organization dedicated to the improvement of health through research that enhances the quality and cost-effectiveness of healthcare.

1050 Wishard Boulevard
RG 6
Indianapolis, IN 46202-2872
Tel: 317-630-7604
www.regenstrief.org

RSNA Radiological Society of North America

To promote and develop the highest standards of radiology and related sciences through education and research. The Society seeks to provide radiologists and allied health scientists with educational programs and materials of the highest quality, and to constantly improve the content and value of these educational activities. The Society seeks to promote research in all aspects of radiology and related sciences, including basic clinical research in the promotion of quality healthcare. The Society seeks to foster closer fellowship among all radiologists and greater cooperation among radiologists and members of other branches of medicine and allied healthcare professionals.

820 Jorie Boulevard
Oak Brook, IL 60523-2251
Tel: 630-571-2670
Fax: 630-571-7837
www.rsna.org

SBU Swedish Council on Technology Assessment in Health Care

Has the mandate of the Swedish Government to comprehensively assess healthcare technology from medical, economic, ethical, and social standpoints. Reports prepared by SBU present the best available scientific evidence on the benefits, risks, and costs associated with different interventions. SBU identifies methods that offer the greatest benefits and the least risk, focusing on the most efficient ways to allocate healthcare resources. However, SBU also identifies methods currently in use that provide no benefits, have not been assessed, or are not cost effective. SBU aims to compile unbiased, scientifically based assessment reports to support decision making in healthcare. Reports by SBU are intended for those who make important choices regarding which healthcare options to use. Target groups include professional caregivers, healthcare administrators, planners, and health policy makers. The findings also concern many patients and their families.

Tyrgatan 7
Box 5650
SE-114 86 Stockholm
Sweden
Tel: +46-8-412-32-00
Fax: +46-8-411-32-60
http://www.sbu.se/en/

SCAR The Society for Computer Applications in Radiology
See SIIMS (SCAR is now SIIM).

Scottsdale Institute

To share information and experiences in information technology-enabled performance improvement.

1660 Highway 100, South
Suite 306
Minneapolis, MN 55416
Tel: 952-545-5880
Fax: 952-545-6116
www.scottsdaleinstitute.org

SGNA Society of Gastroenterology Nurses and Associates
A professional organization of nurses and associates dedicated to the safe and effective practice of gastroenterology and endoscopy nursing. SGNA carries out its mission by advancing the science and practice of gastroenterology and endoscopy nursing through education, research, advocacy, and collaboration, and by promoting the professional development of its members in an atmosphere of mutual support.

401 N. Michigan Avenue
Chicago, IL 60611-4267
Tel: 312-321-5165
Toll free: 800-245-7462
Fax: 312-673-6694
www.sgna.org

SHS The Society for Health Systems
A society within International Institute for Education (IIE), SHS exists to contribute to the improvement of healthcare delivery systems through systems engineering, analysis, and process improvement methods.

3577 Parkway Lane
Suite 200
Norcross, GA 30092
Tel: 800-494-0460
Fax: 770-441-3295
www.iienet2.org

SIIM The Society for Imaging Informatics in Medicine
To advance computer applications and information technology in medical imaging through education and research.

19440 GolfVista Plaza
Suite 330
Leesburg, VA 20176-8264
Tel: 703-723-0432
Fax: 703-723-0415
www.siimweb.org

SIR Society of Interventional Radiology
To improve the health of the public through pioneering advances in image-guided therapy.

3975 Fair Ridge Drive
Suite 400 North
Fairfax, VA 22033
Tel: 703-691-1805
Fax: 703-691-1855
www.sirweb.org

SNRS Southern Nursing Research Society
To (1) advance nursing research; (2) promote dissemination and utilization of research findings; (3) facilitate the career development of nurses and nursing students as researchers; (4) enhance communication among members; and (5) promote the image of nursing as a scientific discipline.

10200 W. 44th Avenue
Suite 304
Wheat Ridge, CO 80033
Tel: 877-314-SNRS
ww.snrs.org

TNA Transplant Nurses Association

To advance the education of nurses and allied health professionals involved in the transplant process by promoting, providing and communicating knowledge and current information to those interested in the transplant field and associated areas; to develop a network between members of TNA with a common interest in transplantation and to discuss professional and ethical issues and exchange information; and to provide transplant nurses with standards generally and specially for their specialised field so as to foster the highest attainable level of patient care.

Box M94
Missenden Road
Camperdown. NSW. 2050
Australia
Tel: +(08) 8204 5819
www.tna.asn.au

UCC Uniform Code Council

See GS1 US (UCC is now GS1).

UNECE United Nations Economic Commission for Europe

To promote pan-European economic integration. To do so, UNECE brings together 56 countries located in the European Union, non-EU Western and Eastern Europe, South-East Europe and Commonwealth of Independent States (CIS) and North America. All these countries dialogue and cooperate under the aegis of the UNECE on economic and sectoral issues. To this end, it provides analysis, policy advice and assistance to governments, and it gives focus to the United Nations global mandates in the economic field, in cooperation with other global players and key stakeholders, notably the business community.

Palais des Nations
CH - 1211
Geneva 10
Switzerland
Tel: +41-0-22-917-12-34
Fax: +41-0-22-917-05-05
www.unece.org

VA Department of Veterans Affairs

"To care for him who shall have borne the battle and for his widow and his orphan." These words, spoken by Abraham Lincoln during his second inaugural address, reflect the philosophy and principles that guide the VA in everything we do and are the focus of our endeavors to serve our nation's veterans and their families.

810 Vermont Avenue, NW
Washington, DC 20420
Tel: 800-827-1000
www.va.gov

VATAP VA Technology Assessment Program

To carry out systematic reviews of the medical literature on "what works" in health care for VHA senior managers; promote excellent health care value through evidence-based decision making; and provide impartial, peer-reviewed evidence-based reports to support better resource management in VHA.

Boston VA Healthcare System
150 S. Huntington Avenue
Boston, MA 02130
Tel: 857-364-5939
Fax: 857-364-6587
www.va.gov/vatap/

VNAA Visiting Nurses Association of America

To support, promote and advance the nation's network of VNAs who provide cost-effective and compassionate home healthcare to some of the nation's most vulnerable individuals, particularly the elderly and individuals with disabilities.

8403 Colesville Road
Suite 1550
Silver Spring, MD 20910-6374
Tel: 240-485-1857
Fax: 240-485-1818
www.vnaa.org

WEDI Workgroup for Electronic Data Interchange

To provide leadership and guidance to the healthcare industry on how to use and leverage the industry's collective knowledge, expertise and information resources to improve the quality, affordability and availability of healthcare.

12020 Sunrise Valley Drive
Suite 100
Reston, VA 20191
Tel: 703-391-2716
Fax: 703-391-2759
www.wedi.org

WHO World Health Organization

The directing and coordinating authority for health within the United Nations system. It is responsible for providing leadership on global health matters, shaping the health research agenda, setting norms and standards, articulating evidence-based policy options, providing technical support to countries and monitoring and assessing health trends.

Avenue Appia 20
1211 Geneva 27
Switzerland
Tel: +41-22-791-21-11
www.who.int/en/

Appendix A
Electronic Health Record (EHR) Definitions

Editor's Note

A number of definitions are currently in use for computerized automated health/medical/personal records. This appendix is not a complete list of electronic record definitions, but rather includes the most commonly accepted definitions. It is considered a work in progress as the terminology evolves. The first definition is preferred by HIMSS and the Standards Task Force. The source of each definition is indicated with a reference number; all sources can be found in the References section at the end this dictionary.

1. **Electronic health record.** A longitudinal electronic record of patient health information produced by encounters in one or more care settings. Included in this information are patient demographics, progress notes, problems, medications, vital signs, past medical history, immunizations, laboratory data and radiology reports. The EHR automates and streamlines the clinician's workflow. The EHR has the ability to generate a complete record of a clinical patient encounter, as well as supporting other care-related activities such as decision support, quality management, and outcomes reporting.[45]

2. **Electronic health record.** Electronically maintained information about an individual's lifetime health status and healthcare (across multiple episodes of care), in all pertinent clinical environments, replacing the paper medical record as the primary record of care, meeting all clinical, legal and administrative requirements and providing added value in supporting decisions about patient management.[1]

3. **Electronic health record.** A newer concept of an automated health record. The EHR concept begins by highlighting the comparative difficulty of ever achieving a true, longitudinal, completely paperless, interoperable complete patient record from birth to death. Components include clinical workstation systems, data entry systems, templates or forms, communication (wireless, hardwired, or Internet-enabled), speech recognition, transcription, security, Master Patient Index (MPI), order entry, results reporting and decision support.[1]

4. **Electronic health record.** A medical record or any other information relating to the past, present or future physical and mental health, or condition of a patient which resides in computers which capture, transmit, receive, store, retrieve, link, and manipulate multimedia data for the primary purpose of providing healthcare and health-related services. EHR records includes patient demographics, progress notes, SOAP notes, problems, medications, vital signs, past medical history, immunizations, laboratory data and radiology reports.[7]

5. **Electronic health record.** The current term used to refer to computerization of health record content and associated processes.[62]

6. **Electronic health record.** A term that may be treated synonymously with computer-based patient record and/or EHR; often used in the U.S. to refer to an EHR in a physician office setting or a computerized system of files (often scanned via a document imaging system) rather than individual data elements.[62]

7. **Electronic health record.** The ASTM work group concluded that E1384 offers the best definition for *clinical encounter* and adopted that definition to define the scope for their effort. EHR is the primary repository for information from various sources; the structure of the EHR is receptive to the data that flow from other systems.[63]

8. **Electronic health record.** Also known as computerized patient records (CPR). EHRs allow for entry and storage of a wide variety of patient information in electronic format, and subsequent access to this information by healthcare providers, patients, and other authorized users. In its fullest form, an EHR replaces the paper record, eliminating the need for filing and storage, as well as the risk and inconvenience of misplaced or otherwise inaccessible charts. Lesser versions of an EHR may require some paper to be retained (such as outside consults or hospital reports), but still allow for most clinical transactions to take place on line, speeding transmission of information and reducing the risk of errors.[64]

9. **Electronic health record.** Literally defined, it is the accumulation of medical information concerning the patient.[65]

10. **Electronic medical record.** A computer-based patient medical record. An EMR facilitates access of patient data by clinical staff at any given location; accurate and complete claims processing by insurance companies; building automated checks for drug and allergy interactions; clinical notes; prescriptions; scheduling; and sending and viewing labs. The term has become expanded to include systems which keep track of other relevant medical information. The practice management system is the medical office functions which support and surround the EMR and relevant medical information.[63]

11. **Electronic medical record.** A generic term used to describe computer-based patient medical records. The term has become expanded to include systems which keep track of other relevant medical information.[64]

12. **Electronic health record.** A general term describing computer-based patient record systems. It is sometimes extended to include other functions such as computer practitioner order entry (CPOE).[65]

13. **Electronic health record.** A repository of electronically maintained information about an individual's lifetime health status and healthcare, stored such that it can serve the multiple legitimate users of the record.[69]

14. **Electronic health care record.** Five (http://www.medrecinst.com/) levels of an electronic healthcare record can be distinguished:

   - The automated medical record is a paper-based record with some computer-generated documents.
   - The computerized medical record (CMR) makes the documents of level 1 electronically available.
   - The electronic medical record (EMR) restructures and optimizes the documents of the previous levels ensuring inter-operability of all documentation systems.
   - The electronic patient record (EPR) is a patient-centered record with information from multiple institutions.
   - The electronic health record (EHR) adds general health and disease related information to the EPR.[70]

15. **Electronic medical record.** An electronic medical record encompasses:

   - A longitudinal collection of electronic health information for and about persons.
   - Immediate electronic access to person- and population-level information by authorized users.
   - Provision of knowledge and decision-support systems (that enhance the quality, safety, and efficiency of patient care).
   - Support for efficient processes for healthcare delivery.[71]

16. **Electronic health record.** Provides each individual in Canada with a secure and private lifetime record of their key health history and care within the health system. The record is available electronically to authorized healthcare providers and the individual anywhere, anytime in support of high quality care. The EHR is the central component that stores, maintains and manages clinical information about patients/persons. The extent of the clinical information sustained by the EHR component may vary based namely on the presence or absence of domain repositories in any given jurisdiction.[74]

17. **Electronic patient record.** Electronic set of information about a single patient/person. An EPR system is a system specifically designed to provide patient/person records electronically. This is not necessarily restricted to a single clinical information system.[72]

18. **Patient care record.** A patient care record that is fully computerized. Also may be called an electronic patient record (EPR) or a computerized patient record (CPR). As envisioned by the CPRI-host this would be a lifetime healthcare record for an individual that would be accessible by authorized users including the patient anywhere in the country. It would also include decision support, contain clinical reminders and alerts, and provide links to factual knowledge bases.[11]

19. **Medical record.** Data source; data obtained from the records or documentation maintained on a patient in any healthcare setting (for example, hospital, home care, long term care, practitioner office). Includes automated and paper medical record systems.[31]

20. **Computer-based patient record health care record.** Stored in an electronic format. This framework representing the main healthcare subsystems, their connections, rules, etc., is the basis for the development of information and communication systems.[73]

21. **Continuity of care record.** A patient health summary standard; a way to create flexible documents that contain the most relevant and timely core health information about a patient and to send these electronically from one caregiver to another. The CCR contains various sections—such as patient demographics, insurance information, diagnosis and problem list, medications, allergies, and care plan—that represent a "snapshot" of a patient's health data that can be useful, even lifesaving, if available when that patient has his or her next clinical encounter. CCR is designed to permit easy creation by a physician using an electronic health record (EHR) software program or electronic medical record (EMR) system at the end of an encounter.[61]

22. **Continuity of care record.** The continuity of care record (CCR) is an emerging standard for communicating patient information electronically among providers. The CCR is intended to provide a snapshot of essential patient information, rather than a complete patient record, that will enable a physician to understand a patient context and provide appropriate care. The format of the CCR allows it to be used universally to help bridge the gaps between EHR systems and improve portability of patient information.[74]

23. **Electronic health record for integrated care.** Repository of information regarding the health status of a subject of care, in computer processable form, stored and transmitted securely and accessible by multiple authorized users, having a standardized or commonly agreed logical information model that is independent of EHR systems and whose primary purpose is the support of continuing, efficient and quality integrated healthcare.[75]

24. **Electronic health record.** Basic generic form repository of information regarding the health status of a subject of care in computer processible form.[75]

25. **EHR system.** Set of components that form the mechanism by which electronic health records are created, used, stored and retrieved including people, data rules and procedures, processing and storage devices, and communication and support facilities.[75]

26. **Electronic health record.** An electronic longitudinal collection of personal health information, usually based on the individual, entered or accepted by healthcare providers, which can be distributed over a number of sites or aggregated at a particular source. The information is organized primarily to support continuing, efficient and quality health care. The record is under control of the consumer and is stored and transmitted securely [ISO/TS 18308:2005].[76]

27. **Electronic health record system.** A system for recording, retrieving, and manipulating information in electronic health records [ISO/TC 215:2005]. Note: The EHR system provides functions only which directly relate to the health record. Other functions required to support clinical care delivery, such as order entry, e-prescribing, and scheduling, are provided by additional, complimentary systems collectively called *clinical information systems.*[76]

28. **Personal health record.** An electronic Personal Health Record ("e-PHR") is a universally accessible, layperson comprehensible, lifelong tool for managing relevant health information, promoting health maintenance and assisting with chronic disease management via an interactive, common data set of electronic health information and e-health tools. The e-PHR is owned, managed, and shared by the individual or his or her legal proxy(s) and must be secure to protect the privacy and confidentiality of the health information it contains. It is not a legal record unless so defined and is subject to various legal limitations.[45]

29. **The electronic health record.** A longitudinal electronic record of patient health information produced by encounters in one or more care settings. Included in this information are patient demographics, progress notes, problems, medications, vital signs, past medical history, immunizations, laboratory data, and radiology reports. The EHR automates and streamlines the clinician's workflow. The EHR has the ability to independently generate a complete record of a clinical patient encounter, as well as supporting other care-related activities such as decision support, quality management, and clinical reporting.

30. **Personal health record.** Electronic application(s) through which individuals can maintain and manage their health information (and that of others for whom they are authorized) in a private, secure, and confidential environment.[130]

31. **Electronic medical record.** An electronic medical record is a medical record in digital format. Most EMR solutions also offer the opportunity to receive critical information—such as formulary or drug interaction checks—at the point of care. Using an EMR typically facilitates (1) access of patient data by clinical staff at any given location, (2) accurate and complete claims processing by insurance companies, (3) clinical note composition, (4) prescribing, (5) scheduling, and (6) sending orders to laboratories and receiving and viewing labs.[131]

32. **Personal health record.** A personal health record is the documentation of any form of patient information—including medical history, medicines, allergies, visit history, or vaccinations—that patients themselves may view, carry, amend, annotate, or maintain.[131]

Appendix B
Interoperability Definitions

Editor's Note

Many definitions exist for the word "interoperability." A number of those definitions are included below. The first definition is preferred by HIMSS and the HIMSS Standards Task Force. The source for each definition is indicated with a reference number; all sources can be found in the References section at the end of this dictionary.

1. Interoperability dimensions that comprise a more expansive notion of interoperability include:

   - Uniform movement of healthcare data from one system to another such that the clinical or operational purpose and meaning of the data is preserved and unaltered.

   - Uniform presentation of data: enabling disparate stakeholders to use different underlying systems to have consistent presentation of data when doing so is clinically or operationally important.

   - Uniform user controls, to the extent that a stakeholder is accessing a variety of underlying systems, and the contextual information and navigational controls are presented consistently and provide for consistent actions in all relevant systems.

   - Uniform safeguarding data security and integrity as data moves from system to system such that only authorized people and programs may view, manipulate, create, or alter the data.

   - Uniform protection of patient confidentiality even as stakeholders in different organizations access data that has been exchanged across systems, particularly in order to prevent unauthorized access to sensitive information by people who should not, or do not, need to know.

   - Uniform assurance of a common degree of system service quality (e.g., reliability, performance, dependability), so that stakeholders who rely on a set of interoperable systems can count on the availability and responsiveness of the overall system as they perform their jobs.[45]

2. Data exchange schema and standards should permit data to be shared between clinician, lab, hospital, pharmacy, and patient regardless of application or application vendor.[77]

3. The ability of different operating and software systems, applications, and services to communicate and exchange data in an accurate, effective, and consistent manner.[78]

4. Exchange of information between an electronic health record (EHR) system and another health information technology system.[79]

5. Supports multi-stakeholder efforts at the state, regional, and community levels to link national standards to neighborhood solutions.[80]

6. Supports the electronic exchange of patient summary information among caregivers and other authorized parties via potentially disparate electronic health record (EHR) systems and other systems to improve the quality, safety, efficiency, and efficacy of care delivery.[81]

7. Supports the exchange of information and function together; using an integration profile and process; then demonstrate.[56]

8. Supports the flow; within healthcare industry, using open standards, to reduce costs and improve care quality.[82]

9. The ability of two or more systems or elements to exchange information and to use the information that has been exchanged.[83]

10. In healthcare, interoperability is the ability of different information technology systems and software applications to communicate, to exchange data accurately, effectively, and consistently, and to use the information that has been exchanged.

    The Center for Information Technology Leadership described four different categories ("levels") of data structuring at which healthcare data exchange can take place. While it can be achieved at any level, each has different technical requirements and offers different potential for benefits realization. In real-world settings, there are gradations both within and between the levels described below. The four levels are as follows:

    - Level 1: Non-electronic data. Examples include paper, mail, and phone call.
    - Level 2: Machine transportable data. Examples include fax, e-mail, and un-indexed documents.
    - Level 3: Machine organizable data (structured messages, unstructured content). Examples include indexed (labeled) documents, images, and objects.
    - Level 4: Machine interpretable data (structured messages, standardized content). Examples include the automated transfer from an external lab of coded results into a provider's EHR. Data can be transmitted (or accessed without transmission) by HIT systems without need for further semantic interpretation or translation.[7]

11. Improve healthcare quality through effective, efficient information exchange and management.[85]

12. The CCR may be prepared, displayed, and transmitted on paper or electronically, provided the information required by this specification is included. When prepared in a structured electronic format, strict adherence to an XML schema and an accompanying implementation guide is required to support standards-compliant interoperability. The Adjunct[3] to this specification contains a W3C XML schema and contains an Implementation Guide for such representation.[39]

13. A state which exists between two applications entities when, with regard to a specific task, one application entity can accept data from the other and perform that task in an appropriate and satisfactory manner without the need for extra operator intervention.[86]

14. Functional interoperability: the ability of two or more systems to exchange information.[75]

15. Interoperability: common (inside systems) convergence EHR domain, (outside) disparate domain, data and functional, mapping translation rules, versioning and audit.[70]

16. A second form of interoperability that is frequently emphasized in the literature—and that has played an important role in CanCore's development—is known as "technical" or "syntactic" interoperability. This form of interoperability is concerned with the "technical issues" and "standards" involved in the effective "communication, transport, storage and representation" of metadata and other types of information.[87]

17. In the context of eHealth, interoperability is the way in which reliable data is provided and communicated in a secure, accurate and efficient way. It has to surmount barriers of national policies, culture, language, and systems of medical knowledge representation and use of ICTs.[136]

18. The operational ability to collaborate is a key success factor for networked enterprises, and interoperability is the target result of the enterprises involved in long established as well as ad-hoc or occasional forms of collaborations. The ATHENA Interoperability Framework (AIF) provides a compound framework and associated reference architecture for capturing the research elements and solutions to interoperability issues that address the problem in a holistic way by inter-relating relevant information from different perspectives of the enterprise.[137]

Appendix C
Healthcare Credentials

I. Certifications

Credential	Full Name	Organization Acronym	Organization Full Name
ACRN	AIDS Certified Registered Nurse	ANAC	Association of Nurses in AIDS Care
ANP	Adult Nurse Practitioner	ANCC	American Nurses Credentialing Center
AOCN	Advanced Oncology Certified Nurse	ONCC	Oncology Nursing Certification Corporation
APRN	Advanced Practice Registered Nurse	ANCC	American Nurses Credentialing Center
CAAMA	Credentialed Member of the American Academy of Medical Administrators	AAMA	American Academy of Medical Administrators
BC	Board Certified	ANCC	American Nurses Credentialing Center
CAP	Certification and Accreditation Professional	$(ISC)^2$	International Information Systems Security Certification Consortium
CCA	Certified Coding Associate	AHIMA	American Health Information Management Association
CCM	Certified Case Manager	CCMC	Commission for Case Manager Certification
CCMA	Certified Management Apprentice	CIAC	Call Center Industry Advisory Council
CCMC	Certified Management Consultant	CIAC	Call Center Industry Advisory Council
CCOM	Certified Operations Manager	CIAC	Call Center Industry Advisory Council
CCRN	Critical Care Registered Nurse	AACN	American Association of Critical-Care Nurses
CCP	Certified in Healthcare Privacy	AHIMA	American Health Information Management Association
CCS	Certified Coding Specialist	AHIMA	American Health Information Management Association
CCSL	Certified Strategic Leader	CIAC	Call Center Industry Advisory Council
CCS-P	Certified Coding Specialist – Physician-based	AHIMA	American Health Information Management Association
CDE	Certified Diabetes Educator	NCBDE	National Certification Board for Diabetes Educators
CDMS	Certified Disability Management Specialist	CDMSC	Certification of Disability Management Specialists Commission
CDN	Certified Dialysis Nurse	NNCC	Nephrology Nursing Certification Commission

Credential	Full Name	Organization Acronym	Organization Full Name
CEN	Certified Emergency Nurse	BCEN	Board of Certification for Emergency Nursing
CHE	Certified Healthcare Executive	ACHE	American College of Healthcare Executives
CHESP	Certified Healthcare Environmental Services Professional	AHA-CC	American Hospital Association Credentialing Center
CHFM	Certified Healthcare Facility Manager	AHA-CC	American Hospital Association Credentialing Center
CHFP	Certified Healthcare Financial Professional	HFMA	Healthcare Financial Management Association
HCQM	Health Care Quality Management	ABQAURP	American Board of Quality Assurance and Utilization Review Physicians
CHPS	Certified in Healthcare Privacy and Security	AHIMA	American Health Information Management Association
CISA	Certified Information Systems Auditor	ISACA	Information Systems Audit and Control Association
CISM	Certified Information Security Manager	ISACA	Information Systems Audit and Control Association
CISSP	Certified Information Systems Security Professional	(ISC)^2	International Information Systems Security Certification Consortium
CMA	Certified Management Accountant	IMA	Institute of Management Accountants
CMRP	Certified Materials and Resource Professional	AHA-CC	American Hospital Association Credentialing Center
CMSRN	Certified Medical-Surgical Registered Nurse	AMSN	Academy of Medical-Surgical Nurses
CNM	Certified Nurse Midwife	ACC	American College of Nurse-Midwives Certification
CNN	Certified Nephrology Nurse	NNCC	Nephrology Nursing Certification Commission
CNS	Clinical Nurse Specialist	AACN	American Association of Critical-Care Nurses
CNOR	Certified in Operating Room Nursing	AORN	Competency and Credentialing Institute of the Association of Perioperative Nurses
COHN	Certified Occupational Health Nurse	ABOHN	American Board for Occupational Health Nurses, Inc.
CPA	Certified Public Accountant	AICPA	American Institute of Certified Public Accountants
CPE	Board Certification in Medical Management	CCMM	Certifying Commission in Medical Management
CPHIMS	Certified Professional in Healthcare Information and Management Systems	HIMSS	Healthcare Information and Management Systems Society

Credential	Full Name	Organization Acronym	Organization Full Name
CPHQ	Certified Professional in Healthcare Quality	HQCB	Healthcare Quality Certification Board
CPHRM	Certified Professional in Healthcare Risk Management	AHA-CC	American Hospital Association Credentialing Center
CPNP	Certified Pediatric Nurse Practitioner	NCBPNP/N	National Certification Board of Pediatric Nurse Practitioners and Nurses, Inc.
CRNA	Certified Registered Nurse Anesthetist	AANA	American Association of Nurse Anesthetists
CRNI	Certified Registered Nurse Intravenous	INS	Intravenous Nursing Society
CRRN	Certified Rehabilitation Registered Nurse	ARN	Association of Rehabilitation Nurses
FNP	Family Nurse Practitioner	ANCC	American Nurses Credentialing Center
HCQM	Health Care Quality Management	ABQAURP	American Board of Quality Assurance and Utilization Review Physicians
IIP	Imaging Informatics Professional	SIMM	Society for Imaging Informatics in Medicine
ISSAP	Information Systems Security Architecture Professional	$(ISC)^2$	International Information Systems Security Certification Consortium
ISSEP	Information Systems Security Engineering Professional	$(ISC)^2$	International Information Systems Security Certification Consortium
ISSMP	Information Systems Security Management Professional	$(ISC)^2$	International Information Systems Security Certification Consortium
MCDBA	Microsoft Certified Database Administrator		Microsoft
MCITP	Microsoft Certified IT Professional		Microsoft
MCP	Microsoft Certified Professional		Microsoft
MCSE	Microsoft Certified Systems Engineer		Microsoft
MCTS	Microsoft Certified Technology Specialist		Microsoft
MT (ASCP)	Certified Medical Technologist	ASCP	American Society for Clinical Pathology
NP-C	Certified Adult Nurse Practitioner	AANP	American Academy of Nurse Practitioners
OCN	Oncology Certified Nurse	ONCC	Oncology Nursing Certification Corporation
ONC	Orthopaedic Nurse Certified	NAON	National Association of Orthopaedic Nurses
PA-C	Physician Assistant - Certified	NCCPA	National Commission on the Certification of Physician Assistants
PMP	Project Management Professional	PMI	Project Management Institute

Credential	Full Name	Organization Acronym	Organization Full Name
RHIA	Registered Health Information Administrator	AHIMA	American Health Information Management Association
RHIT	Registered Health Information Technician	AHIMA	American Health Information Management Association
RN, BC	Registered Nurse, Board Certified	ANA	American Nurses Credentialing Center
RNC	Registered Nurse, Certified	ANA	American Association of Neonatal Nurses
SSCP	Systems Security Certified Practitioner	(ISC)^2	International Information Systems Security Certification Consortium
SSCP	Systems Security Certified Professional	(ISC)^2	International Information Systems Security Certification Consortium

II. Healthcare and Related Degrees

Designation	Full Name
B.Comm	Bachelor of Commerce
BA	Bachelor of Arts
BS or BSc	Bachelor of Science
BScN or BSN	Bachelor of Science in Nursing
BSCS	Bachelor of Science in Computer Science
DBA	Doctor of Business Administration
DO	Doctor of Optometry or Doctor of Osteopathy
DNP	Doctor of Nursing Practice
DNS/DNSc	Doctor of Nursing Science
DPH/DrPH	Doctor of Public Health
EdD	Doctor of Education
JD	Doctor of Law
MA	Master of Arts
MBA	Master of Business Administration
MD	Doctor of Medicine
MEd	Master of Education
MHA	Master of Health Administration
MHSA	Master of Health Services Administration
MPH	Master of Public Health
MPharm	Master of Pharmacy
MS of MSc	Master of Science
MSCIS	Master of Science in Computer Information Systems
MSIS	Master of Science in Information Systems
MSN	Master of Science in Nursing

Designation	Full Name
MSNI	Master of Science in Health Informatics
MSW	Master of Social Work
PharmD	Doctor of Pharmacy
PhD	Doctor of Philosophy

III. Professional Memberships

Designation	Full Name
FAAFP	Fellow of the American Academy of Family Physicians
FACC	Fellow of the American College of Cardiology
FACEP	Fellow of the American College of Emergency Physicians
FACHE	Fellow of the American College of Healthcare Executives
FACMPE	Fellow of the American College of Medical Practice Executives
FACP	Fellow of the American College of Physicians
FASCP	Fellow, American Society of Clinical Pathologists
FCAP	Fellow, College of American Pathologists
FHFMA	Fellow of the Healthcare Financial Management Association
FHIMSS	Fellow of the Healthcare Information and Management Systems Society
FIEEE	Fellow of the Institute of Electrical and Electronics Engineers
HIMSS	Health Information and Management Systems Society
LHIMSS	Life Member of the Healthcare Information and Management Systems Society
LFHIMSS	Life Member and Fellow of the Healthcare Information and Management Systems Society
SMIEEE	Senior Member of the Institute of Electrical and Electronics Engineers

IV. Honors Designations

FAAN	Fellow of the American Academy of Nursing
FAAFP	Fellow of the American Academy of Family Physicians
FACC	Fellow of the American College of Cardiology
FACEP	Fellow of the American College of Emergency Physicians
FACHE	Fellow of the American College of Healthcare Executives
FACMI	Fellow, American College of Medical Informatics
FACMPE	Fellow of the American College of Medical Practice Executives
FACP	Fellow of the American College of Physicians
FHAPI	Honorary Fellow, Association for Pathology Informatics

Appendix D
NAHIT's Key Health Information
Technology Terms*

The ambiguity of meaning created by not having a shared understanding of key health IT terms (listed hereafter) could become an obstacle to progress in health IT adoption when questions about a term's definition and application complicate important policy expectations or directives, contractual matters, and product features. Differences in how a term is used can cause confusion and misunderstanding about what is being purchased, considered in proposed legislation, or included in current applicable policies and regulations.

To address these issues and to provide support for increased adoption of health IT, the Office of the National Coordinator for Health Information Technology (ONC) issued a contract to the National Alliance for Health Information Technology (NAHIT, also known as "The Alliance") to reach consensus on definitions for the terms EMR, EHR, PHR, HIE and RHIO. As discussions and public comments took place around the meanings of these terms, it was noted that dual interpretations of HIE existed, as both a process and an entity. As such, there arose a need to clarify the difference between the process of information exchange and the oversight and accountability functions necessary to support that process. To address this need, a sixth term, health information organization (HIO), was added and defined.

Interoperability is so important that it has been defined many ways. However, the Institute of Electrical and Electronics Engineers (IEEE) definition of interoperability has become the gold standard: *The ability of two or more systems or elements to exchange information and to use the information that has been exchanged.* Definitions provide some of the foundation to allow interoperability to occur.

(Editor's note: The consensus-based definitions that follow were developed by two NAHIT-led work groups, two public forums, and two online public comment periods and are excerpted from Defining Key Health Information Technology Terms. The full report can be downloaded at www.nahit.org.)

---

* From the National Alliance for Health Information Technology Report to the Office of the National Coordinator for Health Information Technology on Defining Key Health Information Technology Terms, presented April 28, 2008. Used by permission of the National Alliance for Health Information Technology.

1. Electronic Medical Record (EMR)

An electronic record of health-related information on an individual that can be created, gathered, managed, and consulted by authorized clinicians and staff within one healthcare organization.

The EMR's structure as a store of electronic information capable of being searched, categorized and analyzed makes it superior to the traditional paper chart for informing the care process. Nevertheless, proceeding from its historical basis as the digital version of a patient's chart, the EMR is a provider-focused view of the patient's health history. It comprises health-related information that is created by clinicians or that results from clinician orders and activity on behalf of a patient, such as diagnostic tests or prescriptions for medications. A main objective of an EMR is to improve the ability of a clinician to document observations and findings and to provide more informed treatment of persons in his or her care.

2. Electronic Health Record (EHR)

An electronic record of health-related information on an individual that conforms to nationally recognized interoperability standards and that can be created, managed, and consulted by authorized clinicians and staff across more than one healthcare organization.

An EHR is patient focused in that it is not limited by what a single provider organization is able to accumulate on behalf of a patient under its care. Through the capabilities of interoperability, an EHR becomes an authorized means to access information from whatever sources have chronicled the healthcare experience of a patient over time. The boundaries of an EHR are built not around the organization documenting the information, but around the patient and his or her health-related information. Though it is patient focused, it is managed and used primarily by authorized care providers, as well as by members of his or her staff who have a need to access the EHR to support the process of care.

3. Personal Health Record (PHR)

An electronic record of health-related information on an individual that conforms to nationally recognized interoperability standards and that can be drawn from multiple sources while being managed, shared, and controlled by the individual.

The most salient feature of the PHR, and the one that distinguishes it from the EMR and EHR, is that the information it contains is under the control of the individual. The concise definition above names the individual as the source of control, but that leaves room for others acting in the individual's interest—his or her agent or agents—to have control over access to the PHR. An agent may be expressly designated by the individual but not in all cases; examples of an agent acting for an individual include parents acting for children, or, in the later stages of life, children acting for parents.

4. Health Information Exchange (HIE)

The electronic movement of health-related information among organizations according to nationally recognized standards.

To act as the medium of interoperable exchange between electronic records and organizations, HIE must itself meet nationally recognized interoperability standards. In addition, other classes of standards enabling the flow of information safely, consistently, accurately, and securely must be part of the requirements for HIE. Interoperability, security, and other standards required for HIE are in various stages of being developed and recognized by the U.S. Department of Health and Human Services (HHS). The definition of HIE includes readiness to use these developing information exchange standards; these standards for interoperability and information exchange, used consistently in HIE, will contribute to the foundation of what will become a Nationwide Health Information Network (NHIN).

5. Health Information Organization (HIO)

An organization that oversees and governs the exchange of health-related information among organizations according to nationally recognized standards.

The purpose of an HIO is to perform oversight and governance functions for HIE. Oversight functions of an HIO may include, but are not limited to:

- Facilitation of operations associated with the movement of information—assuring that hardware, software, protocols, standards, stakeholders, and services supporting the interoperable exchange of health-related information are available and engaged.
- Fiduciary responsibility for the assets, accountability for abiding by regulatory requirements for handling personal health information, and adherence to standards enabling interoperable information exchange.
- Maintenance of information sharing agreements, business associate agreements, or other such contracts.
- Adoption and maintenance of standards ensuring interoperability while protecting the confidentiality and security of the information.
- Making decisions regarding certain types of information for which no nationally recognized interoperability standard is available.
- Developing and sharing best practices among organizations.

6. Regional Health Information Organization (RHIO)

A health information organization that brings together healthcare stakeholders within a defined geographic area and governs health information exchange among them for the purpose of improving health and care in that community.

To be designated a RHIO, an entity needs to have certain core features. These attributes distinguish it from other organizations that do not or cannot execute the distinct purpose and responsibilities of a RHIO. An organization designated as a RHIO:

- Must involve data-sharing participants that are separate and distinct legal entities operating within a defined geographic area whose collaboration through the RHIO will cross organizational boundaries.
- Must intend to benefit the population in the community. This requires that stakeholders come from the defined geographic area and that the RHIO provides well-defined and transparent processes to facilitate the interoperable exchange of health information across the range of participating stakeholders.
- Must be inclusive and convene various types of stakeholders in the delineated geographic area who are vested in improving the health of the community.
- Can arrange for the provision of additional technical and operational services supporting its primary purpose. Such services may vary based on stakeholder needs and a range of environmental factors.

References

1. Rognehaugh A, Rognehaugh R. *Healthcare IT Terms.* Chicago: HIMSS; 2001.

2. HIMSS Analytics. 230 East Ohio St., Suite 500, Chicago, IL 60611. www.himssanalytics.com

3. International Organization for Standardization (ISO).1, ch. de la Voie-Creuse; Case postale 56, CH-1211, Geneva 20, Switzerland.

4. GPCG - General Practice Computing Group. Royal Australian College of General Practitioners. South Melbourne, Victoria, Australia 3205.

5. University of Victoria British Columbia (UVIC). http://gateway.uvic.ca/erf/dictionaries.html

6. *Guide to Nursing Informatics.* Chicago: HIMSS; 1996.

7. Wikipedia. www.wikipedia.org

8. Infoway. 1000 Sherbrooke Street West, Suite 1200, Montreal, Québec, Canada. H3A 3G4. www.infoway-inforoute.ca/

9. Behavioral Health Care Services (BHCS). http://bhcs.co.alameda.ca.us/HIPAA/Glossary.htm

10. HIPAA Glossary. www.wedi.org/snip/public/articles/hipaa_glossary.pdf

11. Informatics & Nursing: Opportunities & Challenges. Web supplement; 2003. http://dlthede.net/Informatics/Informatics.htm

12. Microsoft. www.ms.com

13. Coiera E. *Guide to Health Informatics.* 2nd Ed. 2003. www.coiera.com/glossary.htm

14. Agency for Healthcare Research and Quality (AHRQ). Office of Communications and Knowledge Transfer, 540 Gaither Road, Suite 2000, Rockville, MD 20850. www.ahrq.gov

15. CIGNA. www.cigna.com

16. Health Level 7 (HL7). 3300 Washtenaw Avenue, Suite 227, Ann Arbor, MI 48104. www.hl7.org

17. Global Information Grid. www.cnss.gov/Assets/pdf/cnssi_4009.pdf

18. Department of Defense (DoD). Discovery Metadata Standard (DDMS), Version 1.2. June 2, 2003.

19. SNOMED. International Health Terminology Standards Development Organization (IHTSDO). Rued Langgaards Vej. 7, 5 2300 Copenhagen, Denmark. www.ihtsdo.org

20. Military Health System Enterprise Architecture. www.tricare.osd. mil/Architecture

21. U.S. Government Accountability Office. http://www.gao.gov/special.pubs/ bprag/bprgloss.htm

22. Oracle. http://www.orafaq.com/glossary

23. Clinger-Cohen Act of 1996. www.cio.gov/Documents/it_ management_ reform_act_Feb_1996.html

24. 2005 International Council of Nurses (ICN). http://www.icn.ch/icnpupdate. htm#what

25. World Health Organization (WHO). www.who.org

26. University of Iowa College for Nursing Centers. http://www.nursing.uiowa. edu/centers

27. Virginia Saba, EdD, Honorary PhD, RN, FAAN, FACMI, LL, Distinguished Scholar, Georgetown University.

28. Christopher Chute, MD, DrPH, Professor and Chair Medical Informatics, Mayo Clinic College of Medicine.

29. The OMAHA System. www.omahasystem.org/systemo.htm

30. Institute of Medicine (IOM). 500 Fifth Street NW, Washington, DC 20001. www.medterms.com/script/main/hp.asp

31. The Joint Commission (formerly Joint Commission Accreditation of Health-care Organizations). One Renaissance Boulevard, Oakbrook Terrace, IL 60181. www.jcaho.org

32. http://www.merriam-webster.com

33. World Wide Web Consortium (W3C) Portal to Glossaries. www.w3.org/ Glossary

34. International Engineering Consortium. www.iec.org

35. www.answers.com

36. www.bitpipe.com

37. National Cancer Institute – Cancer Biomedical Informatics Grid. https://cabig. nci.nih.gov

38. Canon Group. www.pubmedcentral.nih.gov/articlerender.fcgi?artid=116200

39. ASTM. www.astm.org

40. American Dental Association (ADA). www.ada.org

41. Pearson Software Consulting. http://www.cpearson.com/excel/search.htm

42. whatis.techtarget.com

43. ANSI. American National Standards Institute. www.ansi.org

44. United States Congress.

45. Healthcare Information and Management Systems Society (HIMSS). www.himss.org

46. Centers for Disease Control and Prevention (CDC). www.cdc.gov

47. Gartner Group. www.gartner.com/Init

48. Healthcare Information Technology Standards Panel (HITSP). www.ansi.org

49. International Council of Nurses (ICN). www.icn.ch

50. Logical Observation Identifiers Names and Codes (LOINC). www.regenstrief. org/loinc

51. Lundy KS, Bergamini A. *Essentials of Nursing Informatics*. 2003.

52. American Nursing Association (ANA). www.nursingworld.org

53. Mayo Clinic College of Medicine. www.mayo.edu

54 National Council on Prescription Drug Programs (NCPDP). www.ncpdp.org/ main_frame.htm

55. ECRI (formerly Emergency Research Care Institute). http://www.ecri.org

56. Integrating the Healthcare Enterprise. www.ihe.net

57. National Institute for Standards Technology (NIST). www.itl.nist.gov/div895/ glossary.html

58. www.webopedia.com

59 Public Health Data Standards Consortium. www.cdc.gov/nchs/otheract/phdsc/ phdsc.htm

60 National Security Council. http://www.whitehouse.gov/nsc

61. Developed jointly by ASTM, the Massachusetts Medical Society (MMS), the Healthcare Information and Management Systems Society (HIMSS), the American Academy of Family Physicians (AAFP), and the American Academy of Pediatrics (AAP), along with multiple healthcare IT vendors.

62. American Health Information Management Association (AHIMA). www.ahima.org

63. The ASTM definition from E1384-02a Practice for Content and Structure of the Electronic Health Record (EHR) was adopted by the President's e-Government Consolidated Health Informatics Initiative (CHI).

64. Indian Health Service. www.ihs.gov

65. www.hipaadvisory.com/action/patientconf.htm

66. http://all-free-info.com/electronic-medical-record/

67. www.mywiseowl.com/articles/Electronic_medical_record

68. ISO 14971:2007 Medical devices. Application of risk management to medical devices (terms only). www.iso.org

69. www.cordis.lu/ist/ka1/administrations/publications/glossary.htm

70. Medical Records Institute. www.medrecinst.com

71. Institute of Medicine; 2003.

72. www.infoway-inforoute.ca/ehr/glossary.php?lang=en

73. www.connectingforhealth.nhs.uk/jargonbuster/

74. www.volunteer-ehealth.org/resources/glossary.htm

75. ISO/TR 20514 EHR Definition, Scope and Context (terms only). www.iso.org

76. www.nehta.gov.au

77. www.centerforhit.org/x174.xml

78. H.R. 2458: the E-Government Act of 2002.

79. www.cchit.org

80. http://ccbh.ehealthinitiative.org/news/SecondAnnualSurvey.mspx

81. www.himssehrva.org

82. www.ibm.com

83. www.IEC.org

84. www.nahit.org

85. www.wedi.org

86. CEN/ISSS e-Health Standardization Focus Group. www.who.int/classifications/terminology/prerequisites.pdf

87. Miller, 2000; Hewlett-Packard, 2003. www.cancore.ca/semantic_and_syntactic_interoperability.html

88. Object Management Group. www.omg.org

89. www.cve.mitre.org/cwe

90. www.linktionary.com

91. www.oasis-open.org

92. www.openclinical.org/docs/int/docs/gello.pdf

93. ISO/TR 28380-1. IHE Global Standards Adoption - Part 1: The Process (Publication in process) (terms only). www.iso.org

94. ISO/TR 22221. Good Principles and practices for a clinical data warehouse (terms only). www.iso.org

95. ISO/TS 22220. Identification of Subjects of Health Care (terms only). www.iso.org

96. National Center for Patient Safety, Department of Veterans Affairs, NCPS P.O. Box 486, Ann Arbor, MI 48106-0486. www.va.gov/ncps/

97. Department of Defense (DoD). Information Technology Security Certification and Accreditation Process (DITSCAP) definitions.

98. ISO/TS 17117 (revision). Criteria for the Categorization and Evaluation of Terminological Systems (terms only). www.iso.org

99. Raymond Aller, MD, FHIMSS, FACMI, HFAPI, FCAP, Director of Bioterrorism Preparedness and Response, Los Angeles County, California.

100. Arnold S (ed.). *Guide to the Wireless Medical Practice: Finding the Right Connections for Healthcare.* Chicago: HIMSS, 2008.

101. DMAA: The Care Continuum Alliance, 701 Pennsylvania Avenue NW, Suite 700, Washington, DC 20004-2694. www.dmaa.org

102. Centers for Medicare & Medicaid Services (CMS). www.cms.hhs.gov

103. National Committee on Vital and Health Statistics (NCVHS). www.ncvhs.hhs.gov

104. The City University of New York. www1.cuny.edu/academics/info-central/library.html

105. Kwantlen University College. www.kwantlen.bc.ca/home.html

106. American College of Physicians. www.acponline.org/

107. iHealthBeat.www.ihealthbeat.org/

108. Rosenbloom ST, Miller RA, Johnson KB, Elkin PL, Brown SH. A model for evaluating interface terminologies. *JAMIA.*15:1; 2008; pp 65-76.

109. Auto ID and Bar Code Task Force, HIMSS. 2007.

110. Richesson RL, Krischer J. Data standards in clinical research: Gaps, overlaps, challenges and future directions. *JAMIA.* 14:6; 2007; pp 687-696.

111. Mulyar N, Van der Aalst WMP, Peleg M. A pattern-based analysis of clinical computer–interpretable guideline modeling languages. *JAMIA.* 14:6; 2007; pp 781-797.

112. Van der Aalst WMP, Hofstede AHM, Russell N, Mulyar N. Control Flow Patterns 2003, 2006. http://is.tm.tue.nl/staff/wvdaalst/BPMcenter/reports/2006/BPM-06-22.pdf

113. Wieteck P. www.ncbi.nlm.nih.gov/pubmed/15141497

114. Federal Identity Management. www.cio.gov/ficc/documents

115. www.privacy.gov.au/publications/

116. ISO/IS #13606-1. Electronic health record communication - Part 1: Reference model (terms only). www.iso.org

117. ISO/IS #21549-7. Patient Health Card Data Part 7: E-Prescription to Med Data (terms only). www.iso.org

118. www.dhs.gov/index.shtm

119. Beolphi EUL (ed.). *Telemedicine Glossary.* 5th Ed. 2003.

120. Tufts Health Care Institute. www.tcmi.org

121. ISO/IS #17090-1. Public Key Infrastructure-1 Framework and Overview (terms only). www.iso.org

122. ISO/TS #21298. Functional and Structural Roles (terms only). www.iso.org

123. Quality Assurance Project (QAP) is funded by U.S. Agency for International Development (USAID). www.qaproject.org/

124. Information Security Management Guidelines for Telecommunications, based on ISO/IEC 27002. ITU-T Study Gp 17 TD 2318.

125. ISO/TS 22600-3. HealthCare Information Privilege Management & Access Control P-3 (terms only). www.iso.org

126. ISO/IS #17115. Vocabulary for Terminological Systems (terms only). www.iso.org

127. ISO/IS #22307. Financial services—Privacy impact assessment (under development) (terms only). www.iso.org

128. Lumetra. www.lumetra.com

129. www.ehrva.org/docs/EHRVA_application.pdf

130. U.S. Department of Health and Human Services. www.hhs.gov

131. www.propractica.com/definitions.htm#emr

132. Care Coordination Work Group: MA Consortium for CSHCN - June 2, 2005 ; revised October 6, 2005.

133. www.treatment-now.com/resources/definitions

134. American Academy of Pediatrics. www.medicalhomeinfo.org

135. www.deloitte.com/us/MedicalHomeReport

136. www.etsi.org

137. www.txtgroup.com/newsletter/attachment/Athena_Paper.pdf

138. Robert Wood Johnson Foundation. www.rwjf.org

139. *Mosby's Medical Dictionary.* 8th Ed. St. Louis: Elsevier; 2009.

140. www.creativyst.com/Prod/Glossary

141. www.ncbi.nlm.nih.gov/gquery/?term=glossary

142. www.delos.info/files/pdf/events/2004_Sett_17/Patel.pdf

143. www.mathsisfun.com/definitions/discrete-data.html

144. Federal Health Architecture. http://healthit.hhs.gov/portal/server.pt?open= 512&mode=2&cached=true&objID=1181

145. Organization for Economic Co-operation and Development. http://stats.oecd. org/glossary/about.asp

146. http://people.dbmi.columbia.edu/cimino/Publications/2000%20-%20SCAMC %20%20An%20Infobutton%20for%20Enabling%20Patients%20to%20 Interpret%20On-line%20Pap%20Smear%20Reports.pdf (Infobuttons)

147. http://www.techterms.com/definition/ascii

148. Microsoft Lexicon. http://cinepad.com/borg.htm

149. Professional Review Organization. http://medical.webends.com/kw/ Professional%20Review%20Organizations

150. http://sharea76.fedworx.org/ShareA76/faqs/Glossary.aspx